Schizo-Obsessive Disorder

Schizo-Obsessive Disorder

Michael Poyurovsky

Director of Research, Tirat Carmel Mental Health Center, Tirat Carmel, Israel, and
Associate Professor of Psychiatry at the Rappaport Faculty of Medicine,
Technion, Israel Institute of Technology, Haifa, Israel

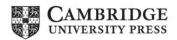

CAMBRIDGE
UNIVERSITY PRESS

CAMBRIDGE
UNIVERSITY PRESS

University Printing House, Cambridge CB2 8BS, United Kingdom

One Liberty Plaza, 20th Floor, New York, NY 10006, USA

477 Williamstown Road, Port Melbourne, VIC 3207, Australia

4843/24, 2nd Floor, Ansari Road, Daryaganj, Delhi - 110002, India

79 Anson Road, #06-04/06, Singapore 079906

Cambridge University Press is part of the University of Cambridge.

It furthers the University's mission by disseminating knowledge in the pursuit of education, learning and research at the highest international levels of excellence.

www.cambridge.org
Information on this title: www.cambridge.org/9781107000124

First published 2013

A catalogue record for this publication is available from the British Library

Library of Congress Cataloging in Publication data
Poyurovsky, Michael.
   Schizo-obsessive disorder / Michael Poyurovsky.
     p.   cm.
   Includes index.
   ISBN 978-1-107-00012-4 (Paperback)
   1. Schizophrenia.   2. Obsessive–compulsive disorder.
   3. Schizophrenia–Treatment.   I. Title.
   RC514.P6834 2013
   616.89'8–dc23

                                                                   2012023162

ISBN 978-1-107-00012-4 Hardback

....

Every effort has been made in preparing this book to provide accurate and up-to-date information which is in accord with accepted standards and practice at the time of publication. Although case histories are drawn from actual cases, every effort has been made to disguise the identities of the individuals involved. Nevertheless, the authors, editors and publishers can make no warranties that the information contained herein is totally free from error, not least because clinical standards are constantly changing through research and regulation. The authors, editors and publishers therefore disclaim all liability for direct or consequential damages resulting from the use of material contained in this book. Readers are strongly advised to pay careful attention to information provided by the manufacturer of any drugs or equipment that they plan to use.

To Arthur and Antinea

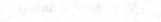

Contents

Foreword

Dear Reader,

You are about to become expert regarding a set of clinical problems that cause great suffering and disability and yet were probably little attended to in your medical education. The focus of this book is the multifaceted interface of schizophrenia and obsessive–compulsive disorder (OCD) across the lifespan. In addition, a middle chapter describes interrelationships between schizophrenia and what are often termed "OCD-spectrum disorders."

In this volume, Dr. Michael Poyurovsky has masterfully brought together the information you will need to understand the evolving conceptualization of these disorders, and our current understanding of their biological underpinnings, psychological manifestations and effects, and of the means available to treat them. With this text as a guide, you can more capably use your power and your privilege as a physician "to cure sometimes, to relieve often, to comfort always."

The focus on the clinical aspects of schizo-obsessive disorder and the various vignettes will be of special interest to multidisciplinary teams of caregivers, including physicians, psychologists, social workers, and occupational therapists. Family members of patients with schizo-obsessive disorder will also benefit. Researchers and physicians interested in the scientific aspects of the schizophrenia–OCD interface will appreciate the novel comprehensive review and discussion of studies focusing on diagnosis and treatment of this challenging subgroup of schizophrenia patients.

I first met Dr. Poyurovsky in 2004 when he came as a Visiting Scholar to the OCD Clinic and Research Program that I directed at Stanford University Medical Center. It was clear from the beginning that he was possessed of a keen mind, new ideas about the clinical conditions covered in this book, and a compassion-driven desire to improve the care given to patients suffering from these conditions. His work has greatly enriched the knowledge base regarding the prevalence, symptoms, and diagnosis of the conditions combining forms of OCD and schizophrenia or *formes frustes* of these disorders, and the pharmacotherapeutic approaches to consider. Even then he was concerned with identifying neurobiological underpinnings and markers, and the genetic and environmental factors that might contribute to the occurrence of these disorders, arguing that understanding these variables could improve our treatment abilities. Our clinical work together has since looked at pharmacotherapy for treatment-resistant OCD, clinical characteristics of OCD patients with schizotypal features, and the diagnostic and therapeutic implications of co-occurrence of symptoms of these two disorders.

Throughout these years of collaboration I have been struck by and been the beneficiary of Dr. Poyurovsky's creativity, drive to uncover clinically helpful new knowledge, his clear thinking, and sound reasoning. Now, dear reader, you, too, can enjoy the results of these characteristics, and through you, so can your patients.

I count Michael Poyurovsky a most valued friend and colleague, and I commend his work to you.

Lorrin M. Koran M.D.
Professor of Psychiatry (Clinical), Emeritus
Stanford University Medical Center

Preface

This book is about individuals who in addition to core symptoms of schizophrenia, also have clinically significant obsessive–compulsive phenomena and form a unique subset of schizophrenia patients. The term "schizo-obsessive" was introduced to delineate the aforementioned subgroup. Although a co-occurrence of schizophrenia and obsessive–compulsive disorder (OCD) was noticed more than a century ago, systematic evaluation of the interface between the two disorders was not pursued until the last two decades. The present book covers historical, epidemiological, clinical, neurobiological, and treatment aspects pertinent to a schizo-obsessive disorder.

The first chapter addresses basic information concerning clinical presentation, etiology, underlying pathophysiology, including structural and functional brain impairment and neurotransmitter alterations, and treatment of schizophrenia and OCD. The analysis of disease expression and neurobiological underpinnings of the two disorders clearly reveals converging trajectories and points toward a plausibility of the coexistence of symptoms of schizophrenia and OCD. Chapter 2 presents a historical perspective of the evolution of views on the co-occurrence and clinical significance of obsessive–compulsive symptoms in schizophrenia. Findings of systematic investigations and meta-analyses on the prevalence of obsessive–compulsive phenomena in schizophrenia, age of onset, and temporal inter-relationship between obsessive–compulsive and schizophrenic symptoms are discussed in Chapter 3. Detailed psychopathological characterization of obsessive–compulsive features in schizophrenia patients is the main focus of Chapter 4. Both typical ego-dystonic obsessive–compulsive symptoms and "atypical" psychotic-related phenomena, such as "obsessive delusions" and "obsessive hallucinations," are described to underscore the complexity of obsessive–compulsive phenomena in schizophrenia. Special attention is given to the assessment of insight into OCD and schizophrenia in schizo-obsessive patients. The next two chapters deal with obsessive–compulsive symptoms in individuals at high risk for psychosis and in the prodromal phase of schizophrenia, as well as across the lifespan. Guidelines for differential diagnosis of a schizo-obsessive disorder from relevant age-related morbidities in adolescent and elderly subgroups are proposed. Chapter 7 covers psychopathological characteristics, differential diagnosis, and treatment strategies in schizophrenia patients with additional OCD-spectrum comorbidities, such as tic disorders and body dysmorphic disorder. A preferential aggregation of these disorders in individuals with a schizo-obsessive disorder is highlighted and underlying mechanisms common to OCD and schizophrenia are discussed. Chapters 8 and 9 deal with the OCD "segment" of the putative schizophrenia–OCD axis of disorders, namely schizotypal OCD and poor-insight OCD. Differential diagnosis from schizophrenia with obsessive–compulsive features is crucial for adequate care of these challenging subgroups; consequently, diagnostic and treatment guidelines are proposed. Results of initial explorative studies of the neurobiology of a schizo-obsessive disorder, including neurocognitive and imaging investigations, as well as the first family and candidate genes association studies are presented in Chapter 10. Chapters 11 and 12 focus on treatment challenges while dealing with this apparently difficult-to-treat subgroup of schizophrenia patients. Treatment strategies are proposed, and the phenomenon of antipsychotic-induced OCD is specifically addressed. The book concludes with a brief summary and suggested diagnostic criteria for a schizo-obsessive disorder.

The reader will notice that some topics, such as epidemiology and clinical characteristics of schizo-obsessive disorder, are now supported by accumulated evidence, while others (e.g., treatment) are solely observational. It is important to keep in mind the limitations of the currently available research findings that are generally cross-sectional design, small sample sizes, and lack of replication. In addition, several issues addressed in this book remain controversial. For example, the distinction between a poor-insight obsession and a delusion is not straightforward and relies on the definition used; the concept of schizotypal OCD is not well established and further research is desperately needed. Even the term "schizo-obsessive" is not universally used; "schizo-OCD" and "OCD–schizophrenia" have also been introduced. Lack of consensus regarding the term that describes the association between the two disorders reflects the uncertainty of what the interface represents – a "simple" comorbidity, a distinct "schizo-obsessive" subtype of schizophrenia, or an obsessive–compulsive dimension of psychopathology in schizophrenia.

With these limitations in mind, I focused primarily on clinical presentation and provided multiple case vignettes to illustrate diagnostic and treatment challenges with patients who have a complex interplay of schizophrenia- and OCD-spectrum disorder symptoms. A majority of the case vignettes are based on personal experience. I chose also to present case reports from the literature to emphasize that the phenomena pertinent to the schizophrenia–OCD association are increasingly observed and documented. A progressively growing number of reports indicate increasing recognition of a schizo-obsessive disorder by clinicians and researchers and the acceptance of its clinical significance. The collected evidence will undoubtedly serve as the basis for the establishment of future consensus regarding the nosological status of a schizo-obsessive disorder. This book represents a step toward this goal. It consolidates current knowledge about a schizo-obsessive subgroup in an effort to "demystify" this complex disorder and to aid in its effective management.

Acknowledgements

I gratefully acknowledge the contributions of my colleagues without whom this book would not have been possible. First and foremost, I am indebted to my dear friends and collaborators Professors Avi and Ronit Weizman from Tel Aviv University. Our collaborative work, continuous discussions that often embraced "devil's advocacy" regarding the very nature of a schizo-obsessive disorder, helped to consolidate the concept of this unique psychiatric condition. Avi with his depth of knowledge in clinical and basic science that goes far beyond the field of psychiatry was a central figure in my research career both as an exceptionally creative thinker and an inspirational model.

Special thanks to Professor Camil Fuchs from Tel Aviv University, an outstanding statistician, who with interest in and knowledge of clinical matters, generously contributed his expertise, time, and passion in planning and analyzing large-scale studies focused on epidemiological, clinical, and neurobiological aspects of schizo-obsessive disorder. Dr. Michael Schneidman, a colleague, a close friend, and a practical guide in clinical practice and life, was instrumental in supporting and encouraging the writing of this book.

I wish to thank the wonderful medical staff of Tirat Carmel Mental Health Center, and particularly the staff of my Department of First-Episode Psychosis for their commitment, support, and cooperation. Special thanks go to my colleague of many years, Dr. Artashez Pashinian, whose enduring assistance in recruiting and interviewing patients was invaluable.

Dr. Sarit Faragian-Rauch, clinical psychologist, began working on the project of schizo-obsessive disorder during its initial stages as a research assistant. She "grew" with the project and her efforts culminated with her receipt of a PhD degree for her work on the neurocognitive deficits in patients with this complex disorder. Sarit's participation was undoubtedly vital to the fruition of this project. Thanks also to Dr. Maya Bleich-Cohen and Professor Talma Hendler from the Functional Brain Center at Tel Aviv Sourasky Medical Center, for their collaboration on the brain imaging studies.

I am grateful to my colleagues from Stanford University (Professors Lorrin M. Koran and Ira Glick). Our collaboration was established during my fellowship sponsored by the Feldman Foundation under the gracious guidance and support of Professor Richard Popp, and later when I was a visiting scholar. Professor Koran is an exceptional friend and supporter, who with his world-renowned expertise in obsessive–compulsive disorder contributed to the challenging endeavor of the delineation of a clinically meaningful interface between obsessive–compulsive disorder and schizophrenia. My sincere appreciation to Larry for agreeing to write the foreword to this book.

I especially would like to thank Rena Kurs, editor, medical librarian, scientific secretary, and truly exceptional person, for her encouragement, relentless support, and professional help during every stage of the preparation of the book. Without her determination and patience this book would not have seen light.

Finally I would like to express gratitude to Cambridge University Press for the goodwill and publication of this book.

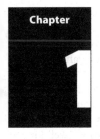

Schizophrenia and OCD: comparative characteristics

According to contemporary psychiatric nomenclature, schizophrenia and obsessive–compulsive disorder (OCD) are distinct nosological entities characterized by non-overlapping diagnostic criteria; they have distinct clinical presentations, treatment, and prognoses. Despite these differences schizophrenia and OCD share some demographic and clinical characteristics, certain aspects of pathophysiology, and treatment strategies (Table 1.1).

Historical perspective

Schizophrenia

Although case descriptions resembling schizophrenia go back hundreds of years, schizophrenia was first described as a disease in the nineteenth century. While searching for basic similarities and dissimilarities in psychotic conditions, Emil Kraepelin, one of the founders of modern psychiatry, noted that a "deteriorating process" was a common denominator for a number of psychotic disorders, such as Kahlbaum's catatonia, Hecker's hebephrenia, Pick's and Sommer's simple deterioration, and paranoid states associated with disorganization (Kraepelin, 1919). Kraepelin found it necessary to retain the above syndromes as

Table 1.1 Schematic comparative characteristics of schizophrenia and OCD

	Schizophrenia	OCD
Prevalence	~1%, narrowly defined 2–3%, broadly defined	2–3%
Gender ratio (M/F)	1/1	1/1
Age of onset	2nd–3rd decade, men earlier than women	1st–2nd decade, men earlier than women
Course	chronic with remissions	chronic, wax and wane
Involved brain regions	cortex: DLPFC, temporal, ACC; thalamus, hippocampus, striatum	cortex: OFC, ACC; thalamus, striatum
Neurotransmitter systems	Dopamine/serotonin/glutamate	Serotonin/dopamine/glutamate
Treatment	Antipsychotic agents (add-on serotonin reuptake inhibitors)	Serotonin reuptake inhibitors (add-on antipsychotic agents)

DLPFC, dorsolateral prefrontal cortex; OFC, orbitofrontal cortex; ACC, anterior cingulate cortex.

subdivisions of the specific disease, "dementia praecox" or premature dementia. Adolescent or early adult onset, deteriorative course, and poor outcome were distinctive characteristics of this disorder. He distinguished dementia praecox from manic-depressive illness characterized by episodic course, lack of deterioration, and relatively favorable outcome.

Eugen Bleuler introduced the term "schizophrenia" and referred to the disorder as the "group of the schizophrenias" to highlight its heterogeneous nature (Bleuler, 1911/1950). He distinguished between basic and accessory schizophrenia symptoms, and determined that disturbances of associations, affect, ambivalence, and autistic isolation (well known as the four As) were the basic symptoms, while hallucinations, delusions, and catatonic symptoms were secondary symptoms, not essential for diagnosis. Bleuler also considered "milder cases" of schizophrenia that developed in patients with a neurosis, a disorder that does not affect rational thinking and reality testing. He ascertained that for some patients who were considered neurotic, obsessive–compulsive symptoms were in fact features of schizophrenia, and emphasized the converging trajectories of the two disorders (see Chapter 2). These views were echoed by Mayer-Gross (1932) who described cases of chronic obsessive–compulsive neurosis associated with "marked autism" as actual schizophrenia.

Kurt Schneider (1959) considered first-rank symptoms (e.g., delusions of control, thought insertion, withdrawal, or broadcasting) pathognomonic to the disorder. He further developed the ideas of Karl Jaspers (1946) who claimed that "un-understandability" of the individual experience was a distinguishing feature of schizophrenia. Over time, however, the elements of un-understandability as defining psychosis have faded and these symptoms have not been found to be specific to schizophrenia (Tandon et al., 2008). Schneider regarded transitory delusional ideas together with obsessive ideas as second-rank symptoms, and differentiated between genuine obsessions and symptomatic obsessions. He doubted whether a genuine obsessional neurosis could develop into schizophrenia (Schneider, 1925). In fact, the proponents of the hierarchical approach in psychiatric classifications viewed successive psychopathological symptoms as "onion-like" hierarchical layers, namely psychopathic–neurotic (including obsessive–compulsive), manic–depressive, schizophrenic, and psycho-organic; disorders of the lower layers that "superseded" disorders of the higher layers (Jaspers, 1946; Schneider, 1987). Thus, this approach to psychiatric disorders did not enable co-occurrence of the two conditions from different "layers."

Current definitions of schizophrenia, including DSM-IV-TR (American Psychiatric Association, 2000) and ICD-10 (World Health Organization, 1992), incorporate Kraepelinian chronicity of illness, Bleulerian negative symptoms, and Schneiderian positive symptoms (Tandon et al., 2008).

Obsessive–compulsive disorder

A unique syndrome characterized by the presence of obsessions and compulsions has been recognized for more than three centuries. This condition has been known as scruples, religious melancholy, folie de doute (insanity of doubt), folie avec conscience (insanity with insight), obsessive–compulsive neurosis, and finally obsessive–compulsive disorder (Berrios, 1989). As the distinction between neurotic and psychotic disorders progressed, the obsessive–compulsive syndrome became one of the prototypic neuroses. An obsession, which is an intrusive, repugnant idea recognized as senseless or irrational and experienced as internal in origin, could thus be distinguished from a delusion, in which the senselessness is not appreciated and the idea is generally attributed to an external source. Although traditionally obsessive–compulsive phenomena have been considered neurotic, earlier descriptions depicted these symptoms with fundamental connections to a psychosis. In perhaps the earliest English language "case report," dated 1660, Jeremy Taylor described a patient whose ego-dystonic intrusive thoughts of having sinned were replaced by a "belief that this scrupulousness of conscience is . . . a punishment of his sins" (cited in Insel and Akiskal, 1986). Similarly, German psychiatrist Westphal who offered one of the most comprehensive descriptions of the obsessive–compulsive syndrome, stressed its similarities with psychosis. He emphasized that the obsession, by its irrational content, represented a basic disorder of thinking, and classified the obsessive–compulsive syndrome as "abortive insanity" (Westphal, 1878).

Henri Legrand du Saulle, a French psychiatrist, was one of the first to recognize that patients who suffered from severe obsessive disorders also had psychotic symptoms. On follow-up some patients with obsessive disorder remained "house-bound, maintaining only a resemblance of insight and harboring darker psychotic attitudes" (cited in Berrios, 1996, p.145). Pierre Janet classified OCD under the term "psychasthenia" and provided precise clinical descriptions of the disorder in his much-cited work *Les Obsessions et la Psychasthénie* (*Obsessions and Psychasthenia*) (Janet, 1903). Among more than 300 cases, 23 patients developed psychosis: patients with primary emotional symptoms and phobias developed melancholia, and those with primary "intellectual obsessions" developed paranoia. Though Janet's psychasthenia included cases other than obsessional neurosis, his observations hinted at the possibility of psychotic (not necessarily schizophrenic) transformation in obsessive–compulsive patients. Psychotic deterioration with affective or paranoid features, rather than schizophrenic disorder, in patients with well-established diagnoses of OCD was later substantiated (Insel and Akiskal, 1986; Eisen and Rasmussen, 1993).

From the historical perspective the consolidation of views on schizophrenia and obsessive–compulsive disorder points toward two independent but partially overlapping psychopathological trajectories. Diagnostic challenges associated with the clinical complexity of the schizophrenia–OCD interface became increasingly evident beginning with the early stages of investigation of the two disorders.

A well-known case of the patient described by Sigmund Freud (1918) in "The History of an Infantile Neurosis" under the pseudonym "Wolfman" called attention to the complex interrelationship between the two disorders and distinct diagnostic approaches of the clinicians. The patient was diagnosed and analyzed as an obsessional neurotic by Freud, but 6 years later his obsessional ideas underwent psychotic transformation into hypochondrial delusions. Before coming to Freud in Vienna, he had been treated in Munich by Emil Kraepelin, who had treated the patient's father for manic–depressive illness and had attributed the same diagnosis to the son. This is not surprising because Kraepelin had a tendency to classify so-called "obsessional insanity" under manic depression. Eugen Bleuler would have classified chronic obsessional neurosis under the umbrella of schizophrenia (Lang, 1997).

Disease expression: signs and symptoms
Schizophrenia

Schizophrenic disorder is characterized by a diverse set of signs and symptoms, including abnormalities of perception, thinking, cognition, motor function, and affect. These disturbances are generally grouped into positive, negative, disorganized, cognitive, mood, and motor symptom dimensions. Psychopathology is differentially expressed across patients and throughout the course of illness. Within the *positive symptom* dimension, delusions of reference and persecution, delusions of control, thought insertion, broadcasting, and withdrawal are traditionally linked to schizophrenia (Schneiderian first-rank symptoms). Although various delusions might occur, in a majority of patients delusional content focuses on a restricted set of typical themes (e.g., reference, persecution, grandeur). Additional positive symptoms, hallucinations, can occur in any of the sensory modalities, though auditory hallucinations – voices commenting or conversing, or imperative voices – are more common. Positive symptoms mark the formal onset of illness, however pathophysiological processes might begin long before. *Formal thought disorders* refer to disorganization of the logical and goal-directed thought process, and range in severity from mild circumstantiality, tangentiality, derailment, and neologisms to severe incoherence and word salad (Andreasen, 1979). According to Bleuler (1911/1950) formal thought disorder, an expression of loosening of associations, is a central deficit in schizophrenia. Disorganized thinking and behavior are prominent, particularly during acute exacerbations and are relatively persistent and associated with poor outcome. *Negative symptoms*, that are intrinsic to schizophrenia, involve restricted and blunted affect, anhedonia, avolition, apathy, and alogia (Andreasen, 1982). Negative symptoms may be detected at every stage of illness; however, they are most prominent in prodromal, post-psychotic, and residual states. Negative symptoms may have distinct pathophysiological mechanisms, remain relatively treatment-resistant, and are strongly associated with functional impairment typical to schizophrenia. *Motor symptoms* can range from simple slowness to complex stereotypic movements, mannerisms, and catatonic symptoms (waxy flexibility, posturing, echolalia, echopraxia, and negativism). *Depressive symptoms*, expressions of affective deregulation in schizophrenia, are common and may be a part of the prodromal or florid phase, follow an acute episode, or occur in remission of schizophrenia. Depressive symptoms substantially contribute to the disease burden, and are strongly associated with suicidality in schizophrenia patients. Similarly, *anxiety symptoms* are prominent features of schizophrenia and may be identified from the early stages and throughout the course of the illness.

There is no single pathognomonic symptom in schizophrenia. According to DSM-IV criteria, the diagnosis is based on a constellation of positive, negative, and disorganized symptoms, illness duration (at least 6 months, including at least 1 month of active-phase symptoms), and functional impairment, after exclusion of mood disorders, and psychoses associated with substance abuse or general medical conditions.

Obsessive–compulsive disorder

Similar to schizophrenia, OCD is associated with disturbances of thoughts, affect, somatosensory perception, and motor function. However, typical presentations of the two disorders are basically different. OCD is most commonly characterized by the occurrence of both obsessions and compulsive rituals, but they can also occur independently (American Psychiatric Association, 2000). There are no objective tests for OCD, and the diagnosis is established based on clinical assessment. According to DSM-IV criteria, a diagnosis of OCD requires either obsessions or compulsions that cause distress, are time-consuming (more than 1 hour per day) and substantially interfere with normal functioning.

Obsessions have the following essential features: recurrent and persistent thoughts, impulses, or images that are experienced as intrusive and cause anxiety; they are not simply excessive worries about real-life issues; the affected individuals attempt to ignore, suppress, or neutralize their obsessions with other thoughts or actions; and the thoughts are recognized as products of their minds. *Compulsions* are repetitive behaviors or mental acts that the affected individuals feel compelled to perform in response to an obsession, or according to rigid rules. Compulsions are aimed at preventing or reducing anxiety and distress associated with obsessions, or at preventing dreaded events. Compulsions are excessive and not realistically connected to what they are intended to prevent (Abramowitz *et al.*, 2009).

The content and character of the obsessions and their relationships to repetitive behaviors sometimes differ. However, akin to delusions with their restricted set of distinctive themes, several typical obsessive themes have been described: contamination, symmetry or exactness, forbidden thoughts (aggressive, sexual, religious, and somatic). Specific obsessions are associated with corresponding compulsions, cleaning, ordering and arranging, checking, and hoarding, and tend to form psychopathological dimensions that are relatively stable over time (Bloch *et al.*, 2008). The content that is characteristic of obsessions and compulsions is usually readily distinguishable from the content of schizophrenic delusions. However, "bizarre" themes exhibited by a subset of otherwise typical OCD patients might complicate the distinction between the two psychopathological phenomena (see Chapter 9). The difference between OCD-related *pathological slowness* (pervasive difficulty initiating and completing routine tasks) and catatonic motor disturbances is not straightforward. *Indecisiveness* (difficulty making decisions about things that other people might not think twice about) and *pathological doubt* (uncertainty about the correctness of performed activities) are common features of OCD. Awareness of the distressful character of these symptoms, usually expressed by OCD patients, distinguishes them from schizophrenia-related ambivalence. Indeed, *insight* into the senseless nature of obsessive–compulsive symptoms is one of the hallmarks of the disorder, in contrast to lack of insight that is a cardinal feature of schizophrenia. According to the DSM-IV, at some point in the course of the illness, the patients must recognize that their obsessions and compulsions are excessive and unreasonable. In typical cases, patients readily acknowledge that their obsessive–compulsive symptoms are illogical and morbid. On the contrary, a significant majority of schizophrenia patients either do not believe that they are ill, or if they do acknowledge symptoms, they misattribute them to other causes (Amador and David, 1998). Notably, a subset of OCD patients presents with poor insight or complete conviction of the true nature of their obsessions, making differential diagnosis from delusions difficult. Nevertheless, cognitive biases that underlie high-conviction beliefs in OCD and delusions (e.g., "jumping to conclusions") are distinct (Jacobsen *et al.*, 2012), and OCD with poor insight differs from a typical psychotic disorder (see Chapter 9). Moreover, though thought processes in OCD are disturbed by intrusive ideas and *magical thinking*, true thought derailment, thought insertion, and thought broadcasting are absent.

In general, OCD and schizophrenia have distinct but partially overlapping psychopathological features. Some, such as delusions and obsessions, most likely represent a continuum of impairments, while others, such as negative and disorganized symptoms, are more disorder-specific (Figure 1.1).

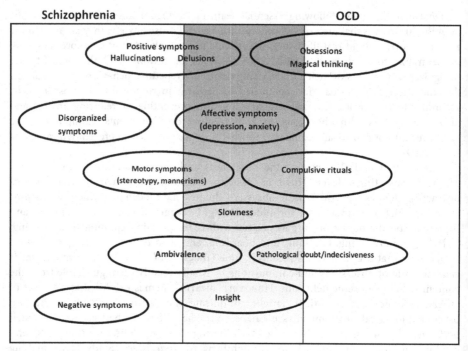

Figure 1.1 Schizophrenia versus OCD: psychopathological features.

Prevalence and demographic and clinical features
Schizophrenia

Schizophrenia is a lifelong condition that affects both men and women, though symptom expression is more severe in men. Men have earlier onset of illness, more negative symptoms, and poorer outcomes. When narrowly defined, the lifetime prevalence of schizophrenia is 0.3–0.66% (McGrath *et al.*, 2008). However, when broader diagnostic categories, such as brief psychotic disorder, delusional disorder, and psychotic disorders not otherwise specified, are included the estimated prevalence approaches 2–3% (Perala *et al.*, 2007). Demarcation between various phases of schizophrenia is imprecise; however, the disorder may be characterized by a sequential trajectory of a *premorbid stage* with non-specific cognitive, motor, and social dysfunction; *prodromal stage* with attenuated positive symptoms and declining function; *first psychotic episode* heralding formal onset of active illness; *initial decade* of illness generally marked by repeated episodes of psychosis with variable degrees of inter-episode remission and finally a *stable phase or plateau*, when psychotic symptoms are less prominent and negative symptoms and stable cognitive deficits become increasingly predominant (Tandon *et al.*, 2008).

Prognosis of the disorder is usually unsatisfactory. Sustained recovery occurs in fewer than 14% within the first 5 years following a psychotic episode, and long-term outcomes are generally only marginally better (Insel, 2010). In Europe, fewer than 20% of people with schizophrenia are employed (Marwaha *et al.*, 2007).

Obsessive–compulsive disorder

The life prevalence of OCD in the general population is estimated at 2–3% (Ruscio et al., 2010), remarkably similar to the estimates of broadly defined schizophrenia. Epidemiological studies in the Americas, Europe, Asia, and Africa have confirmed the rates of occurrence of both disorders across cultural boundaries. Akin to schizophrenia, among adults, men and women are equally affected by OCD, but among adolescents, boys predominate and have an earlier age of onset. The mean age of onset in OCD is about 20 years, and onset of symptoms is before age 30 in about two-thirds of the patients. Late onset is rare. OCD and schizophrenia have similar age-at-onset distribution, with a trend towards earlier age of onset for OCD. There are evident similarities in the course of illness for both disorders: OCD is a chronic, waxing-and-waning disorder. Clinical presentations of both disorders across the lifespan are generally similar. Though the prognosis for OCD is apparently better than for schizophrenia, in comparison to people with anxiety and mood disorders, those with OCD are less likely to be married, more likely to be unemployed, and more likely to report impaired social and occupational functioning (Geller, 2006; Torres et al., 2006; Pallanti, 2008; Ruscio et al., 2010).

Overall, high prevalence, early age of onset, chronic course, and pervasiveness of symptoms render schizophrenia and OCD among the ten leading causes of disability (expressed by the number of years lost due to ill-health, disability, and early death). Noteworthy, when projecting the burden of disease for the year 2020, just as psychiatric disorders, primarily schizophrenia, affective disorders, and OCD, emerged as major contributors to the global disease burden in the 1990 data, mental illnesses are projected to be significant contributors to the 2020 global burden of disease. The proportion of psychiatric disorders in the total global burden of disease is expected to increase from the reported 10.5% in 1990 to 15% by 2020 (Table 1.2).

Genetic and environmental factors

Schizophrenia

Vulnerability for schizophrenia is partly genetic with heritability estimates of roughly 80%, as suggested by twin studies (McGuffin and Gottesman, 1999). Concordance in monozygotic twins is about 50% (not the 100% as might be expected for a Mendelian disorder), and considerably higher than in dizygotic twins or siblings (around 10%). Despite this genetic contribution, the identification of specific genetic associations has been challenging. A small proportion of schizophrenia cases might be explained by rare structural variations (copy-number variants occasioned by small duplications, deletions, or inversions) (Bassett et al., 2010). Combining single-nucleotide polymorphism (SNP) data from several large-scale independent genome-wide studies led to identification of replicable associations with genes, including those involved in neurodevelopment and relevant to the pathophysiology of schizophrenia (Need et al., 2009). Currently, at least 43 candidate genes have been identified, but individual effect sizes are consistently low, especially relative to the evidence for high heritability (Insel, 2010).

Genetic effects and environmental influences that are moderated by genes (gene–environment interaction) account for the established high heritability of schizophrenia. Environmental factors, including perinatal insults (hypoxia, maternal infection, or malnutrition) play a role in accord with genetic vulnerability (Cannon et al., 2002). Advanced paternal age increases the risk of schizophrenia and possibly OCD (Wu et al., 2012). Migrant ethnic groups and children raised in highly urbanized environments are also at increased risk for schizophrenia

Table 1.2 The leading causes of disability worldwide, 1990, as measured by years of life with a disability (YLD): all causes

	Total YLDs (millions)	Percent of total
1. Unipolar major depression	50.8	10.7
2. Iron-deficiency anemia	22.0	4.7
3. Falls	22.0	4.6
4. Alcohol use	15.8	3.3
5. Chronic obstructive pulmonary disease	14.7	3.1
6. Bipolar disorder	4.1	3.0
7. Congenital anomalies	13.5	2.9
8. Osteoarthritis	13.3	2.8
9. *Schizophrenia*	*12.1*	*2.6*
10. *Obsessive–compulsive disorder*	*10.2*	*2.2*

Source: Murray CJL, Lopez AD (1996) The global burden of disease. *Nature Medicine* **4**, 1241–1243. Reprinted with permission.

(van Os *et al.*, 2010). Individuals with pre-existing liability to psychosis are more susceptible to the development of transient psychotic states when exposed to cannabis than healthy controls (van Os *et al.*, 2010). The fact that only a small proportion of those exposed to cannabis, migration, or urban environment develop schizophrenia suggests that some are resilient to these environmental risk factors. The basis for this resilience is not yet clearly understood.

Obsessive–compulsive disorder

Akin to schizophrenia, twin studies have supported strong heritability for OCD, with a genetic influence of 45–65% in studies in children and 27–47% in adults (Carey and Gottesman, 2000; van Grootheest *et al.*, 2005). Monozygotic twins are concordant for OCD (80–87%), compared with 47–50% concordance in dizygotic twins. Furthermore, prevalence of OCD in first-degree relatives of OCD patients is three to five times higher than in relatives of healthy controls, clearly indicating that the disorder runs in families; and there might be a stronger familiarity in childhood-onset OCD than in cases in which the disorder develops later in life (Nestadt *et al.*, 2010). Segregation analyses of OCD implicate a gene of major effect in the etiology of OCD, and reject sporadic and environmental models. Studies of candidate genes selected on the basis of knowledge of the pathophysiology and pharmacology of the condition produced some preliminary leads for the association with the genes relevant to serotonergic, glutamatergic, and dopaminergic systems; however, there have been only few replications of these findings (e.g., the glutamate transporter gene *SLC1A1*) (Nestadt *et al.*, 2010). Large-scale genome-wide association studies that might provide further information about genetic vulnerability to the disorder, are currently underway.

Autoimmune mechanisms may also be involved in OCD. Streptococcal infection and inflammation to the basal ganglia might lead to the development of childhood-onset OCD. Such cases are grouped within a set of clinical conditions called pediatric autoimmune neuropsychiatric disorders associated with streptococcal infection (PANDAS), and are sometimes successfully treated with antibiotics (Swedo *et al.*, 2001).

Cognitive dysfunction

Schizophrenia

Cognitive impairment is one of the core features of schizophrenia. Tandon and colleagues (2008) summarized the major characteristics of cognitive impairment in schizophrenia: (1) cognitive impairment is *highly prevalent* (if not *universal*) in patients with schizophrenia; (2) cognitive impairment distinguishes patients with schizophrenia from healthy comparison subjects to a *robust degree* (i.e., an effect size of approximately 1); (3) the cognitive deficit in schizophrenia is of a *generalized* nature with substantial impairments in specific domains of executive functions and working memory, attention, verbal fluency, processing speed, and episodic memory; (4) cognitive deficits are already present in the premorbid phase of illness and are observed through the long-term course of schizophrenia with a probable deterioration prior to or around the onset of psychotic symptoms, a modest improvement with treatment, and relative stability thereafter; (5) a similar pattern of cognitive impairment of lesser severity is present in non-psychotic relatives and is likely related to patient's *genetic susceptibility* to schizophrenia; (6) cognitive impairment is a *strong predictor* of poor social and vocational outcome.

Obsessive–compulsive disorder

In contrast to generalized and pervasive cognitive impairment in schizophrenia, cognitive deficits in OCD are *more selective* and *less severe* (Table 1.3). Hence, while patients with schizophrenia have generalized deficits in all aspects of executive function, namely a poor sense of planning, impaired decision-making, and response inhibition, patients with OCD share impairment in decision-making and response inhibition, but do not display difficulties with planning (Burdick *et al.*, 2008). Perturbed declarative memory is another example of a transnosological deficit. Of its two basic forms, deficits in semantic memory are mainly restricted to schizophrenia, whereas impairment of episodic memory may also be found in OCD, however in a lesser degree (Table 1.2).

In schizophrenia, faulty social cognition is a crucial issue: it predicts conversion to full psychosis in high-risk asymptomatic individuals. Social withdrawal exacerbates negative symptoms, and false attribution to others of harmful intentions aggravates paranoia and delusions (Brune, 2005). Social cognition must be intact to appropriately decode verbal language, which is compromised in schizophrenia. Disorganization of language, perturbed verbal fluency, and a poor grasp of semantics are core features of schizophrenia. On the contrary, language function and social cognition are generally preserved in OCD (Millan *et al.*, 2012). Moreover, some cognitive domains have opposite directions of change: there is a cardinal loss of focused attention in schizophrenia, and in contrast, there is hypervigilance in OCD. Among the deficits that characterize OCD, impairment of procedural learning is of particular note. Along with other mechanisms, procedural learning underlies the principal failure to "forget" and "inhibit," and thus might account for the occurrence of intrusive thoughts and actions characteristic of OCD (Chamberlain *et al.*, 2005; Burdick *et al.*, 2008).

Certain neurocognitive impairments (e.g., working memory in schizophrenia; response inhibition in OCD) have been found in affected probands and their unaffected first-degree relatives, thus these impairments represent heritable traits (Snitz *et al.*, 2006; Chamberlain *et al.*, 2007). These so-called intermediate phenotypes (because they are between the predisposing genes and the clinical disease phenotype) might be closer to alterations in gene function than the diagnostic category of the corresponding disease. Some of these intermediary

Table 1.3 Comparison of cognitive impairment in patients with schizophrenia and OCD

Cognitive function	Schizophrenia	OCD
Attention and vigilance	+++($\downarrow$)	+++($\uparrow$)
Working memory	+++	+
Executive function	+++	++
Episodic memory	+++	+
Semantic memory	++	0/+
Visual memory	+	+
Verbal memory	+++	0/+
Fear extinction	++	++
Processing speed	++	++
Procedural memory	+	++
Social cognition (theory of mind)	+++	+
Language	+++	0/+

0, essentially absent; 0/+, poorly documented, ambiguous, mid and/or variable; +, consistently present but not pronounced; ++, a common, marked characteristic; +++, a core, severe, and virtually universal characteristic of the disorder; $\uparrow$, increase.
Source: Modified from Millan *et al.* (2012) Cognitive dysfunction in psychiatric disorders: characteristics, causes, and the quest for improved therapy. *Nature Review of Drug Discovery* **11**, 141–168. Reprinted with permission.

phenotypes could be diagnostically relevant: for example the intermediary phenotype of cognitive impairment could have some specificity for the diagnostic category of schizophrenia. Indeed, meta-analytic work has indicated that relatives of patients with bipolar disorder have only minimal cognitive alterations (Arts *et al.*, 2008). Similar comparative evaluations of schizophrenia and OCD patients and their relatives have yet to be performed.

Pathophysiology: structural, functional, and neurotransmitter alterations
Schizophrenia

Structural brain imaging reports demonstrated a subtle but almost universal *decrease* in gray matter, *enlargement* of ventricles, and focal alteration of white-matter tracts in patients with schizophrenia (Glahn *et al.*, 2008; Ellison-Wright and Bullmore, 2009). Reductions have been seen primarily in temporal lobe structures, such as the hippocampus, amygdala, and the superior temporal gyri, as well as in the prefrontal cortex. At least some structural alterations appeared to be present at illness onset and then progressed during the course of illness, supporting the view that brain structural alterations in schizophrenia stem from both early and late developmental derailments (Pantelis *et al.*, 2005; DeLisi, 2008). Medication effects might be involved in some structural brain abnormalities. For example, basal ganglia volume increases might be accounted for by treatment with typical antipsychotic agents, while basal ganglia volume decreases might be attributed to treatment with atypical antipsychotics (Scherk and Falkai, 2006).

Cognitive deficits observed in schizophrenia have been ascribed to reduced activation of the dorsolateral prefrontal cortex, known as *hypofrontality*, revealed in functional magnetic resonance imaging (fMRI) and positron-emission tomography (PET) studies (Millan *et al.*, 2012). Yet other cortical and subcortical structures are also affected with complex patterns of region-dependent hypo- and hyperactivation; increased activity might reflect an attempt to compensate for insufficient performance. It has been suggested that a disturbance of *frontocortical–striatal–thalamic* loops contribute to deficits in attention, working memory, and executive function (Minzenberg *et al.*, 2009). Impaired verbal learning and language in schizophrenia is related to diminished connectivity in the *temporal–frontal* circuitry and reduced left hemispheric lateralization of Broca's area and functionally related regions (Li *et al.*, 2009). Some structural alterations (e.g., hippocampal volume reductions) and abnormalities in prefrontal functioning might be related to a genetic predisposition to the disorder, since qualitatively similar but less severe abnormalities have been found in relatives of patients affected with schizophrenia and subjects in the prodromal phase of the illness (Boos *et al.*, 2007; Fusar-Poli *et al.*, 2007). Taken together, widespread structural alterations and perturbed brain connectivity provide the basis for considering schizophrenia a "disconnection syndrome" (Friston, 1998; Pettersson-Yeo *et al.*, 2011).

Among neurotransmitter systems, abnormal *dopaminergic* neurotransmission is a major contributor to the development of psychosis as reflected by the effectiveness of antipsychotic agents with their dopamine D_2 receptor blockade, and the psychotomimetic effect of dopamine agonists, such as amphetamine. Therefore, psychosis has been linked to a "hyperdopaminergic" state. Neuroimaging studies of the striatum have provided unambiguous evidence for dopamine involvement by showing that patients with schizophrenia have elevated presynaptic dopamine synthesis capacity, and baseline synaptic dopamine levels and dopamine release (Laruelle, 1998; Howes *et al.*, 2012). It has been postulated that while a *hyperactive* mesolimbic dopaminergic system underlies positive symptoms of schizophrenia, a *hypoactive* mesocortical dopaminergic system underlies negative and cognitive symptoms (Weinberger, 1987). In an attempt to fill the gap between neurobiological alterations and patients' subjective experiences, Kapur (2003) theorized that the released dopamine leads to a switch in attention towards the rewarding situation, based on the fact that dopamine neurons fire in response to novel environmental rewards, and thus imbues the stimulus with motivational salience. Aberrant firing of the dopamine system might lead to the aberrant assignment of motivational salience to objects, people, and actions. The mixture of dopamine dysregulation and aberrant assignment of salience to stimuli, together with a cognitive scheme that attempts to grapple with these experiences to give them meaning, might lead to the development of psychotic symptoms. Certain patterns of thinking, such as a tendency to "jump to conclusions," might combine with dopamine dysfunction to increase the risk of delusion formation (Kapur, 2003).

Other neurotransmitters, *such as glutamate* and *gamma-aminobutyric acid* (GABA), which are ubiquitously distributed in the nervous system, apparently play a role in the pathogenesis of the disorder. Schizophrenia might be related to a deficient glutamate-mediated excitatory neurotransmission via *N*-methyl-D-aspartate (NMDA) receptors, based on clinical observations of the emergence of psychotic symptoms triggered by the NMDA antagonists phencyclidine (PCP) and ketamine (Javitt and Zukin, 1991). Reduced levels of GABA in the prefrontal cortex as measured by mRNA levels of glutamic acid decarboxylase, the major determinant of GABA synthesis, was consistently shown in post-mortem studies, as was upregulation of GABA receptors, suggesting a possible compensatory response to reduced GABA levels (Lewis *et al.*, 2005). These changes seem to be disease-specific and account for alterations in neural synchrony and consequently to working memory impairment in schizophrenia (Benes *et al.*, 2007). Finally, although direct evidence of *serotonergic* dysfunction in the pathophysiology of schizophrenia is lacking, marked serotonin antagonism of second-generation antipsychotic agents (e.g., clozapine) points toward complex interaction between serotonin and dopamine systems in the mechanism of antipsychotic drug action and putatively in the pathogenesis of schizophrenia (Kapur and Remington, 1996).

Obsessive–compulsive disorder

Similar to schizophrenia, neurobiological models of OCD have postulated that abnormalities in brain activity underlie the pathogenesis of OCD. To explain an overlap in symptom expression, the concept of parallel neural circuits pertinent to schizophrenia and OCD has been employed (Alexander *et al.*, 1990; Tibbo and Warneke, 1999). According to this concept, there are three circuits that include discrete areas of the prefrontal cortex: the dorsolateral prefrontal cortex (DLPFC), the lateral orbital cortex, and the anterior cingulated cortex. These circuits share anatomic substrates including the frontal lobe, stratum, globus pallidus, and thalamus. Projections from an anatomic region maintain segregation to discrete parts of subsequent anatomic structures in the circuit, maintaining a model of parallel circuits. However, it has been argued that there are open (projections to and from anatomic structures outside the defined circuit) as well as closed (limited to structures of the defined circuit only) properties of these circuits. The DLPFC circuit has been suggested to be predominantly associated with schizophrenia and the lateral orbital cortex circuit with OCD, however this distinction represents an oversimplification of the dysfunctional connectivity underlying both disorders.

The *orbitofrontal–subcortical circuit* (a putative "OCD neural network") is thought to connect regions of the brain that process information involved in the initiation of the behavioral responses that are implemented with limited conscious awareness (Saxena *et al.*, 2001). The classical conceptualization of this circuitry consists of a direct and an indirect pathway (Figure 1.2).

The direct pathway projects from the cerebral cortex to the striatum to the internal segment of the globus pallidus/substantia nigra, pars reticulate complex, then to the thalamus and back to the cortex. The indirect pathway is similar but projects from the striatum to the external segment of the globus pallidus to the subthalamic nucleus before returning to the common pathway. In patients with OCD, overactivity of the direct circuit supposedly leads to obsessions and compulsions. The prevailing functional theory of the OCD circuit is that increased excitatory output from the orbitofrontal/cingulated cortex, or increased caudate activity, causes inhibition of the dorsal thalamus, which in itself can lead to increased activation of the cortex due to loss of inhibition. Note the difference from the putative schizophrenia-related DLPFC circuit that originates in the prefrontal cortical area and projects primarily to the dorsolateral head of the caudate (versus ventromedial head in OCD), the globus pallidus, the ventroanterior and mediodorsal thalamus (as in OCD), and back to the DLPFC (Figure 1.3).

The thalamus seems to be an essential component in both circuits. The multiple nuclei that constitute the thalamus have extensive parallel projections to and from the DLPFC and orbitofrontal cortex, though significant overlap exists (Alexander *et al.*, 1990). It has been argued that the thalamus contributes to filtering or "gating" sensory and motor information, and thus it passes on only relevant information leading to behavioral modification. The assumption of the "input overload" associated with thalamic failure to filter information is

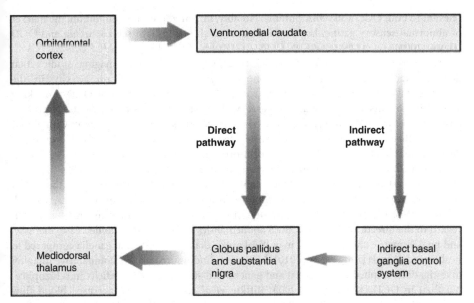

Figure 1.2 Direct (thick arrows) and indirect (thin arrows) pathways of the orbito-subcortical circuit connecting neuroanatomical structures hypothesized to be associated with symptoms of obsessive–compulsive disorder. (From Abramowitz JS, Taylor S, McKay D (2009) Obsessive–compulsive disorder. *Lancet* **374**, 491–499). Reprinted with permission.

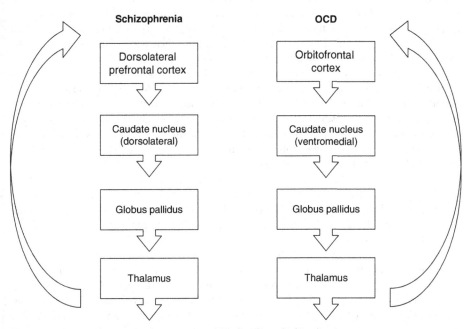

Figure 1.3 Functional circuits in obsessive–compulsive disorder and schizophrenia.

relevant to both OCD and schizophrenia. Notably, impaired pre-pulse inhibition, the marker of abnormal sensory gating, has consistently been shown in both schizophrenia and OCD (Geyer, 2006).

The cortico-striatal model of OCD is consistent with neuroimaging studies that demonstrated abnormal functional connectivity and *increased* brain activity in the orbitofrontal–subcortical circuit during rest and during presentation of OCD-provoking stimuli in patients with OCD as compared with healthy controls and patients with other anxiety disorders (Whiteside *et al.*, 2004). Moreover, successful treatment with either pharmacotherapy or cognitive–behavioral therapy, was associated with a significant decrease in metabolic activity in the orbitofrontal cortex, and caudate that tended to correlate with clinical improvement in symptomatology (Whiteside *et al.*, 2004).

In contrast to compelling evidence pointing to functional hyperactivity in the "OCD neural network," structural imaging studies have yielded non-uniform results. Indeed, though subtle gray matter alterations were detected in OCD, there is inconsistency with regard to the direction of the structural abnormalities in OCD with both decrease, increase, and no volumetric changes found in cortical areas, thalamus, and basal ganglia compared to healthy individuals (Rotge *et al.*, 2010). Moreover, findings from a few comparative imaging investigations implied more robust and generalized structural brain deficits in schizophrenia than in OCD (Kwon *et al.*, 2003; Riffkin *et al.*, 2005). Hence, increased blood flow and metabolism in the fronto-striatal circuitry in patients with OCD are likely to reflect anomalies that are not attributable to abnormal brain volumes; abnormalities in connectivity and/or metabolism may be more robust markers of OCD pathogenesis.

In summary, more similarities than differences emerge when examining the parallel development of the functional-circuit models in OCD and schizophrenia (Tibbo and Warneke, 1999). Anatomically, there is substantial overlap in structures and substructures. If a concept of open circuitry is accepted, thus allowing connections between the various substructures (i.e., between the nuclei of the thalamus) then it could be argued that the circuits described for OCD and schizophrenia are remarkably overlapping. Similarities between the two disorders also emerge when considering the gating or filtering of sensory information in both disorders. The fact that the comparable anatomic structures and parallel cortical–subcortical pathways have been independently documented for both disorders raises the possibility that a common functional aberration can lead to the co-expression of what appear to be completely different symptoms. However, there are many puzzling phenomena in the pursuit of an explanation of the co-occurrence of the two disorders. For example, although similar brain regions have been identified to be functionally and morphologically abnormal in both disorders, they tend to occur in opposite directions, such as the hyperfunctional fronto-striatal systems in OCD, versus the hypofunctional in schizophrenia (Gross-Isseroff *et al.*, 2003; Kwon *et al.*, 2003). For a schematic summary of functional and structural imaging findings in patients with OCD versus schizophrenia see Table 1.4.

Obsessive–compulsive disorder has been linked to a disruption in the brain's *serotonin neurotransmission*, though direct evidence is still sparse. OCD has been associated with hypersensitivity of postsynaptic serotonin receptors. Individuals with the disorder might have a specific dysfunction in the genes encoding for the serotonin transporter and serotonin receptor (5-HT_{2A}), but these have not been consistently identified (Westenberg *et al.*, 2007). Therapeutic efficacy of selective serotonin reuptake inhibitors (SSRIs) and clomipramine, agents that preferentially block the serotonin transporter and through this mechanism

Table 1.4 Simplified schematic summary of structural and functional imaging studies: schizophrenia versus OCD

Brain region	Functional studies		Structural studies	
	OCD	Schizophrenia	OCD	Schizophrenia
Caudate nucleus	↑	↓↑	↑↓	↑↓
OFC	↑	↓↑	↑↓	↓
ACC	↑	↓↑	↑↓	↓
Thalamus	↑	↓	↑	↓
DLPFC	no data	↓	no data	↓

↑, increased activation or volume; ↓, decreased activation or volume.
OFC, orbitofrontal cortex; ACC, anterior cingulate cortex; DLPFC, dorsolateral prefrontal cortex.
Source: Some data extracted from Gross-Isseroff *et al.* (2003).

facilitate serotonin neurotransmission, corroborates a role of serotonin in OCD. Perturbed *dopamine neurotransmission* is also involved. Higher dopamine transporter densities in tandem with a downregulation of the dopamine D_2 receptor suggest higher synaptic concentration of dopamine in the basal ganglia in OCD (Westenberg *et al.*, 2007). Increased midbrain dopamine neurotransmission in OCD echoes that found in schizophrenia; however, whether this is a primary disturbance or a common endpoint of other neurotransmitter pathology underlying each disorder in interest remains unknown. A beneficial effect of the adjunctive dopamine D_2 antagonists is another yet indirect indication for dopamine involvement in the pathogenesis of OCD.

Similar to schizophrenia, the *glutamatergic system* might also be dysfunctional in OCD. Yet contrary to a deficient glutamate-mediated excitatory neurotransmission in schizophrenia, there is likely glutamatergic hyperactivity in OCD. Indeed, elevated levels of a combined measure of glutamate and glutamine in brain regions relevant to OCD were found using magnetic resonance spectroscopy (Whiteside *et al.*, 2006), as were increased glutamate levels in the cerebrospinal fluid of patients with the disorder (Chakrabarty *et al.*, 2005). Preliminary research has implicated glutamate transporter genes, *Sapap3* and *SLC1A1*, in the disorder (Chakrabarty *et al.*, 2005; Arnold *et al.*, 2006).

Treatment
Schizophrenia

All current antipsychotic therapies have been developed on the platform of dopamine D_2 antagonism. Dampening hyperactive dopaminergic mesolimbic neurotransmission is accompanied by a therapeutic effect of antipsychotic agents on positive symptoms of the disorder. The potent serotonin 5-HT$_{2A}$ antagonism characteristic of second-generation antipsychotic agents contributes primarily to a lower risk of motor side effects; however, it does not significantly improve negative and cognitive symptoms. In view of the therapeutic limitations of currently available antipsychotics, a plethora of augmentation strategies are being evaluated in schizophrenia. Among various molecular targets, SSRIs have extensively been studied to address negative symptoms. Unfortunately, there was no global support for an improvement in negative symptoms with SSRI augmentation therapy in schizophrenia

(Sepehry *et al.*, 2007). Quite the opposite: SSRIs show therapeutic efficacy and good tolerability in treating depressive and anxiety symptoms commonly associated with schizophrenia. In addition, agents that moderate glutamatergic neurotransmission, both facilitators of NMDA activity (e.g., glycine, D-cycloserine) and NMDA antagonists (memantine, riluzole), have been administered in an attempt to improve negative and cognitive symptoms of schizophrenia (Tandon *et al.*, 2010). However, benefits of this treatment among clinical populations have not yet been demonstrated.

Obsessive–compulsive disorder

In contrast to their pointed utility in schizophrenia, SSRIs along with clomipramine are the treatment of choice in OCD. Nevertheless, despite therapeutic efficacy roughly 50% of OCD patients fail to respond, indicating that for a substantial number of patients serotonin reuptake inhibition is insufficient to alleviate obsessive–compulsive symptoms. Dopamine D_2 antagonists, the drugs of choice for schizophrenia, exert a positive therapeutic effect for OCD patients as well. Indeed, adjunctive antipsychotic agents, primarily risperidone and haloperidol, in low dose ranges are efficacious in a sizeable proportion of patients who failed to respond to SSRIs (McDougle *et al.*, 2000), pointing to additional areas of overlap between the two disorders. Finally, NMDA antagonists, riluzole and memantine, which showed thus far limited benefits in schizophrenia, seem to have certain therapeutic value in treatment-resistant OCD (Pittenger *et al.*, 2006) (Figure 1.4).

Undoubtedly, schizophrenia and OCD are distinct nosological entities, and typical features of one disorder are readily distinguishable from the other. However, epidemiological and clinical presentations, putative underlying pathogenetic mechanisms, and treatments have been shown to be common to both disorders. This is not to say that all patients with schizophrenia and with OCD share these aberrations, but it helps explain the subset of patients that shares these symptoms and the relative frequency of concurrent schizophrenic and obsessive–compulsive symptoms. In fact, it seems more plausible that symptoms of schizophrenia and OCD can coexist than not.

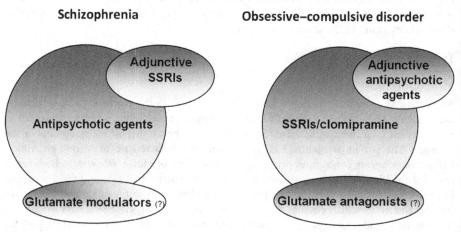

Figure 1.4 Schematic comparison of pharmacotherapy in schizophrenia and obsessive–compulsive disorder.

This book consolidates the current knowledge in the "gray area" of the overlap between two major psychiatric disorders, schizophrenia and OCD. The book pinpoints the relevant aspects of the history, epidemiology, clinical characteristics, neurobiology, and treatment of patients with the complex psychiatric condition "schizo-obsessive" disorder.

References

Abramowitz JS, Taylor S, McKay D (2009) Obsessive-compulsive disorder. *Lancet* **374**, 491–499.

Alexander GE, Crutcher MD, DeLong MR (1990) Basal ganglia-thalamocortical circuits: parallel substrates for motor, oculomotor, "prefrontal" and "limbic" functions. *Progress in Brain Research* **85**, 119–146.

Amador XF, David AS (eds.) (1998) *Insight and Psychosis*. Oxford University Press, New York.

American Psychiatric Association (1994) *Diagnostic and Statistical Manual of Mental Disorders*, 4th edn. American Psychiatric Association, Washington, DC.

American Psychiatric Association (2000) *Diagnostic and Statistical Manual of Mental Disorders*, 4th edn, text revn. American Psychiatric Association, Washington, DC.

Andreasen NC (1979) Thought, language, and communication disorders: I. Clinical assessment, definition of terms, and evaluation of their reliability. *Archives of General Psychiatry* **36**, 1315–1321.

Andreasen NC (1982) Negative symptoms in schizophrenia: definition and reliability. *Archives of General Psychiatry* **39**, 784–788.

Arnold PD, Sicard T, Burroughs E, Richter MA, Kennedy JL (2006) Glutamate transporter gene *SLC1A1* associated with obsessive-compulsive disorder. *Archives of General Psychiatry* **63**, 769–776.

Arts B, Jabben N, Krabbendam L, van Os J (2008) Meta-analyses of cognitive functioning in euthymic bipolar patients and their first-degree relatives. *Psychological Medicine* **38**, 771–785.

Bassett AS, Scherer SW, Brzustowicz LM (2010) Copy number variations in schizophrenia: critical review and new perspectives on concepts of genetics and disease. *American Journal of Psychiatry* **167**, 899–914.

Baxter LR Jr (1992) Neuroimaging studies of obsessive compulsive disorder. *Psychiatric Clinics of North America* **15**, 871–884.

Benes FM, Lim B, Matzilevich D, *et al.* (2007) Regulation of the GABA cell phenotype in hippocampus of schizophrenics and bipolars. *Proceedings of the National Academy of Sciences of the United States of America* **104**, 10 164–10 169.

Berrios GE (1989) Obsessive-compulsive disorder: its conceptual history in France during the 19th century. *Comprehensive Psychiatry* **30**, 283–295.

Berrios GE (1996) *The History of Mental Symptoms: Descriptive Psychopathology since the Nineteenth Century.* Cambridge University Press, Cambridge.

Bleuler E (1911/1950) *Dementia Praecox or the Group of Schizophrenias*, transl. Zinkin J. International Universities Press, New York.

Bloch MH, Landeros-Weisenberger A, Rosario MC, Pittenger C, Leckman JF (2008) Meta-analysis of the symptom structure of obsessive-compulsive disorder. *American Journal of Psychiatry* **165**, 1532–1542.

Boos HB, Aleman A, Cahn W, Hulshaff Pol H, Kahn R (2007) Brain volumes in relatives of patients with schizophrenia: a meta-analysis. *Archives of General Psychiatry* **64**, 297–304.

Brune M (2005) Theory of mind in schizophrenia: a review of the literature. *Schizophrenia Bulletin* **31**, 21–42.

Burdick KE, Robinson DG, Malhotra AK, Szeszko PR (2008) Neurocognitive profile analysis in obsessive-compulsive disorder. *Journal of the International Neuropsychological Society* **14**, 640–645.

Cannon M, Jones PB, Murray RM (2002) Obstetric complications and schizophrenia: historical and meta-analytic review. *American Journal of Psychiatry* **65**, 146–152.

Carey G, Gottesman I (2000) Twin and family studies of anxiety, phobic, and obsessive disorders. In: Klein DF, Rabkin JG (eds.) *Anxiety: New Research and Changing Concepts*. Raven Press, New York.

Chakrabarty K, Bhattacharyya S, Christopher R, Khanna S (2005) Glutamatergic dysfunction in OCD. *Neuropsychopharmacology* **30**, 1735–1740.

Chamberlain SR, Blackwell AD, Fineberg NA, Robbins TW, Sahakian BJ (2005) The neuropsychology of obsessive compulsive disorder: the importance of failures in cognitive and behavioural inhibition as candidate endophenotypic markers. *Neuroscience and Biobehavioral Reviews* **29**, 399–419.

Chamberlain SR, Fineberg NA, Menzies LA, *et al.* (2007) Impaired cognitive flexibility and motor inhibition in unaffected first-degree relatives of patients with obsessive-compulsive disorder. *American Journal of Psychiatry* **164**, 335–338.

DeLisi LE (2008) The concept of progressive brain change in schizophrenia: implications for understanding schizophrenia. *Schizophrenia Bulletin* **34**, 312–321.

Eisen JI, Rasmussen SA (1993) Obsessive-compulsive disorder with psychotic features. *Journal of Clinical Psychiatry* **54**, 373–379.

Ellison-Wright I, Bullmore E (2009) Meta-analysis of diffusion tensor imaging studies in schizophrenia. *Schizophrenia Research* **108**, 3–10.

Friston KJ (1998) The disconnection hypothesis. *Schizophrenia Research* **30**, 115–125.

Fusar-Poli P, Perez J, Broome M, *et al.* (2007) Neurofunctional correlates of vulnerability to psychosis: a systematic review and meta-analysis. *Neuroscience and Biobehavioral Reviews* **31**, 465–484.

Geller D (2006) Obsessive-compulsive and spectrum disorders in children and adolescents. *Psychiatry Clinics of North America* **29**, 353–370.

Geyer MA (2006) The family of sensorimotor gating disorders: comorbidities or diagnostic overlaps? *Neurotoxicity Research* **10**, 211–220.

Glahn DC, Laird AR, Ellison-Wright I, *et al.* (2008) Meta-analysis of gray matter anomalies in schizophrenia: application of anatomic likelihood estimation and network analysis. *Biological Psychiatry* **64**, 774–781.

Gross-Isseroff R, Hermesh H, Zohar J, Weizman A (2003) Neuroimaging communality between schizophrenia and obsessive compulsive disorder: a putative basis for schizo-obsessive disorder? *World Journal of Biological Psychiatry* **4**, 129–134.

Howes OD, Kambeitz J, Kim E, *et al.* (2012) The nature of dopamine dysfunction in schizophrenia and what this means for treatment. *Archives of General Psychiatry* April 2. Epub ahead of print, doi:10.1001/archgenpsychiatry.2012.169

Insel TR (2010) Rethinking schizophrenia. *Nature* **468**, 187–193.

Insel TR, Akiskal HS (1986) Obsessive-compulsive disorder with psychotic features: a phenomenologic analysis. *American Journal of Psychiatry* **143**, 1527–1533.

Jacobsen P, Freeman D, Salkovskis P (2012) Reasoning bias and belief conviction in obsessive-compulsive disorder and delusions: jumping to conclusions across disorders? *British Journal of Clinical Psychology* **51**, 84–99.

Janet P (1903) *Les Obsessions et la Psychasthénie*, vol. 2, Alcan, Paris. (Reprinted: Arno, New York, 1976.)

Jaspers K (1946) *Allgemeine Psychopathologie*. Springer-Verlag, Heidelberg.

Javitt DC, Zukin SR (1991) Recent advances in the phencyclidine model of schizophrenia. *American Journal of Psychiatry* **148**, 1301–1308.

Kapur S (2003) Psychosis as a state of aberrant salience: a framework linking biology, phenomenology, and pharmacology in schizophrenia. *American Journal of Psychiatry* **160**, 13–23.

Kapur S, Remington G (1996) Serotonin-dopamine interaction and its relevance to schizophrenia. *American Journal of Psychiatry* **153**, 466–476.

Kraepelin E (1919) *Dementia Praecox*. Krieger, New York.

Kwon JS, Shin Y-W, Kim C-W, *et al.* (2003) Similarity and disparity of obsessive-compulsive disorder and schizophrenia in MR volumetric abnormalities of the hippocampus–amygdala complex. *Journal of Neurology, Neurosurgery, and Psychiatry* **74**, 962–964.

Lang H (1997) Obsessive-compulsive disorders in neurosis and psychosis. *Journal of the American Academy of Psychoanalysis* **25**, 143–150.

Laruelle M (1998) Imaging dopamine transmission in schizophrenia: a review and meta-analysis. *Quarterly Journal of Nuclear Medicine* **42**, 211–221.

Lewis DA, Hashimoto T, Volk DW (2005) Cortical inhibitory neurons and schizophrenia. *Nature Reviews* **6**, 312–324.

Li X, Branch CA, Delisi LE (2009) Language pathway abnormalities in schizophrenia: a review of fMRI and other imaging studies. *Current Opinion in Psychiatry* **22**, 131–139.

Marwaha S, Johnson S, Bebbington P, *et al.* (2007) Rates and correlates of employment in people with schizophrenia in the UK, France and Germany. *British Journal of Psychiatry* **191**, 30–33.

Mayer-Gross W (1932) *Handbuch der Greistes-Krankenheiten*, vol. 9. Springer-Verlag, Berlin.

McDougle CJ, Epperson CN, Pelton GH, Wasylink S, Price LH (2000) A double-blind, placebo-controlled study of risperidone addition in serotonin reuptake inhibitor-refractory obsessive-compulsive disorder. *Archives of General Psychiatry* **57**, 794–801.

McGrath J, Saha S, Chant D, Wellham J (2008) Schizophrenia: a concise overview of incidence, and mortality. *Epidemiology Review* **30**, 67–76.

McGuffin P, Gottesman II (1999) Risk factors for schizophrenia. *New England Journal of Medicine* **341**, 370–371.

Millan MJ, Agid Y, Brüne M, *et al.* (2012) Cognitive dysfunction in psychiatric disorders: characteristics, causes and the quest for improved therapy. *Nature Reviews Drug Discovery* **11**, 141–168.

Minzenberg MJ, Laird AR, Thelen S, Carter CS, Glahn DC (2009) Meta-analysis of 41 functional neuroimaging studies of executive function in schizophrenia. *Archives of General Psychiatry* **66**, 811–822.

Murray CJL, Lopez AD (eds.) (1996) *The Global Burden of Disease: A Comprehensive Assessment of Mortality and Disability from Diseases, Injuries, and Risk Factors in 1990 and Projected to 2020*, vol. 1. Harvard School of Public Health on behalf of the World Health Organization and the World Bank, Cambridge, MA.

Need AC, Ge D, Weale ME, *et al.* (2009) A genome-wide investigation of SNPs and CNVs in schizophrenia. *PLoS Genetics* **5**, e1000373.

Nestadt G, Grados M, Samuels JF (2010) Genetics of OCD. *Psychiatry Clinics of North America* **33**, 141–158.

Pallanti S (2008) Transcultural observations of obsessive-compulsive disorder. *American Journal of Psychiatry* **165**, 169–170.

Pantelis C, Yücel M, Wood SJ, *et al.* (2005) Structural brain imaging evidence for multiple pathological processes at different stages of brain development in schizophrenia. *Schizophrenia Bulletin* **31**, 672–696.

Perala J, Suvisari J, Saarni SI, *et al.* (2007) Lifetime prevalence of psychotic and bipolar I disorders in a general population. *Archives of General Psychiatry* **64**, 19–28.

Pettersson-Yeo W, Allen P, Benetti S, McGuire P, Mechelli A (2011) Disconnectivity in schizophrenia: where are we now? *Neuroscience and Behaviorial Reviews* **35**, 1110–1124.

Pittenger C, Krystal JH, Coric V (2006) Glutamate-modulating drugs as novel pharmacotherapeutic agents in the treatment of obsessive-compulsive disorder. *NeuroRx* **3**, 69–81.

Rauch SL, Jenike MA, Alpert NM, *et al.* (1994) Regional cerebral blood flow measured during symptom provocation in obsessive-compulsive disorder using oxygen 15-labeled carbon dioxide and positron emission tomography. *Archives of General Psychiatry* **51**, 62–70.

Riffkin J, Yücel M, Maruff P, *et al.* (2005) A manual and automated MRI study of anterior cingulated and orbito-frontal cortices, and caudate nucleus in obsessive-compulsive disorder: comparison with healthy controls and patients with schizophrenia. *Psychiatry Research* **138**, 99–113.

Rotge JY, Langbour N, Guehl D, *et al.* (2010) Gray matter alterations in obsessive-compulsive disorder: an anatomic likelihood estimation meta-analysis. *Neuropsychopharmacology* **35**, 686–691.

Ruscio AM, Stein DJ, Chiu WT, Kessler RC (2010) The epidemiology of obsessive-compulsive disorder in the National Comorbidity Survey Replication. *Molecular Psychiatry* **15**, 53–63.

Saxena S, Bota RG, Brody AL (2001) Brain-behavior relationships in obsessive-compulsive disorder. *Seminars in Clinical Neuropsychiatry* **6**, 82–101.

Scherk H, Falkai P (2006) Effects of antipsychotics on brain structure. *Current Opinion in Psychiatry* **19**, 145–150.

Schneider K (1925) Zwangszustände und Schizophrenie [Compulsive states in schizophrenia]. *Archive für Psychiatrie und Nervenkrankeiten* **74**, 93–107.

Schneider K (1959) *Klinische Psychopathologie*, 12th edn. Georg Thieme, Stuttgart. (Transl. Hamilton MW (1976) *Clinical Psychopathology*. Grune and Stratton, New York).

Schneider K (1987) *Klinische Psychopathologie*, 13th edn. Georg Thieme, Stuttgart.

Sepehry AA, Potvin S, Elie R, Stip E (2007) Selective serotonin reuptake inhibitor (SSRI) add-on therapy for the negative symptoms of schizophrenia: a meta-analysis. *Journal of Clinical Psychiatry* **68**, 604–610.

Snitz BE, MacDonald AW III, Carter CS (2006) Cognitive deficits in unaffected first-degree relatives of schizophrenia patients: a meta-analytic review of putative endophenotypes. *Schizophrenia Bulletin* **32**, 179–194.

Swedo SE, Garvey M, Snider L, Hamilton C, Leonard HL (2001) The PANDAS subgroup: recognition and treatment. *CNS Spectrums* **6**, 419–22, 425–6.

Tandon R, Keshavan MS, Nasrallah HA (2008) Schizophrenia "just the facts" what we know in 2008: II. Epidemiology and etiology. *Schizophrenia Research* **102**, 1–18.

Tandon R, Nasrallah HA, Keshavan MS (2010) Schizophrenia "just the facts": V. Treatment and prevention: past, present, and future. *Schizophrenia Research* **122**, 1–23.

Tibbo P, Warneke L (1999) Obsessive-compulsive disorder in schizophrenia: epidemiologic and biologic overlap. *Journal of Psychiatry and Neuroscience* **24**, 15–24.

Torres A, Prince M, Bebbington P, *et al.* (2006) Obsessive-compulsive disorder: prevalence, comorbidity, impact, and help-seeking in the British National Psychiatric Comorbidity Survey of 2000. *American Journal of Psychiatry* **163**, 1978–1985.

van Grootheest DS, Cath DC, Beekman AT, Boomsma DI (2005) Twin studies on obsessive-compulsive disorder: a review. *Twin Research Human Genetics* **8**, 450–458.

Van Os J, Kapur S (2009) Schizophrenia. *Lancet* **374**, 635–645.

Van Os J, Kenis G, Rutten BF (2010) The environment and schizophrenia. *Nature* **468**, 203–212.

Weinberger DR (1987) Implications of normal brain development for the pathogenesis of schizophrenia. *Archives of General Psychiatry* **44**, 660–669.

Westenberg H, Fineberg N, Denys D (2007) Neurobiology of obsessive-compulsive disorder: serotonin and beyond. *CNS Spectrums* **12** (Suppl. 3), 14–27.

Westphal K (1878) Ueber Zwangsvorstellungen. *Archiv für Psychiatrie und Nervenkrankheiten* **8**, 734–750.

Whiteside SP, Port JD, Abramowitz JS (2004) A meta-analysis of functional neuroimaging in obsessive-compulsive disorder. *Psychiatry Research* **132**, 69–79.

Whiteside SP, Port JD, Deacon BJ, Abramowitz JS (2006) A magnetic resonance spectroscopy investigation of obsessive compulsive disorder and anxiety. *Psychiatry Research* **146**, 137–147.

World Health Organization (1992) *The ICD-10 Classification of Mental and Behavioral Disorders: Clinical Descriptions and*

Diagnostic Guidelines. World Health Organization, Geneva.

Wu Y, Liu X, Luo H, *et al.* (2012) Advanced paternal age increases the risk of schizophrenia and obsessive-compulsive disorder in a Chinese Han population. *Psychiatry Research*, Epub Mar 16.

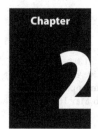

Obsessive–compulsive symptoms in schizophrenia: conceptual history

Obsessive–compulsive symptoms, in contrast to positive, negative, and cognitive symptoms, have not been considered primary features of schizophrenia. However, analysis of clinical presentations and neurobiological underpinnings of schizophrenia and OCD clearly reveal converging trajectories. This chapter evaluates some of the critical stages in consolidation of the concept of schizo-obsessive disorder.

Emil Kraepelin and Eugen Bleuler

Emil Kraepelin and Eugen Bleuler, who laid the foundations for modern conceptualization of schizophrenia, had fairly different views on the interrelationship of schizophrenia and obsessive–compulsive phenomena. Hence, Kraepelin did not consider obsessive–compulsive symptoms a psychopathological component of the disease, but rather believed that the "transition of obsessions into mental afflictions, especially into paranoia is not to be forthcoming" (Slater and Roth, 1969). Eugen Bleuler called attention to the possibility of the development of schizophrenia in some patients with neurotic conditions, such as neurasthenia, hysteria, and especially obsessive–compulsive disorder. Moreover, Bleuler considered obsessive–compulsive symptoms a possible feature of the prodromal phase of schizophrenia, with chronic obsessions an actual manifestation of the disorder. Describing schizophrenic symptoms, he stated that "compulsive thinking (obsession) is the most common of all the automatic phenomena" (Bleuler, 1911/1950). He further depicted obsessive–compulsive symptoms in schizophrenia as "automatisms" that are comparable to auditory or visual hallucinations in that they are "hallucinations of thinking, striving, and wanting" (Bleuler, 1911/1950, p.450). Bleuler also maintained that obsessive–compulsive symptoms are experienced and perceived in schizophrenia as in neurotic conditions, independent of schizophrenia symptoms. However, in some patients they can intertwine with psychosis and pose a substantial diagnostic challenge. Contemporary studies substantiated and expanded these observations by identifying obsessive–compulsive symptoms in schizophrenia patients that are independent of psychosis, as well as psychosis-related complex obsessive–compulsive psychopathological phenomena. Investigations explicitly focused on the prevalence, psychopathology, and clinical significance of obsessive–compulsive symptoms in schizophrenia emerged in the mid twentieth century.

Alfred Gordon

The American psychiatrist Alfred Gordon focused primarily on the psychopathological interrelationship between obsessive and delusional phenomena in patients with schizophrenia and affective disorders (Gordon, 1926). He presented a series of cases and found several putative pathways:

- obsessions form a "point of departure" for development of delusions by a process of "argumentative interpretation";
- direct transformation of obsessions into delusions;
- disappearance of obsessions when delusions unrelated in content to obsessions are developed.

Representative case reports

Case 2.1. Mr. M, 30-year-old clerk, had always been considered a timid and eccentric teenager. He never liked to play with anyone, and preferred to remain alone. He later developed obsessive worries for his child whom he feared was not properly cared for by the nanny. He admitted that his apprehension was baseless and excessive, but could not resist it. Gradually his mental condition changed. His obsessive worries disappeared, but he developed an argumentative attitude toward them. He claimed that in view of the fact that there was never a real reason for his fears concerning the child, there must have been a disturbance in his mental faculties. When attempts were made to confront him with these new ideas, he began to suspect that everyone was trying to deceive him. He developed persecutory delusions toward his physician whom he claimed initiated the falsehood in order to declare his insanity.

Case 2.2. Ms. B, 24-year-old schoolteacher. During childhood she presented with an obsessional fear of behaving badly and of not doing things correctly. She also had obsessive doubts which affected almost all her actions, writing, walking, and speaking. For years the patient's obsessive ideas remained intact, and she continued her studies successfully. However, at age 18 when she became a kindergarten teacher, she gradually developed delusions which incorporated the content of her obsessions. She was convinced of having harmed the children in her kindergarten. Her doubts concerning incorrect teaching became an actual conviction that she taught them the opposite of what she was supposed to and that the children would therefore not be promoted. She feared that she would be accused of misrepresentation, and would be dishonored and dismissed forever. In addition, she started to hear voices on the same theme: she heard pupils' voices reproaching her, and their parents' voices threatening her with violence.

Case 2.3. Mr. O, a 35-year-old musician. As a child he was considered odd and eccentric. From age 19 he began to express obsessive doubts concerning whether what he said to others in conversation was correct, frequently repeating words, sentences, and phrases. For the same reason, he repeatedly went over his letters before sealing them to be mailed. He fully realized the absurdity of these thoughts and rituals but could not resist them. At some point the obsessive phenomena subsided. He began showing paranoid symptoms, claiming that people watched and followed him, and used profane language directed at him. He refused to eat because he feared being poisoned by his doctor. According to him, the latter was in conspiracy with his brother, the maid, and the cook. Previously expressed obsessive symptoms did not re-emerge.

Gordon suggested that obsessions and delusions represent a continuum of the related disorders, rather than discrete psychopathological phenomena. He held the opinion that obsessions might be the basis for the development of delusions (Case 2.1), or may directly transform into delusions (Case 2.2). He also substantiated clinical observations made earlier by Bleuler, indicating that obsessive–compulsive phenomena in schizophrenia typically predated psychosis and in some patients preserve independence from psychotic symptoms (Case 2.3).

Gordon conceived that obsessive–compulsive symptoms were not exclusively associated with schizophrenia, the view shared by A. Lewis, a prominent American psychiatrist of the mid twentieth century (Lewis, 1936). Gordon reported cases pointing towards a close connection between obsessive phenomena and depressive states, corroborating Kraepelin's views on intimate relations between obsessive–compulsive and affective disorders. He noted that obsessive neurosis as an independent clinical entity may exist throughout the entire life of an individual without admixture of manifestations of a psychotic disorder. Individual predisposition determines whether a person is going to develop "pure" obsessive–compulsive neurosis or obsessive–compulsive symptoms in the context of schizophrenia or affective illness (Gordon, 1926; 1950).

Erwin Stengel

The Austrian psychiatrist Erwin Stengel was among the first who systematically evaluated an interface between obsessive–compulsive and psychotic symptoms in schizophrenia patients (Stengel, 1945). Stengel sought to address two key questions: first, whether the interaction of obsessional and psychotic symptoms results in modification of the latter with regard to symptomatology and prognosis; second, the "fate" of obsessions in the course of ensuing psychosis. Based on thorough anamnestic data of patients admitted to the Royal Edinburgh Hospital for Mental and Nervous Disorders (Scotland), direct patient interview, and follow-up, Stengel provided the following clinical characteristics of schizo-obsessive patients:

- obsessive–compulsive symptoms preceded the occurrence of psychosis, and did not follow psychosis in any of the observed cases;
- obsessive–compulsive symptoms preserved their distinguished characteristics throughout the course of illness, usually disappearing during psychotic episodes and re-emerging in remissions;
- there was no direct transformation of an obsession into a delusion, thus delusions could not be regarded as derivates of the obsessions;
- there was frequent emergence of "critical attitudes and doubt" towards the delusions and hallucinations in the presence of obsessions, suggesting their modifying effect on psychotic symptoms. This observation corroborated with Mayer-Gross's (1928) notion of a "pathoplastically veiled" clinical picture of schizophrenia occurring in the presence of an obsessive–compulsive personality;
- no cases of catatonic and hebephrenic schizophrenia were identified, implying that the presence of obsessive–compulsive symptoms "protected against personality disintegration" in schizophrenia;
- a majority of patients revealed a benign course and marked tendency for remission, and "malignant progressive deterioration" did not occur in any of the reported cases;
- the family histories of the presented cases revealed hereditary determinants and constitutional predisposition for both schizophrenia and obsessive–compulsive symptoms anticipating contemporary studies on familial heredity in schizo-obsessive patients.

Representative case reports

Case 2.4. Mrs. S suffered from obsessions ever since childhood. She had always been pedantic and excessively clean. Since puberty she had a washing compulsion. She was voluntarily admitted to a mental hospital for treatment of her obsessive–compulsive symptoms, which had become more severe at age 29. The diagnosis on admission was obsessional neurosis. However, after 2 months she became agitated and expressed numerous delusions. She believed that the chief of the hospital was the King, the matron the Queen, and her husband the heir to the throne. She heard voices telling her that she was a descendant of God. Her mood was elated, and her speech was incoherent. Her condition was regarded as paranoid schizophrenia. About a year after admission the patient gradually improved and she was discharged from hospital, though she still expressed delusions and had some hallucinations. Within a few months of discharge those symptoms disappeared, but then the obsessive–compulsive symptoms, which had been completely absent during the psychotic period, reappeared. The patient had full insight into their morbid nature and tried to resist them. The psychotic period had left behind some degree of emotional flattening . . .

Case 2.5. Mr. C was a normal child and interacted easily with others. At age 10 he developed a compulsive habit of pulling up his socks and a compulsion to touch the door knob repeatedly. He tried to resist those habits, which he regarded as senseless. He also experienced great difficulty in using the school lavatories. He was never sure whether he had shut gates properly, and he had to go back several times to reassure himself. At age 20, he was seen by a psychiatrist, who revealed that the patient was manneristic, and not infrequently a facial grimace was observed. There was no gross formal disorder of thought, but there was a tendency to irrelevancy and over-talkativeness. He felt compelled to touch things, and he explained that by doing this he was making up for not doing things right. He realized that his obsessive thoughts and compulsive acts were senseless and he tried to resist them. No delusions or hallucinations were revealed. There was emotional blunting and social aloofness. The psychiatrist thought the case might be an obsessional neurosis or possibly an early schizophrenia. The patient was not seen again, but a communication from his father revealed that he was much improved, but remained socially disengaged and apathetic.

Stengel's major assumption focused on a "protective effect" exerted by obsessive-compulsive symptoms on psychopathology, course, and prognosis in schizophrenia. He based this hypothesis primarily on a benign course of illness and a favorable prognosis of schizo-obsessive patients, highlighting that "malignant progressive deterioration" did not occur in any of his patients. The author considered these cases intermediate; between constitutional psychasthenia, as described by Janet (1903), and schizophrenia. He offered a psychoanalytic explanation that prevailed in psychiatry in the mid twentieth century, and suggested that the protective effect of obsessive–compulsive symptoms in schizophrenia was due to "a capability of obsessional personality structure to subdue and abort schizophrenic reactions" (Stengel, 1945).

Stengel's contribution was first and foremost in attracting the attention of clinicians to those schizophrenia patients who also exhibit obsessive–compulsive symptoms, and have features distinct from "typical" schizophrenia, rendering them "borderline cases" and thus difficult to diagnose, particularly in the initial stages of illness (Cases 2.4 and 2.5). Anticipating current studies, he drew attention to the clinical heterogeneity within the schizo-obsessive subgroup by showing that some schizo-obsessive patients may have predominant negative symptoms without delusions and hallucinations (Case 2.5), complicating diagnosis even more. He further suggested that these patients may be unfamiliar to hospital psychiatrists, because they are rarely admitted to mental hospitals (Case 2.5).

Ismond Rosen

Ismond Rosen, a psychiatrist who worked in the Maudsley Hospital (London), advanced the examination of the clinical characteristics, course, and outcomes of those schizophrenia patients who also exhibit obsessive–compulsive symptoms (Rosen, 1956). He used case material of schizophrenia patients admitted to the Bethlem Royal Hospital and the Maudsley Hospital from July 1, 1949 to July, 1953, and identified 30 patients (from a total of 5467) who at some point exhibited obsessive–compulsive symptoms. The author presented the following clinical characteristics:

- age at onset of obsessive–compulsive symptoms: there were two peaks, the first in childhood and early adolescence, and the second between 20 and 35 years;
- age at onset of first schizophrenic symptoms was between 15 and 35 years;
- obsessive–compulsive symptoms appeared either prior to, or coincident with, the first schizophrenia symptoms in all cases;
- first psychiatric attention was due to the emergence of schizophrenic but not obsessive–compulsive symptoms in all cases;
- mode of illness onset: four groups of prodromal symptoms were identified – obsessions only, predominant depressive symptoms, both obsessive and schizophrenic symptoms, non-specific behavioral symptoms;
- subtypes of schizophrenia identified: paranoid, schizoaffective, and juvenile;
- content of obsessive–compulsive symptoms: the most frequent obsessions were aggressive, sexual, and counting, the most frequent compulsions were washing, touching, and prayer rituals.

In his analysis of the clinical charts, Rosen found that obsessive–compulsive symptoms were identifiable phenomena in schizophrenia, typical in content, independent of psychotic symptoms, surfaced before or in concert with initial schizophrenia symptoms, and persisted largely unchanged in content and severity after the onset of schizophrenia. Noteworthy, patients tended to seek psychiatric treatment only when schizophrenic symptoms were manifest, despite the fact that in a considerable proportion of patients obsessional symptoms had been present for years. This pattern of help-seeking behavior was consistent with that found in non-schizophrenia OCD patients who were reluctant to seek medical help, "keeping secret" their obsessive symptoms. Lack of catatonic and hebephrenic features among the analyzed cases, episodic course of illness, long remissions associated with relatively high social and occupational functioning in schizo-obsessive patients as compared to their schizophrenia counterparts, led to the conclusion that obsessive–compulsive symptoms are an indicator of beneficial prognosis in schizophrenia. Rosen substantiated Stengel's observations regarding an absence of "malignant schizophrenic development" and "personality disintegration" in schizo-obsessive patients, and the assumption of a "protective effect" of obsessive–compulsive symptoms in schizophrenia. Rosen's input to the field was the description of the two types of obsessive-compulsive phenomena in patients with schizophrenia: typical – similar to obsessional neurosis, and psychotic-related – that seemed to be unique to schizophrenia. The latter represented complex phenomena that are obsessive in content and psychotic in form. He emphasized that in addition to the transition of obsessions into delusions, as previously described by Gordon (1926), a coexistence of both typical and psychotic-related components in the same patient was not uncommon.

The following case extracts exemplify a complexity of obsessive–compulsive phenomena in schizophrenia.

Case 2.6. For years, this patient had obsessional thoughts that she might harm someone. Gradually she began to hear God's voice saying she might harm Him. She later developed bizarre rituals to placate God. She was aware of the unrealistic nature of her voices and the absurdity of the rituals and tried to resist them.

Case 2.7. This patient had repetitive, intrusive, and distressful words such as "Radar," "Sex," and "Crime," which came into her mind from within and which she resisted and felt to be absurd. When schizophrenia developed she felt that someone was manipulating her and putting obscene thoughts and words, including those mentioned above, into her mind.

These vignettes clearly demonstrate that the presence of schizophrenia modifies the phenomenological expression of obsessive–compulsive symptoms and generates diagnostically challenging psychopathological conditions with characteristics of both obsessive–compulsive and psychotic phenomena. Rich clinical material, collected by Ismond Rosen, illustrates that the interrelationship between these two phenomena are bidirectional: obsessive–compulsive symptoms changed the course and the outcome of schizophrenia, while psychotic symptoms of schizophrenia affected the expression of obsessive–compulsive symptoms, accounting for the unique clinical presentation of schizo-obsessive disorder.

Paul Hoch and Phillip Polatin

"Pseudoneurotic schizophrenia" is a term coined by the American psychiatrists Paul Hoch and Phillip Polatin in the 1940s, to describe a subset of patients who presented with "prominent neurotic symptoms that mask a latent psychotic disorder" (Hoch and Polatin, 1949). Retaining phenomenological resemblance to psychoneuroses, these patients, however, differed principally by exhibiting thought, affective, and personality disturbances characteristic of schizophrenia. Absence of delusions, hallucinations, and catatonic symptoms further complicated diagnosis and treatment selection. There were several attempts to delineate this subgroup of patients by highlighting its dissimilarity from typical schizophrenia types, as reflected in the following definitions: ambulatory schizophrenia, latent schizophrenia, borderline schizophrenia, and pseudo-schizophrenic neurosis (as quoted by Hoch and Polatin, 1949).

The diagnosis of pseudoneurotic schizophrenia was warranted in the presence of basic schizophrenia symptoms and accessory symptomatology, the division previously introduced by Bleuler (1911/1950). Though in contrast to Bleuler's accessory symptoms (e.g., delusions, hallucinations), secondary symptoms in psychoneurotic schizophrenia included a broad spectrum of neurotic symptoms (Hoch and Polatin, 1949).

The diagnosis of pseudoneurotic schizophrenia

Primary clinical symptoms:

1. Disorders of thinking and associations: process and content.
2. Disorders of emotional regulation: form and content.
3. Disorders of sensorimotor and autonomic functioning.

Secondary clinical symptoms:

1. Pan-anxiety.
2. Pan-neurosis: neurotic symptomatology, acting-out behavior, and character-disorder symptoms.
3. Pan-sexuality.

From the diagnostic point of view the most distinctive presenting symptoms of the pseudo-neurotic form of schizophrenia were what the writers called pan-anxiety and pan-neurosis. In contrast to psychoneuroses, patients with pseudoneurotic schizophrenia showed "pervading anxiety" which affected all areas of the patients' experiences. Together with diffuse anxiety, simultaneous polymorphous neurotic symptoms (e.g., phobias, conversions), rather than isolated manifestations characteristic of psychoneuroses, were present. Importantly, obsessive–compulsive symptoms were among the central psychopathological features according to the authors' definition of pan-neurosis. "Polymorphous and chaotic" organization of the patients' sexuality also distinguished this schizophrenia subgroup. Although the authors perceived that the basic symptoms of schizophrenia were essential in establishing the diagnosis, they appeared to be less "striking and intense" than in the more gross forms of the disorder. Transient psychotic episodes ("micro-psychosis") were revealed in a substantial proportion of patients with pseudoneurotic schizophrenia, although psychotic symptoms were not critical in establishing the diagnosis.

The following is a case description of a patient with "pseudoneurotic schizophrenia" (Hoch and Catell, 1959):

Case 2.8. Mrs. S, a 21-year-old, dated the onset of her illness to age 15, when obsessive-repetitive cursing words came into her mind interfering with her daily routine. She developed a food phobia fearing that she would be unable to eat and would die that way. She compulsively turned out the light six times before every meal to "prevent the dread event." She also feared "insanity." She acknowledged the absurdity of these thoughts, but felt a compelling urge to think about the psychosis she might develop. She was diagnosed with obsessive-compulsive neurosis. Gradually she began to express hypochondriacal concerns over her "brain cells destroyed by obsessive thoughts." These ideas accounted for repetitive medical consultations with different specialists to rule out her "brain disease." She was constantly anxious. Her school performance progressively declined. She had less interest in friends and leisure activities, and became careless about her dress and hygiene. Her affect was flat, sometimes apathetic. Episodically, she was suspicious about people's attitudes toward her; however there was no evidence of frank delusions or hallucinations. Her primary diagnosis of obsessive-compulsive disorder was changed to schizophrenia, pseudoneurotic type.

Hoch et al. (1962) followed 109 patients with pseudoneurotic schizophrenia to determine the course of illness and the outcome. The follow-up period was 5–20 years (average 9 years). Basic symptoms of schizophrenia were revealed in all patients on follow-up. Notably, approximately 20% of the patients developed overt schizophrenic symptomatology, that is typical catatonic, hebephrenic, and paranoid symptoms. There was a significant incidence of subsequent hospitalization following initial contact, with 40% of the entire sample hospitalized one to nine times. Conversely, a meaningful proportion of patients who did not develop psychotic deterioration revealed good or fair functional outcome, highlighting the clinical diversity of the pseudoneurotic schizophrenia type.

Overall, Hoch and Polatin drew attention to a group of patients who demonstrated clinical symptomatology that was considered to be psychoneurotic by mainstream psychiatrists in the 1940s–1960s. Their scrupulous clinical observations revealed a common denominator between this subgroup and typical schizophrenia patients, the presence of basic schizophrenia symptoms as defined by Bleuler. The authors substantiated the relatedness of the pseudoneurotic subgroup to schizophrenia by a follow-up investigation showing that a considerable number of these patients had short psychotic episodes or alternatively developed frank psychosis. They established diagnostic criteria for the pseudoneurotic subtype, explicitly emphasizing the primacy of basic symptoms of schizophrenia accompanied by secondary symptomatology of pan-neurosis, anxiety, and sexuality. This diagnostic approach was in contrast to the views of those diagnosticians who defined this subgroup as "borderline," "ambulatory," or "latent" schizophrenia, implying that the patient had "neither neurosis nor schizophrenia, but was in some vague, transitional state" (quoted by Hoch and Polatin, 1949). A major limitation, however, was low reliability and validity of the identification of both basic and pseudoneurotic symptoms, and a lack of structured instruments for diagnosis of the pseudoneurotic type. That left clinicians to rely on their professional intuition rather than precise clinical evaluation. Subjective appraisal of symptoms was even more challenging due to a subtle and occasionally atypical expression of the basic schizophrenia symptoms observed in the pseudoneurotic type. Allowing diagnosis of schizophrenia in the presence of basic and pseudoneurotic features, without overt psychotic symptoms, led to a substantial broadening of the diagnostic boundaries of schizophrenia, further limiting both reliability and validity of diagnosis. Although a delineation of a subgroup of schizophrenia patients with prominent pseudoneurotic features was important in the outlying psychopathological diversity of schizophrenia, pseudoneurotic schizophrenia as a diagnostic entity has fallen out of clinical use and is not part of the current classification systems.

An important contribution to research on the schizophrenia–OCD interface was made in a prospective long-term schizophrenia study in an inpatient population diagnosed with schizophrenia, admitted between 1945 and 1959 to the University Psychiatric Clinic in Bonn (Germany) (Huber and Gross, 1989). It was shown that during the prodromal phase of schizophrenia patients may manifest "obsessional perseveration of thoughts" and obsessive–compulsive phenomena per se. These findings clearly corroborated previous observations of Westphal (1872) and Bleuler (1911/1950). Moreover, the authors revealed that obsessive–compulsive symptoms may appear during both early and late stages, including residual states of schizophrenia (Huber and Gross, 1989).

In conclusion, identification and psychopathological description of obsessive–compulsive phenomena in patients with schizophrenia early in the history of schizophrenia research helped to raise awareness of the linkage between the two disorders. Obsessive–compulsive phenomena appeared to be clinically meaningful and diagnostically challenging in schizophrenia patients. Substantial heterogeneity within the schizo-obsessive subgroup was also acknowledged as reflected in the different "proximity" between obsessive–compulsive and psychotic symptoms. Early research in this area, however, was characterized by the observational nature and lack of diagnostic criteria and structured diagnostic instruments for both schizophrenia and obsessive–compulsive disorder. Cross-sectional evaluation prevailed and served as a basis for conclusions regarding the interrelationship between the two disorders. Many patients diagnosed with schizophrenia by early diagnosticians showed prominent affective features and would probably not be considered schizophrenic according to modern diagnostic criteria. These factors along with the predominance of psychoanalytic thinking in mid-twentieth century psychiatry accounted at least in part, for the consideration of obsessive–compulsive symptoms as protective factors and predictors of a positive course and good prognosis in schizophrenia patients.

Contemporary studies

Major attempts to classify psychiatric conditions were undertaken after the Second World War. In 1952 the Diagnostic and Statistical Manual: Mental Disorders – now known as DSM-I – was first published (American Psychiatric Association, 1952). At that time, mental disorders were considered maladaptive neurotic reactions to the environment. DSM-II, published in 1968 (American Psychiatric Association, 1968) retained the psychoanalytical focus on neurosis and adaptation. The nine types of schizophrenia recorded in DSM-I were divided into 15 in DSM-II in order to capture a wide range of symptoms associated with the disorder. Among these 15 types, latent schizophrenia referred to pseudoneurotic and other non-psychotic variants of the disorder. However, the revision did little to standardize diagnosis. Over a decade later, DSM-III (American Psychiatric Association, 1980) revolutionized psychiatry by making it evidence-based. The DSM-III eschewed psychoanalytical theory and hypothetical causes of the disorders in order to establish diagnostic reliability and validity. The standards in DSM-III were also aligned with the World Health Organization's International Classification of Diseases (ICD) manual used in Europe. Schizophrenia subtypes lacking validity, including the latent type, were collapsed to five types and two main symptom domains: the positive, which included delusions and hallucinations, and the negative, which included impaired emotional, cognitive, and social functions.

One of the principles underlining psychiatric classification in DSM-III was the exclusion rule, based on the assumption regarding the hierarchical nature of psychiatric disorders. According to this rule, obsessive–compulsive symptoms and other secondary syndromes revealed in patients with schizophrenia were not diagnosed in the presence of schizophrenia because they were thought to be "better accounted for" by, caused by, or part of the schizophrenia, a disorder higher on the hierarchy. Hierarchical assumptions were considered a useful convention to achieve parsimony of diagnosis among psychiatric patients, even when they had symptoms of a variety of disorders (Jaspers, 1972). These exclusion criteria, however, temporarily delayed research on a co-occurrence of schizophrenia and other psychiatric syndromes, primarily OCD.

A seminal work by Fenton and McGlashan (1986), based on the Chestnut Lodge Follow-Up Study, played an important role in renewing the interest of clinicians and researchers in the interrelationship between schizophrenia and obsessive–compulsive symptoms. This pioneering research included the following features: operationally defined diagnostic criteria; adequate predictor characterization of samples; an outcome that was measured multidimensionally; independence of follow-up data collection from the diagnostic/predictor data collection; and reliability testing of all measures. The authors were concerned with the application of the DSM-III definitions for obsessions and compulsions to schizophrenia, particularly the requirement that the patient show insight into the nature of, and resistance to, the symptoms. They found these distinctions nebulous and elected to describe and classify obsessive–compulsive symptoms behaviorally. One of the major findings of this investigation was a higher than previously considered rate of obsessive–compulsive symptoms in schizophrenia; roughly 13% (21/163) of the patients had clinically meaningful obsessive–compulsive symptoms. The most striking result, however, was that the schizo-obsessive patients had substantially worse outcomes in multiple domains than their schizophrenia counterparts. These results challenged the previously predominant "positive" views of obsessive–compulsive symptoms in schizophrenia as a predictor of better prognosis. Hence, the schizo-obsessive group's duration of index hospitalization was twice that of patients without obsessive–compulsive symptoms; they spent about 50% of the post-discharge period hospitalized, compared to about 37% of the comparison group. Highly significant differences emerged in the area of occupational functioning. Only 7% of the schizo-obsessive–compulsive group was employed during the follow-up period, compared to 33% of the schizophrenia patients. Similarly, though both groups demonstrated persistent and marked impairment in social functioning and psychopathology, the schizo-obsessive patients had significantly poorer functioning. Noteworthy, foreseeing the results of subsequent investigations with more rigorous research methodology, Fenton and McGlashan (1986) revealed that obsessive–compulsive symptoms preceded psychotic symptoms and are typical in content. Only two patients exhibited delusional transformation of obsessions.

This pivotal study prompted further research to evaluate the prevalence and clinical significance of obsessive–compulsive phenomena in schizophrenia. Additional impetus for research in this area was associated with the introduction of the latest edition of DSM. DSM-IV accepted the possibility of co-occurrence of schizophrenia and OCD and stated that "if another Axis I disorder is present, the content of the obsessions or the compulsions should not be restricted to it," i.e., paranoid delusions in paranoid schizophrenia. By permitting multiple Axis I diagnoses, DSM-IV drew attention to the presence of additional and potentially treatable "non-schizophrenic" syndromes, such as obsessive–compulsive disorder, depression, and panic disorder, in patients with a primary diagnosis of schizophrenia (Bermanzohn et al., 2000). This conceptual change motivated research on the prevalence and clinical characterization of additional psychopathological syndromes, including OCD, in schizophrenia patients.

References

American Psychiatric Association Committee on Nomenclature and Statistics (1952) *Diagnostic and Statistical Manual of Mental Disorders*. American Psychiatric Association, Washington DC.

American Psychiatric Association Committee on Nomenclature and Statistics (1968) *Diagnostic and Statistical Manual of Mental Disorders*, 2nd edn. American Psychiatric Association, Washington DC.

American Psychiatric Association Task Force on Nomenclature and Statistics, Task Force on DSM-III (1980) *Diagnostic and Statistical Manual of Mental Disorders*, 3rd edn. American Psychiatric Association, Washington DC.

Bermanzohn PC, Porto L, Arlow PB, *et al.* (2000) Hierarchical diagnosis in chronic schizophrenia: a clinical study of co-occurring syndromes. *Schizophrenia Bulletin* **26**, 517–525.

Bleuler E (1911/1950) *Dementia Praecox or the Group of Schizophrenias*, transl. Zinkin J. International Universities Press, New York.

Fenton WS, McGlashan TH (1986) The prognostic significance of obsessive-compulsive symptoms in schizophrenia. *American Journal of Psychiatry* **143**, 437–441.

Gordon A (1926) Obsessions in the relation to psychoses. *American Journal of Psychiatry* **82**, 647–659.

Gordon A (1950) Transition of obsessions into delusions: evaluation of obsessional phenomena from the prognostic standpoint. *American Journal of Psychiatry* **107**, 455–458.

Hoch P, Polatin P (1949) Pseudoneurotic forms of schizophrenia. *Psychiatric Quarterly* **23**, 248–276.

Hoch PH, Cattell JP (1959) The diagnosis of pseudoneurotic schizophrenia. *Psychiatric Quarterly* **33**, 17–43.

Hoch PH, Cattell JP, Strahl MO, Pennes HH (1962) The course and outcome of pseudoneurotic schizophrenia. *American Journal of Psychiatry* **119**, 106–15.

Huber G, Gross G (1989) The concept of basic symptoms in schizophrenic and schizoaffective patients. *Schizophrenia Bulletin* **6**, 592–605.

Janet P (1903) *Les Obsessions et la Psychasthénie*, vol. 2. Alcan, Paris. (Reprinted: Arno, New York, 1976.)

Jaspers K (1972) *Subjective Phenomena of Morbid Psychic Life in General Psychopathology.* University of Chicago Press, Chicago.

Kraepelin E (1919) *Dementia Praecox and Paraphrenia.* E. & S. Livingstone, Edinburgh. (Reprinted: Thoemmes Press, Bristol, 2002.)

Lewis A (1936) Problems of obsessional illness. *Proceedings of the Royal Society of Medicine* **29**, 325–336.

Mayer-Gross W (1928) Psychopathologie und Klinik der Trugwahrnehmungen. In: Bumke O (ed.) *Handbuch der Geisteskrankheiten, vol. 1, part 1, Allgemeiner.* Springer, Berlin.

Rosen I (1956) The clinical significance of obsessions in schizophrenia. *Journal of Mental Science* **103**, 773–785.

Slater E, Roth M (1969) *Clinical Psychiatry,* 3rd edn. Ballière, Tindall and Cassell, London.

Stengel EA (1945) A study of some clinical aspects of the relationship between obsessional neurosis and psychotic reaction types. *Journal of Mental Science* **91**, 166–187.

Westphal C (1872) Ueber Zwangsvorstellungen. *Berliner Klinischen Wochenschrift* **3**, 390–397.

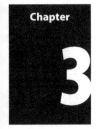

Obsessive–compulsive symptoms in schizophrenia: epidemiological and clinical aspects

Prevalence

Prevalence studies are essential to estimate the extent of obsessive–compulsive phenomena in schizophrenia, their clinical significance, and the burden of illness, and to plan effective forms of intervention. Prevalence studies may also facilitate understanding the mechanisms that underlie the association between the two disorders. Several assumptions were put forward to explain the interrelationship between OCD and schizophrenia (Buckley *et al.*, 2009):

- OCD co-occurs with schizophrenia simply by chance;
- OCD manifests secondary to the core disorder, schizophrenia;
- obsessive–compulsive symptoms manifest because schizophrenia is more common in patients with OCD;
- co-occurrence of OCD and schizophrenia is a consequence of some underlying shared liability to both sets of disorders.

Prevalence of OCD in schizophrenia

Initially, obsessive–compulsive symptoms were thought to occur in a minority of patients with schizophrenia (1.1–3.5%), and were considered a positive prognostic indicator (Stengel, 1945; Rosen, 1956). Early investigations, as discussed in the previous chapter, suffered from their observational character, small sample sizes, and lack of operationally defined diagnostic criteria for both disorders. Contemporary studies challenged this "positive" view. Suspending diagnostic hierarchy rules and applying operationally defined behavioral criteria, Fenton and McGlashan (1986) and later Berman and colleagues (1995) found a significantly higher rate of obsessive–compulsive symptoms in schizophrenia (12.8–25%) and a poorer prognosis for schizo-obsessive patients. These investigations prompted further research to evaluate the prevalence of obsessive–compulsive features in schizophrenia.

A majority of contemporary prevalence studies of obsessive–compulsive phenomena in schizophrenia used the Structured Clinical Interview and rigorous DSM criteria for both schizophrenia and OCD. In general, there was a striking consistency among these reports in revealing a considerably higher rate of OCD in schizophrenia patients than initially suggested. Epidemiological surveys and studies based on clinical samples estimate that roughly 3.7–45% of schizophrenia patients also exhibit OCD (Table 3.1). The wide estimate range is accounted for by variations in the definition of obsessive–compulsive features (disorder vs. symptoms), diagnostic criteria applied (categorical vs. dimensional), the patient population studied (inpatients vs. outpatients vs. community residents), research methodologies (chart review vs. direct interview; lay vs. clinician assessments), assessment instruments, and the phase of the schizophrenic illness (first admission vs. chronic stage).

Table 3.1 Rate of occurrence of OCD in schizophrenia

Reference	Country	Study sample	Study design, diagnostic criteria for schizophrenia and OCD	Prevalence of OCD/OCS in schizophrenia
Epidemiological sample				
Bland et al. (1987)	USA	N = 20; random community residents	DSM-III for OCS	OCS = 59.2%
Karno et al. (1988)	USA	N = 18 500; community residents	Survey interview; DSM-III	12.2%
Regier et al. (1990)	USA	N = 20 861; community residents	Survey interview	23.7%
Kessler et al. (2005)	USA	N = 2322; community residents	National household survey; SCID for DSM-IV NAP; CIDI for DSM-IV OCD	13.3%
Van Dael et al. (2011)	Netherlands	N = 7076; community residents	CIDI	13.1%
First-episode or recent-onset schizophrenia				
Strakowski et al. (1993)	USA	N = 10; inpatients	SCID; DSM-III-R	20%
Poyurovsky et al. (1999)	Israel	N = 50; inpatients	SCID; DSM-IV	14%
Craig et al. (2002)	USA	N = 225; inpatients	SCID; DSM-III-R	3.8%; OCS = 16.2%
de Haan et al. (2005)	Netherlands	N = 113; inpatients	SCID-P; DSM-IV	29.2%; OCS = 15%
Sim et al. (2006)	Singapore	N = 142; inpatients	SCID; DSM-IV	6.3%
Sterk et al. (2011)	Netherlands	N = 194; inpatients	CASH; DSM-III-R	1.5%; OCS = 9.3%
Chronic schizophrenia				
Fenton and McGlashan (1986)	USA	N = 163; inpatients	Operational criteria for OCS	12.9%
Berman et al. (1995)	USA	N = 108; outpatients	Operational criteria for OCS	26.5%
Eisen et al. (1997)	USA	N = 77; outpatients	SCID; DSM-IV	7.8%
Porto et al. (1997)	USA	N = 50; outpatients	SCID-P; DSM-IV	26%; OCS = 20%
Cassano et al. (1998)	Italy	N = 31; inpatients	SCID; DSM-III-R	29%
Meghani et al. (1998)	USA	N = 192; outpatients	SCID and self-report measures	31.7%
Cosoff and Hafner (1998)	Australia	N = 60; inpatients	SCID; DSM-III-R	13%
Dominguez et al. (1999)	Mexico	N = 52; outpatients	Chart review, self-rated MOCI for OCS	OCS = 32.7%
Higuchi et al. (1999)	Japan	N = 45; inpatients/outpatients	SCID; DSM-III-R	20%
Kruger et al. (2000)	Germany	N = 76; inpatients	SCID; DSM-III-R	15.8%

Study	Country	Sample	Instrument/Criteria	Prevalence
Tibbo et al. (2000)	Canada	N = 52; outpatients	SCID; DSM-IV	25%
Lysaker et al. (2000)	USA	N = 46; outpatients	Chart review	45%
Bermanzohn et al. (2000)	USA	N = 37; outpatients	SCID; DSM-IV	29.7%
Poyurovsky et al. (2000)	Israel	N = 68; inpatients	SCID; DSM-IV	23.5%
Fabisch et al. (2001)	Austria	N = 150; inpatients	Operational criteria for OCS	OCS = 10%
Baylé et al. (2001)	France	N = 40; inpatients/outpatients	Clinical diagnosis	35%
Goodwin et al. (2003)	USA	N = 184; inpatients	DIGS; DSM-III-R	5.4%
Ohta et al. (2003)	Japan	N = 71; inpatients/outpatients	SCID; DSM-IV	18.3%
Pallanti et al. (2004)	Italy	N = 80; outpatients	SCID; DSM-IV	22.5%
Kayahan et al. (2005)	Turkey	N = 100; outpatients	SCID; DSM-IV	30%; OCS = 64%
Byerly et al. (2005)	USA	N = 100; outpatients	SCID; DSM-IV	23%; OCS = 30%
Ongur and Goff (2005)	USA	N = 118; outpatients	SCID; DSM-IV	8.8%
Braga et al. (2005)	Brazil	N = 53; outpatients	SCID; DSM-IV	15.1%
Ciapparelli et al. (2007)	Italy	N = 42; outpatients	SCID; DSM-IV	23.8%
Seedat et al. (2007)	South Africa	N = 70; inpatients	MINI	4.3%
Ndetie et al. (2008)	Kenya	N = 691; inpatients	SCID; DSM-IV	12.2%
Owashi et al. (2010)	Japan	N = 92; inpatients	MINI	14.1%; OCS = 51.1%
Üçok et al. (2011)	Turkey	N = 184; outpatients	SCID; DSM-IV	17%; OCS = 17.6%
Adolescent schizophrenia				
Nechmad et al. (2003)	Israel	N = 50; inpatients	SCID; DSM-IV	26%
Ross et al. (2003)	USA	N = 83; outpatients	Kiddie-SADS-PL; DSM-IV	20%
Elderly schizophrenia				
Poyurovsky et al. (2006)	Israel	N = 50; inpatients	SCID; DSM-IV	16%

SCID, Structured Clinical Interview for DSM-Patient Edition; CASH, Comprehensive Assessment of Symptoms and History Schedule; MOCI, Maudsley Obsessive–Compulsive Inventory; DIGS, Diagnostic Interview for Genetic Studies; Kiddie-SADS-PL, the Schedule for Affective Disorders and Schizophrenia for school-age children-present and lifetime version; MINI, Mini International Neuropsychiatric Interview; CIDI, Composite International Diagnostic Interview; OCD/OCS, obsessive–compulsive disorder/symptoms; NAP, non-affective psychoses.

Achim and colleagues (2011) performed an extensive systematic review and meta-analysis that produced a methodological explanation for the reported variation of rates of OCD and other anxiety disorders in patients with non-affective psychoses. The authors included relevant articles (published prior to May 2009) focusing on the prevalence of anxiety disorders, particularly OCD, in patients with schizophrenia-spectrum psychotic disorder. Standardized DSM-III-R or DSM-IV diagnostic criteria were used in all studies to diagnose both schizophrenia-spectrum and comorbid anxiety disorders. Based on an analysis of 34 studies with more than 3000 participants that explicitly focused on the assessment of OCD in patients with schizophrenia, an estimated pooled prevalence of OCD in schizophrenia was *12.1%* (95% confidence interval [CI], 7.0–17.1%) (Achim *et al.*, 2011). It is of note, however, that there was evidence of significant heterogeneity in OCD rates across the individual studies (heterogeneity $\chi^2 = 317.98, p < 0.001$), which called for cautious interpretation of this prevalence rate. Several moderating variables contribute to the documented heterogeneity, and some of them are of particular relevance to clinicians. *First*, the greater OCD rate in studies that supplemented the Structured Clinical Interview for DSM with additional instruments, such as Yale–Brown Obsessive–Compulsive Scale (Y-BOCS) (Goodman *et al.*, 1989), suggests that there is a benefit of inquiring about typical OCD obsessions and compulsions while detecting whether a schizophrenia patient presents with a co-occurring OCD. *Second*, for patients with acute psychosis evaluated during hospitalization, it is worthwhile to reassess the presence of OCD after resolution of psychosis, since OCD symptoms might then be more easily detectable, which could explain the higher rates of OCD found in outpatients. *Third*, a somewhat higher prevalence of OCD in patients with repeated episodes of psychosis compared to first-episode patients suggests that factors related to a core disorder (e.g., antipsychotic treatment) along with temporal fluctuations of OCD, may account for the "influx" of incident OCD cases over time. This in turn stipulates detection of obsessive–compulsive phenomena during the entire course of schizophrenia. Noteworthy, no significant moderating effect of gender, age, or type of schizophrenia-spectrum disorder (schizophrenia vs. schizoaffective vs. schizophreniform disorder) on the rate of OCD was identified. Importantly, when the diagnostic threshold is relaxed from DSM-IV OCD to subthreshold obsessive–compulsive symptoms, an even higher proportion of schizophrenia patients exhibit clinically significant obsessions and/or compulsions. A weighted average of the available data crudely estimates a *25%* prevalence of obsessive–compulsive symptoms in schizophrenia (Buckley *et al.*, 2009). This figure echoes a high prevalence of subthreshold obsessive–compulsive symptoms revealed in the general population in the National Comorbidity Survey Replication, a nationally representative survey of US adults (28.2%) (Ruscio *et al.*, 2010), suggesting that the health burden of obsessive–compulsive phenomena is significantly greater than the DSM-IV OCD prevalence implies. *Fourth*, a complexity of obsessive–compulsive phenomena in schizophrenia goes beyond the typical OCD obsessive–compulsive symptoms, since unique psychotic-related obsessive–compulsive psychopathological complexes (e.g., compulsive hand-washing due to command auditory hallucinations; ego-dystonic[1] obsessions experienced as thought insertions) have repeatedly been discovered in schizo-obsessive patients (Rosen, 1956; Porto *et al.*, 1997; Poyurovsky *et al.*, 2004; Burgy, 2007). In view of the fact that these complex psychopathological features are not captured by currently used diagnostic instruments for the assessment of

---

[1] Ego-dystonic, as opposed to ego-syntonic, is defined as anything that is unacceptable to the part of the psyche that mediates reality testing, impulse control, and thought content (Ayd, 1995).

obsessive–compulsive phenomena, it is plausible that at present the overall prevalence of obsessive–compulsive features in schizophrenia is underestimated.

Determining whether the reported rates of occurrence of OCD in schizophrenia differ from those in the general population is crucial to appraise potential etiological links between OCD and schizophrenia. A systematic review of literature published between 1980 and 2004 reporting findings of the prevalence of anxiety disorders in the general population, estimated international pooled lifetime prevalence for OCD at 1.3% (95% CI, 0.86–1.80%) (Somers *et al.*, 2006). A comparable lifetime prevalence estimate for DSM-IV OCD (2.3%, standard error 0.3%) was found in the National Comorbidity Survey Replication (Ruscio *et al.*, 2010). A comparison of the OCD rates in patients with schizophrenia and those in the general population, reported in a meta-analyses by Achim *et al.* (2011) and Somers *et al.* (2006), respectively, demonstrated that the rate for OCD is significantly higher in schizophrenia than the lifetime rate found in the general population, as supported by the revealed non-overlapping 95% CIs (12.1% [95% CI, 7.0–17.1%] vs. 1.3% [95% CI, 0.86–1.80%]).

A critical question is whether the high prevalence of OCD in schizophrenia results solely from the reported OCD-inducing potential of second-generation antipsychotics (Lykouras *et al.*, 2003), or from yet to be identified causes associated with the core disorder, schizophrenia. First-episode research methodology addresses this issue by estimating obsessive–compulsive phenomena in drug-naïve schizophrenia patients experiencing their first psychotic episode. Indeed, a comparable rate of OCD was noted in first-episode, predominantly drug-naïve patients, indicating that OCD is not consequent to primary schizophrenia-related factors (Table 3.1). These findings are substantiated by the detection of obsessive–compulsive symptoms in a meaningful proportion of individuals at ultra-high risk for psychosis and in patients in the prodromal phase of illness (Rosen *et al.*, 2006; Niendam *et al.*, 2009). The identification of comparable rates of obsessive–compulsive symptoms across the lifespan in adolescent (Nechmad *et al.*, 2003), adult, and elderly (Poyurovsky *et al.*, 2006) schizophrenia patients further highlights the extent of these phenomena in schizophrenia (Table 3.1).

A cross-cultural aspect of the problem is worth mentioning. As in "pure" OCD, there is a remarkable consistency in the reported rates of OCD in schizophrenia samples across the globe (e.g., North America, Australia, Europe, Africa, India, Japan). It appears that cross-cultural prevalence rates of OCD are stable in patients with and without schizophrenia. Notably, a study by Niehaus *et al.* (2005) evaluating the prevalence of OCD in Xhosa-speaking schizophrenia patients in South Africa seems to stand alone. The authors found that only three (0.5%) of 509 patients met criteria for OCD. These findings starkly contrast most OCD comorbidity data in schizophrenia patients of Caucasian ethnicity. Both schizophrenia and OCD are disorders with significant commonality across different cultures and ethnic groups. Nevertheless, a variation in the phenomenology of schizophrenia across ethnic groups, and a lower prevalence of OCD in some ethnic communities were also reported (Weissman *et al.* 1994; Emsley *et al.*, 2002). If replicated, Niehaus *et al*'s provoking findings might support the hypothesis that cultural and/or genetic factors play a role in protecting against comorbid OCD in schizophrenia in certain ethnic groups.

Prevalence of schizophrenia in OCD

Contrary to the substantial aggregation of obsessive–compulsive phenomena in patients with schizophrenia, the development of full-blown schizophrenia in patients with a well-established diagnosis of OCD is extremely rare (Table 3.2). Indeed, early studies found that patients with

Table 3.2 Rate of occurrence of schizophrenia in patients with OCD

Reference	Study sample	Study design and diagnostic criteria	Prevalence of schizophrenia-spectrum disorders in OCD
Goodwin et al. (1969)	13 follow-up studies on obsessive neurosis	Descriptive analysis	Low risk for development of schizophrenia
Eisen and Rasmussen (1993)	475 OCD patients	Semistructured interview, DSM-III-R criteria	4% (18/475)
Reddy et al. (2000)	54 OCD children and adolescents	SCID, DSM-III-R criteria	None
De Haan et al. (2009)	757 OCD patients in specialized clinic	SCID, DSM-IV criteria	1.7% (13/757)

SCID, Structured Clinical Interview for DSM.

full-blown obsessive neurosis were at no greater risk for developing schizophrenia than the general population. Some early investigators who described psychotic transformation in OCD patients were unwilling to call this schizophrenia and used the term "doubtfully schizophrenic" (Rudin, 1953; Ingram, 1961; Rosenberg, 1968). Roth (1978) similarly noted the emergence of psychosis in patients with long-standing neurosis and distinguished this state from nuclear schizophrenia. Because conversion of obsessive–compulsive symptoms to psychosis is brief and reversible among obsessive–compulsive patients, the author invoked the Scandinavian concept of reactive psychosis. After reviewing 13 early follow-up studies, Goodwin and colleagues (1969) concluded that patients with a well-established diagnosis of obsessive–compulsive disorder developed schizophrenia at a rate that was not significantly different from that in the general population. This was later supported by Eisen and Rasmussen (1993) who, after evaluating a large cohort of patients with DSM-III-R diagnosis of OCD, found that 4% (18 of 475) met criteria for both OCD and schizophrenia. Recently, using the SCID and DSM-IV criteria for Axis I disorders, de Haan and colleagues (2009) reported the results of an extensive cross-sectional clinical evaluation of the largest to date group of 757 patients consecutively referred to an academic clinic that specializes on the diagnosis and treatment of OCD. Only 13 (1.7%) of 757 adult OCD patients were diagnosed with a psychotic disorder (eight with schizophrenia, two with schizoaffective disorder, three with psychotic disorder not otherwise specified). Similarly, explicit assessment of psychiatric comorbidity in adolescent patients with a primary diagnosis of OCD showed that in contrast to a substantial prevalence of comorbid affective, anxiety, and tic disorders, none of the 54 children and adolescents with OCD satisfied DSM-III-R criteria for schizophrenia or other psychotic disorder (Reddy et al., 2000).

Overall, in contrast to a substantial prevalence of obsessive–compulsive phenomena in patients with schizophrenia, patients with a primary diagnosis of OCD are not at particular risk for developing schizophrenia. The underlying mechanism of this "asymmetric" inter-relationship between the two disorders remains to be discovered.

Despite methodological differences and substantial heterogeneity between the reports, there is compelling evidence indicating that the odds for obsessive–compulsive phenomena in schizophrenia patients are considerably higher than would be expected in random co-occurrence between the two disorders. Instead, the most parsimonious conclusion at the present time is that their common co-occurrence is a consequence of some underlying pathophysiological mechanisms shared by both disorders.

Age of onset

Discernment of disorder-specific age of onset is important for targeting early interventions, and focusing research on the underlying mechanisms of mental disorders. Generally, younger age of onset is associated with greater severity and persistence of illness, as well as poorer response to treatment and poorer prognosis (Kessler *et al.*, 2007).

Schizophrenia vs. OCD

Extensive research on age of onset in schizophrenia and OCD clearly demonstrates its clinical and prognostic significance. Patients with earlier age of onset of schizophrenia are more likely to be men, have poor premorbid adjustment, lower educational achievement, more evidence of structural brain abnormalities and greater cognitive impairments, increased severity of functional disabilities, less responsiveness to antipsychotic medications, and greater likelihood of relapse and rehospitalization (Angermeyer and Kuhn, 1988; DeLisi, 1992; Hafner, 2000; Ongur *et al.*, 2009). Early onset of psychiatric symptoms may also predict conversion to psychosis in help-seeking individuals at ultra-high risk for schizophrenia (Amminger *et al.*, 2006). Similar to patients with schizophrenia, patients with early-onset OCD have some potentially important differences in the course of illness, comorbidity, neuroimaging findings, and treatment response compared to those with adult-onset OCD (Leckman *et al.*, 2010). Early-onset OCD has been associated with male predominance, tic disorders, higher frequency of tic-like compulsions, compulsions not triggered by obsessions, greater symptom severity, and treatment resistance (Geller *et al.*, 1998; Rosario-Campos *et al.*, 2001; de Mathis *et al.*, 2009; Lomax *et al.*, 2009).

The finding that patients with early onset are more likely to have relatives with the same illness (Wickham *et al.*, 2002) suggests that early age at onset may be related to genetic vulnerability. The pattern of familial transmission with higher family loading of the disorder in early-onset subgroups has repeatedly been shown for both schizophrenia and OCD (Byrne et al., 2002; Pauls, 2008). In addition to evidence of familiality of age at onset, there is a preliminary indication for genetic linkage to certain chromosomal regions and polymorphisms, based on age of onset in both schizophrenia and OCD (Cardno *et al.*, 2001; Numata *et al.*, 2006; Walitza *et al.*, 2010). It is therefore important to examine patterns of age at onset for further clues to the neurobiology of both disorders and their comorbidity.

Reliable determination of age of onset is challenging. A long-term prospective community survey to estimate incidence of a disorder and its age of onset is the ideal approach. However, prospective birth-cohort studies in schizophrenia that cover the entire age range of risk for the onset of the disorder are sparse (Jones *et al.*, 1994; Lauronen *et al.*, 2007). Analogous birth-cohort studies in OCD are lacking. As a result, we have to rely largely on retrospective cross-sectional community and clinical studies that estimate age-of-onset distributions of the two disorders.

The definition of age of onset poses an additional challenge. The onset of positive symptoms of schizophrenia is clearly more relevant to the determination of etiological factors than, for example, age when a patient was first hospitalized (DeLisi, 1992). However, this information, which is usually obtained subjectively from the patient or a close relative and depends largely on recall, may not be accurate. Moreover, the onset of more subtle negative symptoms such as withdrawal from friends, lack of energy, or diminished interests, are even more difficult to define, although they may be more relevant in determining the onset of the pathological process. Similarly, for a substantial proportion of OCD patients the onset of obvious obsessions and/or compulsions precedes the onset of functional impairment required for DSM-IV diagnosis of OCD by many years. In addition, the typically insidious onset of symptoms in both schizophrenia and OCD, the non-specific character of initial symptoms in a vast majority of patients with schizophrenia, and the "secretive" nature of OCD symptoms due to patients' embarrassment or lack of insight, substantially complicate determination of age of onset.

Despite these methodological difficulties, we now know that age of onset of schizophrenia ranges from mid adolescence to late adult life, and characteristically peaks in early adulthood (DeLisi et al., 1994; Tandon et al., 2009). Age of onset of OCD appears to be earlier with fully half of all cases beginning in childhood and adolescence (Millet et al., 2004; Pinto et al., 2006; Ruscio et al., 2010). In addition, OCD has a narrower age-of-onset range and there are fewer new onsets after the early thirties (Ruscio et al., 2010). Importantly, the two disorders have a remarkably similar earlier age of onset in men than in women (Angermeyer and Kuhn, 1988; Castle et al., 1993; Ruscio et al., 2010).

Schizophrenic vs. obsessive–compulsive symptoms in schizo-obsessive patients

Comparative evaluation of age at onset of first schizophrenic and obsessive–compulsive symptoms is imperative to facilitate understanding of their temporal interrelationship in schizo-obsessive patients. Devulapalli et al. (2008) analyzed the temporal sequence of schizophrenic and obsessive–compulsive symptoms reported in studies focusing on the clinical characteristics of schizo-obsessive patients. A meta-analysis of studies that documented ages of onset, found that the mean age of OCD onset was earlier than the mean age of schizophrenia onset (Table 3.3). Remarkably, all studies reported a lower mean age of onset for OCD. When data were pooled and analyzed collectively an unstandardized mean difference of 1.04 years was calculated (95% CI, 0.67–2.15). This mean difference of age of onset between the two disorders falls short of statistical significance ($p = 0.07$), most likely due to small sample sizes and the resulting insufficient power to detect a difference. Other limitations of this meta-analysis included small number of studies, and a failure to indicate whether or not obsessive–compulsive symptoms developed after initiation of treatment with second-generation antipsychotic agents which may induce or exacerbate OCD in schizophrenia patients.

Several additional reports substantiated the revealed tendency towards earlier age of onset of obsessive–compulsive symptoms compared to schizophrenia symptoms in patients who met diagnostic criteria for both disorders. Hence, Seedat et al. (2007) conducted a genetic study of schizophrenia, and identified 53 (of 400) patients who in addition to schizophrenia or schizo affective disorder also had OCD. The mean age of onset of obsessive–compulsive symptoms was found to be significantly earlier than the mean age of onset of schizophrenia (18.5 vs. 22.0 years, respectively, $p < 0.0001$). Likewise, Sterk et al. (2011) reported a trend toward earlier mean age of onset of obsessive–compulsive symptoms in a small group of 18 patients with first-episode schizophrenia or a related psychotic disorder (18.5 ± 5.6 vs. 19.9 ± 3.7 years).

Our group conducted a systematic assessment of age of onset of schizophrenic and obsessive–compulsive symptoms among patients who were consecutively hospitalized at

Table 3.3 Mean age of schizophrenia and OCD onset

Reference	Mean age OCD onset (SD)	Mean age schizophrenia onset (SD)	Sample size	Effect size (Cohen's d)	p
Poyurovsky et al. (1999)[a]	16.6 (8.7)	23.4 (5.9)	7	0.91	NA
Tibbo et al. (2000)	25.6 (10)	28.9 (6)	13	0.40	0.31
Ganesan et al. (2001)	21.5 (1.7)	22.5 (3.8)	12	0.34	0.30
Nechmad et al. (2003)[a]	14.3 (2.8)	15.1 (2.4)	13	0.31	NA
Meta-analysis	19.8	22.4	45	1.04[b]	0.066[c]

[a] Study did not provide sufficient data for the calculation of p value.
[b] Unstandardized mean difference given in years.
[c] Random effects model.
Source: From Devulapalli KK, Welge JA, Nasrullah HA (2008) Temporal sequence of clinical manifestation in schizophrenia with comorbid OCD: review and meta-analysis. *Psychiatry Research* **161**, 105–108. Reprinted with permission.

Tirat Carmel Mental Health Center (Israel) during the years 1999–2010 and who met DSM-IV criteria for both schizophrenic or schizoaffective disorder and OCD (Faragian et al., 2012). The total sample of 133 patients included 97 men and 36 women, mean age 31.1 ± 8.7 years, with mean duration of illness 10.3 ± 7.9 years and mean number of hospitalizations 2.9 ± 2.6. We also recruited 113 schizophrenia patients without OCD, hospitalized at the same institution during the same time period, who matched the schizo-obsessive group for gender, age, and number of hospitalizations. The enrollment of the two schizophrenia groups matched for key demographic and clinical characteristics other than obsessive–compulsive symptoms made it possible to examine the putative modifying effect of OCD on age of onset of schizophrenia.

Determination of age of onset was based on analysis of retrospective reports obtained from both patients and their first-degree relatives. To improve accuracy of the assessment a series of questions was designed to avoid unlikely response patterns attained when using the standard age-of-onset question (Simon and Von Korff, 1995). The sequence began with a question designed to emphasize the importance of accurate responses: "Can you remember the exact age of the very first time you had psychotic symptoms, like hearing voices and a feeling of persecution, and symptoms of OCD, that is repetitive thoughts and/or compulsive rituals?" Respondents who answered "No" were encouraged to try and pinpoint the emergence of initial symptoms by moving up the age range incrementally (e.g., "Was it before you first started school? Was it before you became a teenager?"). Age of onset was set at the higher age. Experimental research has shown that this sequence of questions yields responses with a much more plausible age-of-onset distribution than the standard age-of-onset question (Knauper et al., 1999). A similar memory-priming method was employed for the interviews of patients' relatives.

We showed that the mean age of onset of the first psychotic symptoms, was 20.4 ± 5.9 years (median 19, range 10–40 years), while mean age of onset of the first clinically significant obsessions and/or compulsions was 19.1 ± 7.7 years (median 17, range 6–36 years). The difference was statistically significant (paired t-test $= 2.03$, $p = 0.044$). When gender was considered, there was a significantly earlier age of onset of obsessive–compulsive symptoms than schizophrenic symptoms in men (18.3 ± 6.5 vs. 19.8 ± 4.8 years, $p < 0.05$), but not in women (21.2 ± 9.2 vs. 22.1 ± 7.9 years, $p = 0.55$). Since there was a considerable time gap (roughly 10 years) between the mean age at diagnostic assessment and age of onset of schizophrenic and obsessive–compulsive symptoms, increasing the likelihood of recall bias, we reanalyzed the data focusing on a subgroup of 54 first-episode schizophrenia patients. This sub-analysis revealed that clinically significant obsessive–compulsive symptoms emerged approximately 3 years earlier than schizophrenic symptoms (18.2 ± 6.2 vs. 21.6 ± 6.2, $p = 0.003$). Notably, patients who were drug-naïve prior to admission made up a majority of the first-episode group, limiting the possibility of an occurrence of obsessive–compulsive symptoms due to antipsychotic drug treatment. Temporal proximity between the mean age at diagnostic assessment (22.4 ± 2.3 years) and the revealed mean age of onset of the initial schizophrenic and obsessive–compulsive symptoms in this subgroup of young first-episode schizophrenia patients minimized recall bias and increased the validity of the assessment. Indeed, our earlier study on an independent but substantially smaller sample of first-episode schizophrenia patients found a comparable difference in age of onset between obsessive–compulsive and schizophrenic symptoms (16.6 ± 8.7 and 23.4 ± 5.9 years, respectively) (Poyurovsky et al., 1999). Splitting the age range at diagnostic assessment into 10-year periods clearly shows that the earlier the age at assessment, the stronger the evidence for earlier age at onset of obsessive–compulsive symptoms compared to schizophrenia symptoms (Table 3.4). There was an inverse relationship between the analyzed parameters only in the oldest group (>45 years), with mean age of onset of schizophrenic symptoms lower than mean age of onset of obsessive–compulsive symptoms. One possible explanation is recall bias, which positively correlated with the age of assessment. Alternatively, patients with longer duration of schizophrenic disorder may well develop obsessive–compulsive symptoms due to antipsychotic drug treatment, chronic course of illness, or as yet unknown causes.

Similar to "pure" forms of the disorders, men with schizo-obsessive disorder had earlier age of onset of both schizophrenic (19.8 ± 4.8 vs. 22.1 ± 7.9 years, $p < 0.05$) and obsessive–compulsive (18.3 ± 6.5 vs. 21.2 ± 9.2 years, $p < 0.05$) symptoms compared to women. The age at onset of OCD for nearly 20% of the men was before age 10. In contrast, women have a much more rapid accumulation of new cases after age 10, with the highest slope during adolescence. Onset among men and women after the mid thirties was rare.

Table 3.4 Relationship between age at assessment (in 10-year periods) and age of onset of schizophrenic and obsessive–compulsive symptoms in schizo-obsessive patients

Age at assessment (years)	Number of patients	Age of onset		p
		Obsessive–compulsive	Schizophrenic	
<25	41	15.1 ± 3.5	16.9 ± 2.8	0.011
26–35	69	19.2 ± 6.8	21.1 ± 5.5	0.073
36–45	12	23.2 ± 9.0	25.0 ± 8.2	0.61
>45	10	29.9 ± 12.1	25.1 ± 6.6	0.49

Source: Faragian S, Fuchs C, Pashinian A, et al. (2012) Age-of-onset of schizophrenic and obsessivecompulsive symptoms in patients with schizo obsessive disorder. Psychiatry Research **197**, 19–22.

Comparison between the two schizophrenia groups with and without OCD revealed that the average age of onset of first psychotic symptoms was significantly earlier in schizo-obsessive patients than in their non-OCD schizophrenia counterparts (20.4 ± 5.9 vs. 23.4 ± 6.7 years, $p < 0.001$). Again, this difference was accounted for by an earlier age of onset in men (19.8 ± 4.8 vs. 23.9 ± 7.1, $p < 0.01$), but not in women (22.1 ± 7.9 vs. 22.3 ± 5.5, $p = 0.73$) (Faragian et al., 2012).

What can be learned from the systematic evaluation of age of onset of schizophrenic and obsessive–compulsive symptoms in patients who meet diagnostic criteria for both disorders?

- Average age of onset of obsessive–compulsive symptoms precedes average age of onset of first psychotic symptoms. The earlier average age of onset of obsessive–compulsive symptoms indicates that in a sizeable proportion of schizophrenia patients they are independent of psychosis and are not consequent to primary schizophrenia-related factors (e.g., antipsychotic treatment).
- There are substantial gender-related differences in age-of-onset distributions of schizophrenic and obsessive–compulsive symptoms in patients who meet criteria for both disorders. Compared to women, men have an earlier onset of both sets of symptoms. Moreover, an earlier age of onset of obsessive–compulsive symptoms relative to schizophrenic symptoms was detected only in men.
- The presence of obsessive–compulsive symptoms is associated with earlier age of onset of psychosis, and this effect seems to be gender-specific. A similar effect of comorbid panic disorder associated with an almost 4-year earlier age of onset of psychosis has also been reported, suggesting that early occurrence of obsessive–compulsive disorder and anxiety disorders may herald earlier emergence of psychosis in susceptible individuals (Ongur et al., 2009). Noteworthy, in a large group of 500 patients enrolled in the Systematic Treatment Enhancement Program for Bipolar Disorder (STEP-BPD), anxiety disorders, particularly OCD, were associated with significantly earlier mean age of onset of bipolar disorder in patients with lifetime comorbid anxiety disorders than in patients without anxiety disorders (15.6 vs. 19.4 years, respectively) (Simon et al., 2004). Although the mechanism underlying this effect is not yet known, the fact that OCD is typically an early-onset disorder means that it might be a useful marker of youth at high risk for progression to later psychotic and bipolar disorder (Kessler et al., 2011).

The role of familial loading of schizophrenia- and OCD-spectrum disorders on age of onset of schizo-obsessive disorder is yet to be clarified. According to a recent meta-analysis, only non-familial forms of schizophrenia are sexually dimorphic in terms of age of onset, since the presence of family history of schizophrenia was associated with the disappearance of any sex differences in age-of-onset distributions (Esterberg et al., 2010). An additional potential etiological factor that deserves consideration is cannabis. Growing evidence indicates that cannabis may play a causal role in the development of psychosis in some patients (Ongur et al., 2009; Leeson et al., 2011), accounting for roughly 2.7 years earlier age of onset of the disorder (Large et al., 2011). There is a substantial overlap between obsessive–compulsive and addictive behaviors on phenomenological and neurobiological levels (Fontenelle et al., 2011). An interacting effect of obsessive–compulsive symptoms and cannabis on age of onset of schizophrenia merits further investigation.

Course of illness

The course of schizo-obsessive disorder is chronic and lifelong. The two psychopathological trajectories, obsessive–compulsive and schizophrenia, persist from the early stages of illness throughout the lifespan. Symptom severity fluctuates over time and there are several patterns of onset and progression of the illness.

Temporal interrelationship between schizophrenic and obsessive–compulsive symptoms

Obsessive–compulsive symptoms may precede, co-occur with, or follow the emergence of schizophrenia symptoms. A meta-analysis of studies that focused on the temporal onset sequence of obsessive–compulsive and schizophrenic symptoms in patients suffering from both disorders identified eight studies that reported the psychiatric history of patients diagnosed with OCD first, schizophrenia first, or both disorders simultaneously (Devulapalli *et al.*, 2008). When the samples of these studies were analyzed collectively, the following results emerged: 71 (48%) of 148 patients were diagnosed with OCD prior to schizophrenia, 45 (30.4%) were diagnosed with schizophrenia first, and the remaining 32 (21.6%) were diagnosed with both disorders concurrently (Table 3.5). It is notable that all but one study reported the occurrence of obsessive–compulsive symptoms prior to or concomitantly with the onset of a psychotic disorder.

Two recent studies extend and substantiate earlier reports of the emergence of obsessive–compulsive symptoms prior to schizophrenia symptoms in a meaningful proportion of schizo-obsessive patients (Tiryaki and Ozkorumak, 2010; Üçok *et al.*, 2011). In a majority of cases in both reports (18/31 [59.5%] and 19/22 [86.4%], respectively) obsessive–compulsive symptoms were detected before the emergence of psychotic symptoms. A more modest variation in distribution of the time of onset of OCD as compared to schizophrenia, however, was found in a group of 18 recent-onset schizophrenia patients (Sterk *et al.*, 2011). OCD emerged prior to or simultaneously with schizophrenia in ten (55.6%) patients, and followed the onset of schizophrenia in eight (44.4%) patients.

In our group including 133 schizo-obsessive patients, roughly half of the sample (64 [48.1%]) presented with OCD prior to schizophrenia, one-third of the participants (37 [27.8%]) presented with OCD after the occurrence of schizophrenia and in the remaining 32 (24.2%) patients both disorders co-occurred (Faragian *et al.*, 2012). Though the time interval between the occurrence of the two set of symptoms ranged from 1 to 21 years, in two-thirds of the sample the interval was 5 years or less. The temporal onset sequence was similar for men and women.

Representative clinical vignettes are given below.

Case 3.1. Mr. B, a 22-year-old man, had clear-cut schizoid personality traits from adolescence, and was characterized as shy, detached from his peers, and a "strange person." By the eighth grade he began to exhibit difficulties concentrating and in social functioning. He eventually stopped doing his schoolwork, and cut all social relationships. He admitted to occasionally hearing a whispering noise "inside his head," and a "frustrating feeling" that he is being watched by his neighbors. In addition, he developed a fear of contracting AIDS, and recently began washing hands after touching objects that he thought would expose him to AIDS. In an effort to reduce anxiety associated with fears of contamination, he also repeatedly checked his clothes and the things in his room. Mr. B's health-related and contamination fears were not of delusional intensity and the severity of his obsessive–compulsive symptoms did not meet criteria for OCD. Roughly 1 year after his first psychotic and obsessive–compulsive symptoms

Table 3.5 Temporal data regarding diagnostic history of comorbid OCD–schizophrenia patients

Reference	Total sample	Analysis sample	OCD first	Schizophrenia first	Concurrence	Symptom induction
Poyurovsky et al. (1999)	50	7	4	2	1	No mention of antipsychotic-induced OCD
Tibbo et al. (2000)	52	13	6	5	2	Two cases of antipsychotic-induced OCD
Krüger et al. (2000)	76	12	10	0	2	No mention of antipsychotic-induced OCD
Ganesan et al. (2001)	12	12	4	3	5	No mention of antipsychotic-induced OCD
Poyurovsky et al. (2004)	55	55	26	15	14	Antipsychotic-induced OCD exclusion
Ohta et al. (2003)	71	12	9	3	0	Antipsychotic-induced OCD exclusion
Byerly et al. (2005)	100	29	8	13	8	No mention of antipsychotic-induced OCD
Poyurovsky et al. (2006)	50	8	4	4	0	No mention of antipsychotic-induced OCD
Total	466	148	71 (48.0%)	45 (30.4%)	32 (21.6%)	

Source: From Devulapalli KK, Welge JA, Nasrullah HA (2008) Temporal sequence of clinical manifestation in schizophrenia with comorbid OCD: review and meta-analysis. *Psychiatry Research* **161**, 105–108. Reprinted with permission.

became evident, Mr. B developed a full-blown psychotic episode characterized by auditory imperative hallucinations, aggressive behavior, and delusions of reference and persecution, unrelated to the content of OCD. He met DSM-IV criteria for schizophrenic disorder, paranoid type. Obsessive–compulsive symptoms did not re-emerge during the 3-year follow-up.

Case 3.2. Mr. R is a 19-year-old high-school graduate. His father suffers from schizophrenic disorder. R's fist clinically significant obsessive–compulsive symptoms were identified at age 17, and were characterized by repetitive, intrusive, and distressful thoughts of symmetry and order, accompanied by checking, ordering, and touching rituals. He felt an irresistible urge to touch his glasses in order to keep them "just right" in the middle of his face. A notable duration of rituals lasted for as long as 4 hours per day and interfered significantly with his daily routine. He was referred to a psychiatric evaluation and was diagnosed with DSM-IV

OCD, based on the presence of typical ego-dystonic obsessions and compulsions. Treatment with fluvoxamine was initiated and gradually titrated up to 200 mg/day. Three months of treatment led to a clinically significant attenuation of OCD symptoms (Yale–Brown Obsessive–Compulsive Scale [Y-BOCS] score decreased from 33 to 19). A substantial change in the clinical picture was observed during the following 2 months. Gradually increased anxiety, agitation, and insomnia followed by an acute psychotic episode characterized by delusions of persecution, auditory hallucinations, and first-rank Schneiderian symptoms prompted hospitalization. He met DSM-IV criteria for schizophreniform disorder. No signs of OCD were noted during an acute psychotic episode. He had pervasive delusions and hallucinations unrelated to the content of OCD. Eight weeks after the resolution of psychosis, OCD symptoms re-emerged. Subsequently, he developed two additional psychotic episodes and the diagnosis was changed to schizophrenic disorder, paranoid type, in addition to DSM-IV OCD.

Case 3.3. Mr. F, a 27-year-old student, exhibited contamination fears and washing rituals from age 11. By age 15 multiple obsessions and compulsions emerged: contamination obsessions, fear of AIDS, and compulsive checking, hand-washing, and counting to deal with anxiety associated with obsessions. Distressful, intrusive, and time-consuming obsessions and compulsions that lasted more than 3 hours a day were typical to OCD. Mr. F had a fair degree of insight into the senseless nature of these symptoms. DSM-IV OCD diagnosis was established. His academic achievements and social functioning were preserved. He successfully completed military service, and started his own computer business. At age 25, 14 years after the first obsessive–compulsive symptoms and 10 years after the formal DSM diagnosis of OCD, he began to complain of fatigue, and lack of concentration and motivation. Suspiciousness, social withdrawal, and increasing anxiety culminated in an acute psychotic episode requiring hospitalization. At admission, he revealed clear-cut delusional content focused on contracting AIDS by "exposure to alien forces" accompanied by auditory hallucinations of hearing voices commenting on his "AIDS-related appearance." Formal thought disorders were prominent and were associated with disorganized behavior and affect. At that point Mr. F met DSM-IV criteria for schizophrenic disorder, undifferentiated type.

Case 3.4. Ms. H, a 36-year-old woman, was diagnosed with DSM-IV schizophrenic disorder, paranoid type, at age 22 when she was hospitalized due to auditory hallucinations and delusions of grandeur and persecution. She held a firm conviction that God marked her uniqueness and sent her special messages. She had been treated for the past 3 years with haloperidol decanoate (50 mg for 4 weeks). She recently began to report a repetitive aggressive obsession, that she would blurt out obscenities while praying in the synagogue. She was afraid that people would know she was cursing God in her mind, and was therefore convinced that they were following her. Every day she spent hours cleaning and arranging things in order to "please God" whom she was repeatedly cursing. Ms. H was aware that this behavior was excessive but felt a compelling urge to perform rituals.

Case 3.5. Mr. S, a 36-year-old single man, had a 15-year history of DSM-IV schizophrenic disorder, undifferentiated type, and was repeatedly hospitalized for psychotic exacerbations. At the time of his assessment, negative schizophrenic symptoms were the most prominent clinical feature. There was no previous history of OCD. Clozapine was initiated after adequate consequent trials with typical and atypical antipsychotic agents failed. There *was substantial improvement in the intensity of negative symptoms and social functioning after 12 weeks of treatment (clozapine 350 mg/day). Nevertheless, he recently began to exhibit ritualistic touching and checking behaviors. He was often preoccupied with stereotyped repetitive questions: "What if I have AIDS?", "What if I am a homosexual?". He was completely aware of the senselessness and offensiveness of his repeated questions and checking rituals but was unable to contain them.*

Several patterns of onset sequence of obsessive–compulsive and schizophrenic symptoms, as portrayed in the clinical vignettes, point toward the existence of more than one underlying mechanism of their temporal interrelationship. Echoing Bleuler's belief that obsessive–compulsive symptoms may be a feature of the prodromal phase of schizophrenia, contemporary studies found obsessive–compulsive symptoms along with attenuated psychotic symptoms in a substantial proportion of individuals with prodromal signs of schizophrenia. In this scenario obsessive–compulsive symptoms, usually expressed as subthreshold OCD, can be considered early symptoms of the psychotic illness (Case 3.1). Alternatively, obsessive–compulsive symptoms may precede schizophrenia in the form of full-scale DSM-IV OCD. At least some of these patients will be treated with serotonin reuptake inhibitors (SRIs). It is plausible that the use of SRIs, while ameliorating obsessive–compulsive symptoms, may accelerate the emergence of psychotic symptoms of schizophrenia in susceptible individuals (Case 3.2). Personal and/or family history of schizophrenia-spectrum disorders in patients with OCD (Cases 3.1 and 3.2) should also alert clinicians to increased odds for transition to psychosis.

Another putative underlying mechanism is the direct transformation of an obsession into a delusion, along with the occurrence of core schizophrenia symptoms, such as formal thought disorders and negative symptoms (Case 3.3). Persons prone to OCD show a cognitive style characterized by unsuccessful thought suppression and negative interpretations including the idea that the person's choice can result in harm, which needs to be neutralized (Salkovskis, 1999). Consequent to this cognitive style, occasional intrusive thoughts tend to recur, cause distress, and become symptomatic. In severe cases of OCD, insight can become tenuous as obsessions progress. At some point, an obsessional concern may be regarded as justified and beyond reasonable question, thereby corresponding to the definition of a delusion. It is possible that the development of a delusional appraisal or belief of an intrusive thought, particularly in the presence of this obsession-prone cognitive style, may predispose for psychosis, which is in line with psychological models of psychosis (Maher, 1988).

When obsessive–compulsive symptoms followed the occurrence of schizophrenia, the hypothesis that they might be associated with presumed pathophysiological and psychological changes related to schizophrenia (Case 3.4), or antipsychotic treatment (Case 3.5), is conceivable. During the enduring course of schizophrenia, psychotic experiences may become a "focus of obsessive preoccupation," giving rise to the appearance of complex psychopathological phenomena psychotic in content and obsessive in form (Jaspers, 1972; Bermanzohn et al., 2000). These cases, further support the presence of a psychopathological continuum between obsessive–compulsive and psychotic phenomena (Case 3.4). Finally, obsessive–compulsive symptoms in schizophrenia may be a consequence of antipsychotic treatment, given that there is ample evidence pointing toward a propensity of atypical antipsychotic agents to induce *de novo* or exacerbate pre-existing obsessive–compulsive symptoms in schizophrenia patients (Case 3.5).

Obsessive–compulsive symptom trajectories in schizophrenia

The course of OCD unrelated to schizophrenia has been typically divided into the following categories (Goodwin et al., 1969): episodic course with periods of incomplete remission, phasic course with periods of complete remission between exacerbations, continuous and unremitting course associated with fluctuations in severity of symptoms, and a minority experiencing a chronic and deteriorative course. Studies showed differing rates among the categories, with estimates of the continuous course at approximately 50–80%, with a minority (roughly 10%) experiencing a deteriorating course (Attiullah et al., 2000). The Brown Longitudinal Obsessive–Compulsive Disorder Study (Eisen et al., 2010), the largest prospective study to date, which included 293 OCD patients, corroborates the existence of diverse course trajectories in OCD. In this study, roughly two-thirds of the participants had a continuous course (with mild variations in intensity of symptoms but without remission), 23% waxing and waning (with periods of at least 3 months' duration of only subclinial symptoms), 8% episodic (with periods of complete remission of 3 months or more), and 2% deteriorative (OCD continues to deteriorate even with treatment). Importantly, distinction between these categories is not straightforward and it may differ depending on the criteria set applied in a particular study.

Comparable to OCD, large-scale studies that prospectively evaluate the course of obsessive–compulsive symptoms in schizophrenia patients are still lacking. Based on clinical experience, Hwang et al. (2009) describe some of the potential obsessive–compulsive symptom trajectories in schizophrenia. As already mentioned, obsessive–compulsive symptoms may occur during the prodromal phase, preceding the acute phase of schizophrenia, and may resolve or attenuate after the onset of psychosis. Alternatively, OCD that predates the onset of schizophrenia may persist or worsen regardless of the progress of the schizophrenic illness, as an independent coexisting disorder. Patients in this category may have initially met criteria for OCD, and subsequently developed psychosis that meets criteria for schizophrenia. In some patients obsessive–compulsive symptoms develop as a part of an acute psychosis and usually resolve with overall improvement in psychosis. As the psychotic symptoms improve, the obsessive–compulsive symptoms may attenuate and present as obsessive rumination or obsessive doubt.

In a prospective short-term study Fabish et al. (2001) revealed a temporal stability of obsessive–compulsive symptoms over the period of acute exacerbation of schizophrenia. In contrast, a substantial influx of new cases of obsessive–compulsive disorder was observed by Craig et al. (2002) in first-admission schizophrenia patients followed for 24 months, suggesting that the lifetime occurrence rate of obsessive–compulsive phenomena in schizophrenia may be associated with the age of onset or duration of illness. The high attrition rate in this study limits the interpretation of the longitudinal course of obsessive–compulsive phenomena in schizophrenia.

Adopting the Eisen et al. (2010) course definitions, we retrospectively analyzed the course of obsessive–compulsive symptoms in 133 schizophrenia patients using all information available from the treating physicians, caregivers, and patients (unpublished data). The distribution of course trajectories in schizo-obsessive patients was remarkably similar to that found in OCD patients. Thus, 52.6% (70 of 133) of the schizo-obsessive patients had a continuous course of obsessive–compulsive symptoms with mild variation in intensity of symptoms, 35.3% (47 of 133) a waxing-and-waning course with periods of 3 months or longer of mild or subclinical obsessive–compulsive symptoms, and only 12.1% (15 of 133) an episodic course with periods of complete remission of at least 3 months' duration. Applying the DSM-IV definition for the course of schizophrenia, approximately half of the sample had an episodic course (54% [72 of 133]) while the remaining 46% (61 of 133) had a continuous course of illness. Comparison between the two trajectories revealed that patients with a continuous course of schizophrenia tend to have a continuous course of obsessive–compulsive symptoms, while episodic schizophrenia was more likely to be associated with an episodic course of obsessive–compulsive symptoms.

Representative clinical vignettes are given below.

Case 3.6. Mr. T, a 29-year-old student, developed his first clinically significant obsessive–compulsive symptoms at age 11. He repeatedly washed his hands and spent hours in the shower due to contamination fears. He also cleaned his room for hours to avoid contamination by "polluted agents from the atmosphere." At age 14 he was diagnosed with DSM-IV OCD based on his typical clinical presentation of obsessions and compulsions associated with a fair degree of insight. At age 17 the prodromal symptoms of psychosis, suspiciousness, social isolation, and increased anxiety, surfaced and peaked 8 months later with an acute psychotic episode characterized by delusions of reference and persecution, disorganized speech and affect, and thought disorders. He met DSM-IV criteria for schizophrenic disorder, disorganized type. No signs of OCD were detected during the acute psychotic episode. A few weeks after the resolution of psychosis, previously observed OCD symptoms resurfaced. He subsequently experienced three additional psychotic episodes with intermittent full symptomatic remissions. Though OCD symptoms persisted during the remission of schizophrenia, they were undetectable during the acute phases of psychosis.

Case 3.7. Ms. Z, 33 years old, a single mother of a 7-year-old child. She first reported a preoccupation with being contaminated by dirt, germs, and bodily fluids at age 19. She spent hours a day checking that she was not contaminated, and washed her hands compulsively, holding her hands in a position that mimicked surgeons after scrubbing up for surgery, in order to protect herself from contamination. She expressed good insight into the excessive and senseless nature of OCD symptoms and recognized them as a product of her own imagination. Her first prodromal psychotic symptoms, namely social anxiety, isolation, irritability, insomnia, and suspiciousness, developed at age 26. She was hospitalized 1 year later due to delusions of grandeur and persecution along with imperative auditory hallucinations that met DSM-IV criteria for schizophrenic disorder, paranoid type. Importantly, her repetitive hand-washing intensified during an acute psychotic phase and resulted in irritant contact dermatitis. In contrast to the pre-psychotic phase, she now believed that hand-washing was "essential to protect her from alien forces she felt surrounded by." She regained insight into her ritualistic behavior after resolution of psychosis. During the following 7 years, an episodic course of schizophrenia with two additional psychotic exacerbations was paralleled by a waxing-and-waning course of OCD. The observed pattern of insight into OCD, namely fair insight during a remission of schizophrenia and a delusional transformation of insight during psychotic exacerbations, was maintained during the entire course of follow-up.

Case 3.8. Mr. A, a 30-year-old unmarried man with no previous psychiatric hospitalizations. When he was 17, Mr. A began feeling lonely and detached, and felt that his parents did not respect him and perhaps even wanted to harm him. He sometimes reported hearing voices of peers who were laughing at his physical appearance. Gradually he restricted social contacts to only one person, his oldest brother, with whom he shared his worries. He believed that "he was losing his body every time he left a room." This repetitive and intrusive thought prompted him to repeatedly check to make sure that "he did not lose his body" and to ask for reassurance that he was still intact. In response to these thoughts, he performed repetitive behaviors to reduce anxiety, including arranging and rearranging items and ritualistically touching his parents to ensure their safety. These repetitive behaviors often took up to 3 hours a day. He recognized that these thoughts were a product of his own mind but was otherwise unaware of their unreasonable and excessive nature. In addition, he had typical contamination obsessions associated with washing and cleaning rituals that were intrusive, distressful, and time-consuming, taking up to 2 hours a day. His functioning level decreased substantially, and during the last 3 years he abandoned all social contacts and locked himself in his room and accepted food only from his parents. Gradually increasing self-neglect and lack of hygiene, as well as an increase in obsessive–compulsive symptom severity, prompted his referral for psychiatric evaluation. On examination, he had poor eye contact, blunted affect, and lack of interpersonal relatedness. He had prominent thought disorders, thought-blocking, derailments, and tangentiality, as well as delusional ideas of reference. He confirmed occasionally hearing voices to which he "became accustomed." He admitted having repetitive and intrusive thoughts of contamination and compulsive urges to wash his hands and clean items around him to prevent himself from contracting infectious diseases. He understood that these behaviors were unreasonable and excessive but could not resist performing the rituals. In contrast, he completely lacked insight into his fears of "losing his body" and the need to perform checking and touching rituals to decrease associated anxiety. He met DSM-IV diagnoses of schizophrenia, undifferentiated type, and OCD. Mr. A did not respond to several trials of antipsychotic agents. Treatment with clozapine with and without anti-obsessive medications was not associated with any meaningful changes in symptom severity, functional status, or chronic deteriorating course of both schizophrenic and obsessive–compulsive symptoms.

These case vignettes illustrate some of the possible courses of obsessive–compulsive symptoms and their relation to schizophrenia symptom trajectories. The two disorders may progress as independent coexisting disorders, as exemplified in Cases 3.6 and 3.7. In this course scenario, OCD typically precedes schizophrenia. Psychotic exacerbations are accompanied by attenuation or disappearance of obsessive–compulsive symptoms, while symptomatic remissions in schizophrenia are associated with resurfacing of obsessive–compulsive symptoms. With repeated assessments the diagnoses of both disorders are straightforward, despite a possibility that during psychotic exacerbations obsessive–compulsive symptoms may undergo "psychotic transformation" incorporating into the delusional themes typical to schizophrenia (Case 3.7). Conversely the two sets of symptoms may progress concurrently in a chronic unremitting and deteriorating course (Case 3.8). From clinical experience, this small subgroup of schizo-obsessive patients with predominantly negative symptoms and diagnostically challenging, psychotic-related, obsessive–compulsive symptoms is usually less responsive to treatment interventions and has a less favorable prognosis.

Longitudinal prospective studies with comparative assessment of obsessive–compulsive symptoms and positive, negative, and disorganized schizophrenia symptom severity in conjunction with functional status are desperately needed to fully account for a diversity of symptom trajectories in schizo-obsessive disorder. Lysaker and Whitney (2009) underscored that prospective studies could address the following questions: Do changes in one set of symptoms precede or accompany changes in others? Are obsessive–compulsive symptoms more stable or less stable over time than core schizophrenia symptoms? Does severity of obsessive–compulsive symptoms increase or decrease when there are exacerbations or remission of positive and negative schizophrenia symptoms? Do obsessive–compulsive symptoms persist among persons who meet strict criteria for remission or recovery in schizophrenia?

Until prospective longitudinal studies are performed, repeated clinical assessments over time are essential to improve identification of both sets of symptoms and their temporal interrelationships in schizo-obsessive patients.

References

Achim AM, Maziade M, Raymond E, et al. (2011) How prevalent are anxiety disorders in schizophrenia? A meta-analysis and critical review on a significant association. *Schizophrenia Bulletin* 37, 811–821.

Amminger GP, Leicester S, Yung AR, et al. (2006) Early onset of symptoms predicts conversion to nonaffective psychosis in ultra-high risk individuals. *Schizophrenia Research* 84, 67–76.

Angermeyer MC, Kuhn L (1988) Gender differences in age at onset of schizophrenia. *European Archives of Psychiatry and Neurological Sciences* 237, 251–364.

Attiullah N, Eisen JL, Rasmussen SA (2000) Clinical features of Obsessive-compulsive disorder. *Psychiatric Clinics of North America* 23, 469–491.

Baylé FJ, Krebs MO, Epelbaum C, Levy D, Hardy P (2001) Clinical features of panic attacks in schizophrenia. *European Psychiatry* 16, 349–353.

Berman I, Kalinowski A, Berman S, Lengua J, Green AI (1995) Obsessive-compulsive symptoms in chronic schizophrenia. *Comprehensive Psychiatry* 36, 6–10.

Bermanzohn PC, Porto L, Arlow PB, et al. (2000) Hierarchical diagnosis in chronic schizophrenia: a clinical study of co-occurring syndromes. *Schizophrenia Bulletin* 26, 517–525.

Bland RC, Newman SC, Orn H (1987) Schizophrenia: lifetime co-morbidity in a community sample. *Acta Psychiatrica Scandinavica* 75, 383–391.

Bottas A, Cooke RG, Richter MA (2005) Comorbidity and pathophysiology of obsessive-compulsive disorder in schizophrenia: is there evidence for a schizo-obsessive subtype of schizophrenia? *Journal of Psychiatry and Neuroscience* 30, 187–193.

Braga RJ, Mendlowicz MV, Marrocos RP, Figueira IL (2005) Anxiety disorders in outpatients with schizophrenia: prevalence and impact on the subjective quality of life. *Journal of Psychiatric Research* 39, 409–414.

Buckley PF, Miller BJ, Lehrer DS, Castle DJ (2009) Psychiatric comorbidities and schizophrenia. *Schizophrenia Bulletin* 35, 383–402.

Burgy M (2007) Obsession in the strict sense: a helpful psychopathological phenomenon in the differential diagnosis between obsessive-compulsive disorder and schizophrenia. *Psychopathology* 40, 102–110.

Byerly M, Goodman W, Acholonu W, Bugno R, Rush AJ (2005) Obsessive compulsive symptoms in schizophrenia: frequency and clinical features. *Schizophrenia Research* 76, 309–316.

Byrne M, Agerbo E, Mortensen PB (2002) Family history of psychiatric disorders and age at first contact in schizophrenia: an epidemiological study. *British Journal of Psychiatry* 181, s19–s25.

Cardno AG, Holmans PA, Rees MI, et al. (2001) A genomewide linkage study of age at onset in schizophrenia. *American Journal of Medical Genetics* 105, 439–445.

Cassano GB, Pini S, Saettoni M, Rucci P, Dell'Osso L (1998) Occurrence and clinical correlates of psychiatric comorbidity in patients with psychotic disorders. *Journal of Clinical Psychiatry* 59, 60–68.

Castle DJ, Wessely S, Murray RM (1993) Sex and schizophrenia: effects of diagnostic stringency, and associations with and premorbid variables. *British Journal of Psychiatry* 162, 658–664.

Ciapparelli A, Paggini R, Marazziti D, et al. (2007) Comorbidity with axis I anxiety disorders in remitted psychotic patients 1 year after hospitalization. *CNS Spectrums* 12, 913–919.

Cosoff SJ, Hafner RJ (1998) The prevalence of comorbid anxiety in schizophrenia, schizoaffective disorder and bipolar disorder. *Australian and New Zealand Journal of Psychiatry* 32, 67–72.

Craig T, Hwang MY, Bromet EJ (2002) Obsessive-compulsive and panic symptoms in patients with first-admission psychosis. *American Journal of Psychiatry* 159, 592–598.

de Haan L, Hoogenboom B, Beuk N, van Amelsvoort T, Linszen D (2005) Obsessive-compulsive symptoms and positive, negative, and depressive symptoms in patients with recent-onset schizophrenic disorders. *Canadian Journal of Psychiatry* 50, 519–524.

de Haan L, Dudek-Hodge C, Verhoeven Y, Denys D (2009) Prevalence of psychotic disorders in patients with obsessive-compulsive disorder. *CNS Spectrums* 14, 415–417.

de Mathis MA, Diniz JB, Shavitt RG, et al. (2009) Early onset obsessive-compuslvie disorder with and without tics. *CNS Spectrums* 14, 362–370.

DeLisi LE (1992) The significance of age-of-onset for schizophrenia. *Schizophrenia Bulletin* 18, 209–215.

DeLisi LE, Bass N, Boccio A, Shields G, Morganti C (1994) Age of onset in familial schizophrenia. *Archives of General Psychiatry* 51, 334–335.

Devulapalli KK, Welge JA, Nasrallah HA (2008) Temporal sequence of clinical manifestation in schizophrenia with comorbid OCD: review and meta-analysis. *Psychiatry Research* 161, 105–108.

Dominguez RA, Backman KE, Lugo SC (1999) Demographics, prevalence, and clinical features of the schizo-obsessive subtype of schizophrenia. *CNS Spectrums* 4, 50–56.

Eisen JL, Rasmussen SA (1993) Obsessive-compulsive disorder with psychotic features. *Journal of Clinical Psychiatry* 54, 373–379.

Eisen JL, Beer DA, Pato MT, Venditto TA, Rasmussen SA (1997) Obsessive compulsive disorder in patients with schizophrenia and schizoaffective disorder. *American Journal of Psychiatry* 154, 271–273.

Eisen JL, Pinto A, Mancebo MC, et al. (2010) A 2-year prospective follow-up study of the course of obsessive-compulsive disorder. *Journal of Clinical Psychiatry* 71, 1033–1039.

Emsley RA, Roberts MC, Rataemane S, et al. (2002) Ethnicity and treatment response in schizophrenia: a comparison of 3 ethnic groups. *Journal of Clinical Psychiatry* 63, 9–14.

Esterberg ML, Trotman HD, Holtzman C, Compton MT, Walker EF (2010) The impact of a family history of psychosis on age-at-onset and positive and negative symptoms of schizophrenia: a meta-analysis. *Schizophrenia Research* 120, 121–130.

Fabish K, Fabish H, Langs G, Huber HP, Zapotoczky HG (2001) Incidence of obsessive-compulsive phenomena in the course of acute schizophrenia and schizoaffective disorder. *European Psychiatry* 16, 336–341.

Faragian S, Fuchs C, Pashinian A, et al. (2012) Age-of-onset of schizophrenic and obsessive-compulsive symptoms in patients with schizo-obsessive disorder. *Psychiatry Research* 197, 19–22.

Fenton WS, McGlashan TH (1986) The prognostic significance of obsessive-compulsive symptoms in schizophrenia. *American Journal of Psychiatry* 143, 437–441.

Fontenelle LF, Oostermeijer S, Harrison BJ, Pantelis C, Yücel M (2011) Obsessive-compulsive disorder, impulse control disorders and drug addiction: common features and potential treatments. *Drugs* 71, 827–840.

Ganesan V, Kumar TC, Khanna S (2001) Obsessive-compulsive disorder and psychosis. *Canadian Journal of Psychiatry* 46, 750–754.

Geller D, Biederman J, Jones J, et al. (1998) Is juvenile obsessive-compulsive disorder a developmental subtype of the disorder? A review of the pediatric literature. *Journal of the American Academy of Child and Adolescent Psychiatry* 37, 420–427.

Goodman WK, Price LH, Rasmussen SA, et al. (1989) The Yale–Brown obsessive-compulsive Scale: I. Development, use, and reliability. *Archives of General Psychiatry* 46, 1006–1011.

Goodwin DW, Guze SB, Robins E (1969) Follow-up studies in obsessional neurosis. *Archives of General Psychiatry* 20, 182–187.

Goodwin RD, Amador XF, Malaspina D, *et al.* (2003) Anxiety and substance use comorbidity among inpatients with schizophrenia. *Schizophrenia Research* **61**, 89–95.

Hafner H (2000) The epidemiology of onset and course of schizophrenia. *European Archives of Psychiatry and Clinical Neuroscience* **250**, 292–303.

Higuchi H, Kamata M, Yoshimoto M, Shimisu T, Hishikawa Y (1999) Panic attacks in patients with chronic schizophrenia: a complication of long-term neuroleptic treatment. *Psychiatry and Clinical Neurosciences* **53**, 91–94.

Hwang MY, Kim S-W, Yum SY, Opler LA (2009) Management of schizophrenia with obsessive-compulsive features. *Psychiatry Clinics of North America* **32**, 835–851.

Ingram IM (1961) Obsessional illness in mental hospital patients. *Journal of Mental Science* **107**, 382–402.

Insel TR, Akiskal HS (1986) Obsessive compulsive disorder with psychotic feature: a phenomenological analysis. *American Journal of Psychiatry* **143**, 1527–1533.

Jaspers K (1972) Subjective phenomena of morbid psychic life. In: *General Psychopathology*, transl. Hoenig J, Hamilton MW. University of Chicago Press, Chicago, pp.55–57.

Jones P, Rodgers B, Murray R, Marmot M (1994). Child development risk factors for adult schizophrenia in the British 1946 birth cohort. *Lancet* **344**, 1398–1402.

Karno M, Golding JM, Sorenson SB, Burnam MA (1988) The epidemiology of obsessive-compulsive disorder in five US communities. *Archives of General Psychiatry* **45**, 1094–1099.

Kayahan B, Ozturk O, Veznedaroglu B, Eraslan D (2005) Obsessive-compulsive symptoms in schizophrenia: prevalance and clinical correlates. *Psychiatry and Clinical Neurosciences* **59**, 291–295.

Kessler RC, Chiu WT, Demler O, Merikangas KR, Walters EE (2005) Prevalence, severity, and comorbidity of 12-month DSM-IV disorders in the National Comorbidity Survey Replication. *Archives of General Psychiatry* **62**, 617–627. Erratum *Archives of General Psychiatry* **62**, 709.

Kessler RC, Amminger GP, Aguilar-Gaxiola S, *et al.* (2007) Age of onset of mental disorders: a review of recent literature. *Current Opinion in Psychiatry* **20**, 359–364.

Kessler RC, Petukhova M, Zaslavsky AM (2011) The role of latent internalizing and externalizing predispositions in accounting for the development of comorbidity among common mental disorders. *Current Opinion in Psychiatry* **24**, 307–312.

Knauper B, Cannell CF, Schwartz N, Bruce ML, Kessler R (1999) Improving accuracy of major depression age-of-onset reports in the US National Comorbidity Survey. *International Journal of Methods in Psychiatry Research* **8**, 39–48.

Krüger S, Bräunig P, Höffler J, *et al.* (2000) Prevalence of obsessive-compulsive disorder in schizophrenia and significance of motor symptoms. *Journal of Neuropsychiatry and Clinical Neurosciences* **12**, 16–24.

Large M, Sharma S, Compton MT, Slade T, Nielssen O (2011) Cannabis use and earlier onset of psychosis: a systematic meta-analysis. *Archives of General Psychiatry* **68**, 555–561.

Lauronen E, Miettunen J, Veijola J, *et al.* (2007) Outcome and its predictors in schizophrenia with the Northern Finland 1966 Birth Cohort. *European Psychiatry* **22**, 129–136.

Leckman JF, Denys D, Simpson HB, *et al.* (2010) Obsessive-compulsive disorder: a review of the diagnostic criteria and possible subtypes and dimensional specifiers for DSM-V. *Depression and Anxiety* **27**, 507–527.

Leeson VC, Harrison I, Ron M, Barnes TR, Joyce EM (2011) The effect of cannabis use and cognitive reserve on age at onset and psychosis outcomes in first-episode schizophrenia. *Schizophrenia Bulletin* Mar 9 [Epub ahead of print].

Lomax CL, Oldfield VB, Salkovskis PM (2009) Clinical and treatment comparisons between adults with early and late-onset obsessive-compulsive disorder. *Behaviour Research and Therapy* **47**, 99–104.

Lykouras L, Alevizos B, Michalopoulou P, Rabavilas A (2003) Obsessive-compulsive symptoms induced by atypical antipsychotics: a review of the reported cases. *Progress in Neuropsychopharmacology and Biological Psychiatry* **27**, 333–346.

Lysaker PH, Whitney KA (2009) Obsessive-compulsive symptoms in schizophrenia: prevalence, correlates and treatment. *Expert Review of Neurotherapeutics* **9**, 99–107.

Lysaker PH, Marks KA, Picone JB, et al. (2000) Obsessive and compulsive symptoms in schizophrenia: clinical and neurocognitive correlates. *Journal of Nervous and Mental Disease* **188**, 78–83.

Maher BA (1988) Anomalous experience and delusional thinking: the logic of explanations. In: Maher BA, Oltmanns TF (eds.) *Delusional Beliefs.* John Wiley, Oxford, pp.15–33.

Meghani SR, Penick EC, Nickel EJ, et al. (1998) Schizophrenia patients with and without OCD. In: *Proceedings of the 151st Annual Meeting of the American Psychiatric Association,* Toronto.

Millet B, Kochman F, Gallarda T, et al. (2004) Phenomenological and comorbid features associated in obsessive-compulsive disorder: influence of age of onset. *Journal of Affective Disorders* **79**, 241–246.

Nechmad A, Ratzoni G, Poyurovsky M, et al. (2003) Obsessive-compulsive disorder in adolescent schizophrenia patients. *American Journal of Psychiatry* **160**, 1002–1004.

Ndetei DM, Pizzo M, Ongecha FA, et al. (2008) Obsessive-compulsive (oc) symptoms in psychiatric in-patients at Mathari Hospital, Kenya. *African Journal of Psychiatry (Johannesburg)* **11**, 182–186.

Niehaus DJ, Koen L, Muller J, et al. (2005) Obsessive-compulsive disorder: prevalence in Xhosa-speaking schizophrenia patients. *South African Medical Journal* **95**, 120–122.

Niendam TA, Berzak J, Cannon TD, Bearden CE (2009) Obsessive-compulsive symptoms in the psychosis prodrome: correlates of clinical and functional outcome. *Schizophrenia Research* **108**, 170–175.

Numata S, Ueno S, Iga J, et al. (2006) Brain-derived neurotrophic factor (BDNF) Val66Met polymorphism in schizophrenia is associated with age at onset and symptoms. *Neuroscience Letters* **401**, 1–5.

Ohta M, Kokai M, Morita Y (2003) Features of obsessive-compulsive disorder in patients primarily diagnosed with schizophrenia. *Psychiatry and Clinical Neurosciences* **57**, 67–74.

Ongür D, Goff DC (2005) Obsessive-compulsive symptoms in schizophrenia: associated clinical features, cognitive function and medication status. *Schizophrenia Research* **75**, 349–362.

Ongür D, Lin Lewei, Cohen BM (2009) Clinical characteristics influencing age at onset in psychotic disorders. *Comprehensive Psychiatry* **50**, 13–19.

Owashi T, Ota A, Otsubo T, Susa Y, Kamijima K (2010) Obsessive-compulsive disorder and obsessive-compulsive symptoms in Japanese inpatients with chronic schizophrenia: a possible schizophrenic subtype. *Psychiatry Research* **179**, 241–246.

Pallanti S, Quercioli L, Hollander E (2004) Social anxiety in outpatients with schizophrenia: a relevant cause of disability. *American Journal of Psychiatry* **161**, 53–58.

Pauls DL (2008) The genetics of obsessive-compulsive disorder: a review of the evidence. *American Journal of Medical Genetics Part C Seminars in Medical Genetics* **148**, 133–139.

Pinto A, Mancebo MC, Eisen JL, Pagano ME, Rasmussen SA (2006) The Brown Longitudinal Obsessive Compulsive Study: clinical features and symptoms of the sample at intake. *Journal of Clinical Psychiatry* **67**, 703–711.

Porto L, Bermanzohn PC, Pollack S (1997) A profile of Obsessive-compulsive symptoms in schizophrenia. *CNS Spectrums* **2**, 21–25.

Poyurovsky M, Fuchs K, Weizman A (1999) Obsessive-compulsive symptoms in patients with first episode schizophrenia. *American Journal of Psychiatry* **156**, 1998–2000.

Poyurovsky M, Dorfman-Etrog P, Hermesh H, et al. (2000) Beneficial effect of olanzapine in schizophrenic patients with obsessive-compulsive symptoms. *International Clinical Psychopharmacology* **15**, 169–173.

Poyurovsky M, Weizman A, Weizman R (2004) Obsessive-compulsive disorder in schizophrenia: clinical characteristics and treatment. *CNS Drugs* **18**, 989–1010.

Poyurovsky M, Bergman J, Weizman R (2006) Obsessive-compulsive disorder in elderly schizophrenia patients. *Journal of Psychiatric Research* **40**, 189–191.

Poyurovsky M, Faragian S, Shabeta A, Kosov A (2008) Comparison of clinical characteristics, co-morbidity and pharmacotherapy in adolescent schizophrenia patients with and without obsessive-compulsive disorder. *Psychiatry Research* **159**, 133–139.

Reddy YC, Reddy PS, Srinath S, *et al.* (2000) Comorbidity in juvenile obsessive-compulsive disorder: a report from India. *Canadian Journal of Psychiatry* **45**, 274–278.

Regier DA, Narrow WE, Rae DS (1990) The epidemiology of anxiety disorders: the Epidemiologic Catchment Area (ECA) experience. *Journal of Psychiatric Research* **24** (Suppl. 2), 3–14.

Rosario-Campos MC, Leckman JF, Mercadante MT, *et al.* (2001) Adults with early-onset obsessive-compulsive disorder. *American Journal of Psychiatry* **158**, 1899–1903.

Rosen I (1956) The clinical significance of obsessions in schizophrenia. *Journal of Mental Science* **103**, 773–785.

Rosen JL, Miller TJ, D'Andrea JT, McGlashan TH, Woods SW (2006) Comorbid diagnoses in patients meeting criteria for the schizophrenia prodrome. *Schizophrenia Research* **85**, 124–131.

Rosenberg CM (1968). Complications of obsessional neurosis. *British Journal of Psychiatry* **114**, 477–478.

Ross RG, Novins D, Farley GK, Adler LE (2003) A 1-year open-label trial of olanzapine in school-age children with schizophrenia. *Journal of Child and Adolescent Psychophamacology* **13**, 301–309.

Roth M (1978) Psychiatric diagnosis in clinical and scientific settings. In: Akiskal HS, Webb WL (eds.) *Psychiatric Diagnosis: Exploration of Biological Predictors*. Spectrum Publications, New York.

Rudin G (1953) Ein Beitrag zur Frage der Zwangskrankheit. *Archiv für Psychiatrie und Nervenkrankheit* **191**, 14–54.

Ruscio AM, Stein DJ, Chiu WT, Kessler RC (2010) The epidemiology of obsessive-compulsive disorder in the National Comorbidity Survey Replication. *Molecular Psychiatry* **15**, 53–63.

Salkovskis PM (1999) Understanding and treating obsessive-compulsive disorder. *Behaviour Research and Therapy* **37** (Suppl. 1), S29–S52.

Seedat F, Roos JL, Pretorius HW, Karayiorgou M, Nel B (2007) Prevalence and clinical characteristics of obsessive-compulsive disorder and obsessive-compulsive symptoms in Afrikaner schizophrenia and schizoaffective disorder patients. *African Journal of Psychiatry (Johannesburg)* **10**, 219–224.

Sim K, Chan YH, Chua TH, *et al.* (2006) Physical comorbidity, insight, quality of life and global functioning in first episode schizophrenia: a 24-month, longitudinal outcome study. *Schizophrenia Research* **88**, 82–89.

Simon GE, Von Korff M (1995) Recall of psychiatric history in cross-sectional surveys: implications for epidemiologic research. *Epidemiologic Reviews* **17**, 221–227.

Simon NM, Otto MW, Wisniewski SR, *et al.* (2004) Anxiety disorder comorbidity in bipolar disorder patients: data from the first 500 participants in the Systematic Treatment Enhancement Program for Bipolar Disorder (STEP-BD). *American Journal of Psychiatry* **161**, 2222–2229.

Somers JM, Goldner EM, Waraich P, Hsu L (2006) Prevalence and incidence studies of anxiety disorders: a systematic review of the literature. *Canadian Journal of Psychiatry* **51**, 100–113.

Stengel EA (1945) A study of some clinical aspects of the relationship between obsessional neurosis and psychotic reaction types. *Journal of Mental Science* **91**, 166–187.

Sterk B, Lankreujer K, Linzen DH, de Haan L (2011) Obsessive-compulsive symptoms in first episode psychosis and in subjects at ultra high risk for developing psychosis: onset and relationship to psychotic symptoms. *Australian and New Zealand Journal of Psychiatry* **45**, 400–467.

Strakowski SM, Tohen M, Stoll AL, *et al.* (1993) Comorbidity in psychosis at first hospitalization. *American Journal of Psychiatry* **150**, 752–757.

Tandon R, Nasrallah HA, Keshavan MS (2009) Schizophrenia, "just the facts" 4. Clinical features and conceptualization. *Schizophrenia Research* **110**, 1–23.

Tibbo P, Kroetsch M, Chue P, Warneke L (2000) Obsessive-compulsive disorder in schizophrenia. *Journal of Psychiatric Research* **34**, 139–146.

Tiryaki A, Ozkorumak E (2010) Do the obsessive-compulsive symptoms have an effect in schizophrenia? *Comprehensive Psychiatry* **51**, 357–362.

Üçok A, Ceylan ME, Tihan AK, *et al.* (2011) Obsessive-compulsive disorder and symptoms may have different effects on schizophrenia. *Progress in Neuropsychopharmacology and Biological Psychiatry* **35**, 429–433.

Van Dael F, van Os J, de Graaf R, *et al.* (2011) Can obsessions drive you mad? Longitudinal evidence that obsessive-compulsive symptoms worsen the outcome of early psychotic experiences. *Acta Psychiatrica Scandinavica* **123**, 136–146.

Walitza S, Wendland JR, Gruenblatt E, *et al.* (2010) Genetics of early-onset obsessive-compulsive disorder. *European Child and Adolescent Psychiatry* **19**, 227–235.

Weissman MM, Bland RC, Canino GJ, *et al.* (1994)The Cross National epidemiology of obsessive-compulsive disorder: The Cross National Collaborative Group. *Journal of Clinical Psychiatry* **55** (Suppl.), 5–10.

Wickham H, Walsh C, Asherson P, *et al.* (2002) Familiality of clinical characteristics in schizophrenia. *Journal of Psychiatric Research* **36**, 325–329.

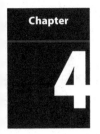

Chapter

Obsessive–compulsive symptoms in schizophrenia: psychopathological characteristics

A major difficulty in identifying obsessive–compulsive phenomena in schizophrenia is in distinguishing between obsessions and delusions or formal thought disorders and compulsions from schizophrenic mannerisms and stereotypic behavior.

According to DSM-IV criteria, OCD is characterized by recurrent, persistent, and intrusive thoughts, images, or impulses (obsessions), and repetitive actions (compulsions) or mental rituals that aim to prevent or reduce anxiety and distress that arise from obsessions (American Psychiatric Association, 1994). Obsessive thoughts are "a product of the patients' own mind," and are recognized to be unreasonable and excessive.

Obsessions can usually be distinguished from delusions by their *content* (e.g., contamination, aggressive/sexual obsessions vs. delusions of reference, persecution), *insight* into the nature of the impairment (present vs. absent), *affect* (obsession-associated anxiety vs. delusion-associated paranoid affect), *perception* (intact vs. delusional), and *associated actions* (e.g., repetitive rituals vs. delusional persecutory behavior) (Table 4.1). Notably, "bizarreness" of thoughts does not distinguish between obsessions and delusions (see Chapter 9). Compulsions can be distinguished from movement disorders in schizophrenia by typical *movement expression* (e.g., checking, washing vs. stereotypy, mannerisms), *driven agency* (obsession vs. autonomous), *purpose* (reducing distress/anxiety vs. purposeless), and *insight* (present vs. absent) (Table 4.2). British psychiatrist, Frank Fish, made a beginning toward this differential diagnosis more than 40 years ago in his careful descriptions of psychiatric signs and symptoms (Fish, 1967). Fish noted differences in the degree of insight preserved in the obsessive compared to the schizophrenia patient, the absence of the experience of "thought alienation" ("the experience that his thoughts are under the control of an outside agency or that others are participating in this thinking": Fish, 1967, p.39) in the obsessive patient, and differences in the content of schizophrenic delusions compared to obsessions (e.g., themes of persecution, jealousy, love, grandiosity, nihilism, and poverty may be present in schizophrenia, but are not seen in OCD).

In clinical reality, however, there is an overlap between obsessive–compulsive and schizophrenic symptoms that poses a significant diagnostic challenge.

Typical obsessive–compulsive symptoms in schizophrenia
Insight
Insight has consistently been considered one of the key distinguishing features between obsessive–compulsive and psychotic phenomena. Historically, from the description of a patient with obsessive–compulsive disorder (Esquirol, 1838), two primary characteristics emerged: (1) a "continuous fight" against obsessive thoughts and (2) accompanying

57

Table 4.1 Obsessions vs. delusions: distinctive features

Characteristic	Obsessions	Delusions
Cognitive domain	Thoughts, images, urges	Thoughts
Content	Contamination, aggressive, sexual, order/symmetry	Reference, persecution, grandeur, jealousy, guilt
Form	Recurrent, persistent, intrusive, distressful	Systematic delusion
Accompanying affect	Anxiety	Delusional affect
Accompanying perception	Intact	Delusional perception with or without hallucinations
Associated behavior	Repetitive rituals	Delusion-driven behavior (e.g., persecutory behavior)
Insight	Present	Absent

Table 4.2 OCD-related rituals vs. schizophrenia-related movement disorders

Characteristic	OCD-related rituals	Schizophrenia-related movement disorders
Typical expression	Checking, washing, cleaning, touching, ordering	Stereotypy, mannerisms
Driven agency	Obsession; or according to rules that must be applied rigidly	Autonomous; or driven by delusions and/or hallucinations
Aim	Preventing or reducing distress/anxiety; or preventing some dreaded event	Purposeless; or acting upon delusions and/or hallucinations
Insight	Patient recognizes compulsions as excessive and unreasonable	Lack of awareness

awareness of their "ridiculous nature." According to Esquirol, OCD is characterized by a "recurrent or persistent idea, thought, image, feeling or movement which is accompanied by a sense of subjective compulsion and a desire to resist it, the event being recognized by the individual as foreign to his personality, and into the abnormality of which he has insight" (cited by Pollitt, 1956, p.842). Westphal's (1878) definition of obsessive phenomena is "those which, with intelligence being otherwise intact . . . , step into the foreground of consciousness against the respective person's will . . . which the person affected always acknowledges as abnormal and alien to him and which he faces with his sane consciousness" (cited by Berrios, 1996, p.669). Kurt Schneider's (1939) core definition of obsession shares a similar emphasis on its senseless nature: "Obsession is when someone can not repress contents of consciousness although he judges them as being nonsensical or dominating for no reason." With usual methodological and terminological clarity, Karl Jaspers defined obsessions "in the strict sense": first, the ego assesses the contents of consciousness as being unfounded, nonsensical, and incomprehensible, and second, the ego defends itself against them (cited by Burgy, 2007, p.104).

Based on clinical observations that some patients with OCD do not consider their symptoms unreasonable or excessive, empirical evaluations challenged the traditional association of insight and OCD. Contemporary studies convincingly demonstrate that patients with OCD may exhibit varying degrees of insight into the validity of their beliefs ranging from total lack of insight to full insight (Lelliott *et al.*, 1988; Eisen and Rasmussen, 1993). Poor insight was found in a substantial proportion (10–36%) of OCD patients (Kozak and Foa, 1994; Catapano *et al.*, 2001; Matsunaga *et al.*, 2002). DSM-IV acknowledges this phenomenon and specifies "with poor insight" for individuals who "for most of the time during the current episode, do not recognize that the obsessions or compulsions are excessive or unreasonable."

The idea that the beliefs' conviction is broadly distributed, and that a continuum more accurately describes insight than "present or absent" categories, is not specific to OCD; similar suggestions are valid for delusions in patients with schizophrenia. Karl Jaspers (1923) defined a delusion as "a judgment made which is held on to with full conviction, not only with a consciousness of validity but with a sense of absolute certainty" (p.135). DSM-IV defines a delusion as "a false belief based on incorrect inference about external reality that is firmly sustained despite what almost everyone else believes and despite what constitutes incontrovertible and obvious proof or evidence to the contrary" (American Psychiatric Association, 1994, p.765). Nevertheless, the concept of delusion as a complete loss of insight has been challenged by the observation that delusions in schizophrenia form and resolve gradually, rather than in an "all or nothing" manner. Similarly, Strauss (1969) described a range of conviction in the delusions of schizophrenia, noting that certain delusions are held with less than complete conviction; and the term "recovering delusion" (Spitzer, 1990) was used to highlight the possibility of the patients' partial awareness of the falsity of a delusional idea.

The "all or nothing" character of delusions is debatable not only because of the evident continuum of beliefs' conviction, but also because there are several dimensions to delusions (Kendler *et al.*, 1983; Appelbaum *et al.*, 1999). Conviction, self-evidence, resistance to reason, unlikely content, and absence of cultural support are commonly ascribed dimensions of delusions (Mullen, 1979). Using the Dimensions of Delusional Experience rating scale that measured several aspects of delusional beliefs (conviction, preoccupation, bizarreness, systematization, extension), Kendler and colleagues (1983) found low correlations among the dimensions in a group of delusional patients substantiating the finding that delusional experience has various components.

Considering the existing psychopathological complexity and overlap between obsessive–compulsive and delusional symptoms, the relevance of such OCD criteria as insight and resistance in schizophrenia patients has been questioned (Fenton and McGlashan, 1986). Moreover, multiple deficits in self-awareness exhibited by roughly half of all schizophrenia patients (Amador *et al.*, 1993) can obscure the identification of insight into OCD in schizophrenia even more. Despite these pitfalls, explicit evaluation of insight clearly demonstrated that a substantial proportion of schizo-obsessive patients possess good or fair insight into their obsessive–compulsive symptoms (Poyurovsky *et al.*, 2007).

The Brown Assessment of Beliefs Scale (BABS) (Eisen et al., 1998) was used to address different aspects of insight into obsessive–compulsive symptoms in schizo-obsessive patients. In addition, the Scale to Assess Unawareness of Mental Disorder (SUMD) (Amador et al., 1994) was administered to compare insight into obsessive–compulsive symptoms with general awareness of illness in schizophrenia.

BABS is a seven-item, semistructured, clinician-administered scale that was used to measure insight in patients with psychiatric disorders, primarily OCD. The BABS assesses insight dimensionally and includes the following components: conviction, perception of others' views, explanation of differing views, fixity of beliefs, attempts to disprove beliefs, insight (recognition that the belief has a psychiatric/psychological cause), and referential thinking (this item is not included in the total score). Each item is rated from 0 to 4, with higher scores indicating poorer insight. A sum of the six items represents a total score (range, 0–24). A cut-off score of 18 and a score of 4 on the "conviction" item are used to classify patients as having a lack of insight into obsessive–compulsive symptoms. Good psychometric properties of the scale, including internal consistency, inter-rater reliability, and sensitivity to change, has consistently been demonstrated in patients with OCD and OCD-related disorders (e.g., body dysmorphic disorder) (Eisen et al., 1998; 2000).

The SUMD enables assessment of the awareness of mental disorder ("Does the subject believe that he has a mental disorder?"), awareness of the consequences of mental disorder ("What is the subject's belief regarding the reasons he has been unemployed, evicted, hospitalized?"), and awareness of the effects of medication ("Does the subject believe that medications have diminished the severity of his symptoms?"). In addition, the patient's awareness of delusions subscale is incorporated in the SUMD ("Does the subject believe that he experiences delusions as such, that is, as internally produced erroneous beliefs?"). Scores for each of the SUMD items range from 1 ("aware") to 5 ("severely unaware"). Assessment of inter-rater reliability using this scale has been in the excellent to good range with intra-class correlations ranging from 0.82 to 0.91 (Lysaker et al., 2006)

When OCD-related beliefs of each schizophrenia patient were identified (e.g., "If I check the distance between my eyes repeatedly, I will never go blind"), and specific BABS probes and anchors were used to assess subdimensions of insight into these beliefs, the mean BABS total score was 9.9 ± 6.9, that is substantially lower than the cut-off score of 18 used to identify patients with lack of insight into obsessive–compulsive symptoms (Table 4.3). Indeed, the majority (85%, 48 of 57) of schizo-obsessive patients exhibited good or fair insight into OCD. These patients were aware of the unrealistic nature of their OCD-related beliefs; admitted that most people consider their beliefs inaccurate; they usually tried to disprove beliefs and expressed certainty that these beliefs were illness-related and could be cured. Only a few patients (15%, 9 of 57) revealed lack of insight. Unlike the patients with good insight, these patients were convinced of the veracity of their beliefs; they expressed certainty that others condoned their OCD-related beliefs and were reluctant to consider the option that their beliefs were unfounded and had no insight into the possible psychiatric or psychological basis of the belief. The proportion of poor insight schizo-obsessive patients in this study is within the 10–36% range observed in the DSM-IV field trial of "pure" OCD without schizophrenia (Foa et al., 1995), and corresponds to 12% reported in the large-scale Brown Longitudinal OCD Study (Pinto et al., 2006). Furthermore, correlation analysis revealed some noteworthy associations. First, there was a positive correlation between insight into OCD (BABS total score) and global awareness of schizophrenia (SUMD subscales scores) (r values $= 0.29$–0.37, p values $= 0.005$–0.009). This suggests that cognitive ability for general awareness of illness and a more specific awareness of obsessive–compulsive phenomena in schizo-obsessive patients are interdependent, and patients with poor insight into OCD are those that lack awareness of schizophrenia, and vice versa. Second, in contrast to the above-mentioned association, there was a lack of correlation between insight into OCD and awareness of delusions in schizophrenia

Table 4.3 Insight into obsessive–compulsive symptoms and awareness of illness in schizophrenia patients with and without obsessive–compulsive symptoms

Variable	Schizophrenia with OCD ($N=57$)	Schizophrenia without OCD ($N=80$)
Sex (M/F)	42/12	63/17
Age (y)	31.8 (9.1)	30.4 (9.5)
Education (y)	11.6 (2.2)	12.1 (1.7)
Age at onset of schizophrenia (y)[a]	20.2 (5.3)	23.0 (5.7)
Age at onset of OCD (y)	18.7 (7.5)	—
Duration of schizophrenia (y)[a]	11.6 (8.4)	7.3 (8.6)
Number of hospitalizations	3.2 (2.5)	3.5 (3.9)
Scale scores		
SAPS/SANS		
Positive	7.9 (3.6)	7.4 (3.8)
Negative	11.3 (4.3)	11.9 (4.4)
Disorganized	5.4 (3.2)	5.8 (2.6)
CGI	4.1 (0.9)	4.0 (0.9)
SUMD		
Awareness of mental disorder	2.0 (0.9)	2.0 (0.9)
Awareness of social consequences	1.8 (0.8)	2.0 (0.9)
Awareness of medication response	1.9 (0.9)	2.0 (0.9)
Y-BOCS		
Obsessions	10.7 (4.8)	
Compulsions	9.4 (4.4)	
Total	20.2 (8.2)	
BABS		
Conviction	1.8 (1.4)	
Perception of others' views	1.1 (1.3)	
Explanation of different views	1.5 (1.4)	
Fixity of ideas	1.7 (1.4)	
Attempt to disprove beliefs	2.3 (1.3)	
Insight	1.5 (1.5)	
Total	9.8 (7.0)	

Figures in parantheses, SD. SAPS, Schedule for the Assessment of Positive Symptoms; SANS, Schedule for the Assessment of Negative Symptoms; CGI, Clinical Global Impression scale; Y-BOCS, Yale–Brown Obsessive–Compulsive Scale; BABS, Brown Assessment of Beliefs Scale.
[a] $p < 0.001$ schizo-obsessive vs. non-OCD schizophrenia.
Source: Poyurovsky M, Faragian S, Kleinman-Balush V, Pashinian A, Kurs R, Fuchs C (2007) Awareness of illness and insight into obsessive–compulsive symptoms in schizophrenia patients with obsessive–compulsive disorder. *Journal of Nervous and Mental Disease* **195**, 765–768. Reprinted with permission.

($r = -0.18$, $p = 0.26$). This is consistent with clinical experience with the schizo-obsessive subgroup: while a majority of these patients refers to obsessive–compulsive symptoms as senseless and distressful, they may be fully convinced of the "true" nature of their delusional ideas (e.g., persecution, control, grandeur). *Third*, the BABS total score did not correlate with any of the clinical variables, including severity of schizophrenia symptoms, as assessed by the Schedule for the Assessment of Positive (SAPS) (Andreasen, 1984) and Negative (SANS) (Andreasen, 1983) Symptoms (r values $= 0.09$–0.45, p values > 0.10). This lack of correlation lends additional support to the independent nature of obsessive–compulsive symptoms in schizophrenia.

Considering that 85% of the schizo-obsessive patients exhibited satisfactory insight into OCD, it was conceivable to assume that a comparable proportion of patients would exhibit sufficient awareness of schizophrenia. This was not the case. In fact, awareness of schizophrenia was low in the schizo-obsessive group and almost half of the schizo-obsessive patients failed to fully acknowledge that they had mental impairment. Moreover, the multiple deficits in self-awareness revealed in the schizo-obsessive group were remarkably similar to those found in the comparison group of non-OCD schizophrenia patients (Table 4.3). Thus, OCD does not considerably improve the awareness of schizophrenia in schizo-obsessive patients.

The following case vignettes portray schizo-obsessive patients with different degrees of insight into OCD-related beliefs.

Case 4.1. Schizophrenia patient with good insight into obsessive–compulsive symptoms.

Mr E, a 35-year-old man, has a 10-year history of DSM-IV schizophrenic disorder, paranoid type. During psychotic exacerbations at age 25 and 29 he exhibited delusions of reference and persecution, auditory hallucinations, and formal thought disorders. After resolution of psychosis he regained a satisfactory level of functioning and was employed as a clerk in a government office. Initial clinically significant obsessive–compulsive symptoms emerged at age 15 before the occurrence of his first psychotic symptoms, when he began to complain of intrusive and distressful thoughts of contamination and a fear of contracting a lethal disease. He developed multiple cleaning, washing, and checking rituals to deal with anxiety associated with contamination fears. E revealed good insight into the excessive, unrealistic, and senselessness nature of his intrusive thoughts; however, he could not resist performing rituals he felt driven to perform in response to distress associated with obsessions. A DSM-IV diagnosis of OCD was established at age 17. These typical obsessive–compulsive symptoms had a continuous course and were present during active and remitted phases of schizophrenia, although in different degrees of severity. He underwent several structured clinical interviews during acute and remitted stages of schizophrenia using rating scales for the assessment of a severity of both schizophrenic and obsessive–compulsive symptoms, including the BABS and the SUMD. According to the BABS assessment during the remitted phase of schizophrenia, he was certain that his contamination fears were false ("My mind is contaminated by thoughts, but I can not uproot them"), and that others also believed that his thoughts and fears were unrealistic; he was easily willing to consider the professional explanation of the falsity of his beliefs, and usually tried to disprove them by himself. E was certain that his obsessions and compulsions had a medical origin, after reading about OCD on the internet. BABS subscale scores (conviction, perception of others views of beliefs, explanation of differing views, fixity of ideas, attempts to disprove ideas, insight) ranged from 0 to 1 (total BABS score 4), indicating good insight. Remarkably, E maintained a fair degree of insight into his obsessive–compulsive symptoms (total BABS score 8) during an exacerbation of psychosis. At the same time, he showed a lack of insight for his delusional beliefs, and was completely convinced that he was watched and followed by CIA agents who implanted listening devices in his room to monitor his behavior (SUMD "insight into delusion" subscale score 5 "severely unaware"). After resolution of psychosis, E exhibited satisfactory insight in both components of the disorder, and was able to acknowledge that he had a mental illness, schizophrenia, that was accompanied by OCD. His high awareness was coupled with treatment compliance and a favorable prognosis.

Case 4.2. Schizophrenia patient with poor insight into obsessive–compulsive symptoms.

Mr. G, a 21-year-old man. His first clinically significant obsessive–compulsive symptoms were identified at age 14, and were characterized by repetitive, intrusive, and distressful thoughts of a possible eye penetration by an acute object accompanied by checking and touching rituals. He also felt an urge to ask questions repeatedly for reassurance that his eye was not damaged. Rituals lasted for as long as 6 hours per day and interfered substantially with his scholastic performance and daily routine. During his first psychiatric assessment at age 18, a DSM-IV diagnosis of OCD was established owing to the presence of typical repetitive intrusive and distressful thoughts and associated rituals. A distinctive feature of G's mental condition was poor insight into OCD-related beliefs. G was convinced that an acute object might indeed enter his eye and that others shared his belief; he was reluctant to consider the option that this belief was unfounded and had no insight whatsoever into its possible psychiatric or psychological cause. A "poor insight" qualifier was added to his OCD diagnosis. At that point he denied any referential thinking, claiming that others were not aware of his beliefs. BABS subscale scores ranged from 3 to 4 (total BABS score 21), indicating poor insight. One year later, social withdrawal and substantial functional decline emerged along with initial psychotic symptoms. He now claimed that voices of unknown individuals made obnoxious remarks about his beliefs concerning acute objects. He verbally assaulted his parents because they "deliberately harm his eyes using acute objects." This delusional idea prompted him to intensify performance of checking and touching rituals that by now resembled stereotypic movements of schizophrenia. At that point G met DSM-IV criteria for schizophrenic disorder, paranoid type. BABS assessment yielded the highest total score – 24, and conviction score – 4, indicating lack of insight. In addition, referential thinking and complete transformation of thought content from obsessional into delusional was also acknowledged in the BABS delusions of reference additional subscale (score 4). After resolution of psychosis and disappearance of delusions and hallucinations, prominent negative symptoms and cognitive impairment surfaced, as did intrusive thoughts of the same pre-psychotic content and corresponding checking rituals. Poor insight into obsessive–compulsive symptoms was allied with lack of awareness of schizophrenia, and need for treatment.

The following conclusions can be drawn based on the evaluation of insight into obsessive–compulsive symptoms in schizophrenia.

- Satisfactory insight into obsessive–compulsive symptoms in a majority of schizo-obsessive patients unambiguously shows that obsessive–compulsive symptoms represent an *identifiable* dimension of psychopathology independent of core schizophrenia symptoms. Their autonomous character is further substantiated by a lack of association between insight into OCD-related beliefs and any of the clinical parameters related to schizophrenia. It is essential to explicitly inquire into different aspects of insight into obsessive–compulsive symptoms in the differential diagnosis between obsessive–compulsive and psychotic phenomena in schizophrenia patients.
- Lack of correlation between insight into obsessions and delusions, along with distinctive behavioral, cognitive, and affective features, suggests that obsessions in schizophrenia

are distinguishable from delusions. During the course of illness a lack of awareness of the delusional experience may well co-occur with a reasonable understanding of the unrealistic character of an obsession (Case 4.1). In some cases, however, poor insight into an obsession predominates (Case 4.2). These patients pose a particular diagnostic challenge. Poor insight obsessions can be differentiated from delusions based on the typical OCD content, accompanying compulsions, intact perception, and lack of delusional affect. During psychotic exacerbations, obsessions might transform into referential delusional content and form complex psychopathological phenomenon that incorporate both obsessive–compulsive and psychotic elements.

- In a majority of schizophrenia patients, high awareness of obsessive–compulsive symptoms apparently does not translate into high awareness of the primary schizophrenic disorder. In fact, no difference in multiple self-awareness indices was found between the schizophrenia groups with and without OCD, implying that the presence of obsessive–compulsive symptoms does not significantly modify patients' awareness of schizophrenia. Considering that poor awareness of schizophrenia is often associated with poor treatment compliance and poorer outcome, improvement of general illness awareness is critical for improving the prognosis of schizophrenia patients with or without OCD.

- Satisfactory insight into OCD observed in a substantial proportion of schizo-obsessive patients implies potential clinical utility of a cognitive–behavioral approach together with pharmacotherapy to target the obsessive–compulsive component in schizophrenia.

Obsessive–compulsive symptom characteristics

The pervasive character of psychosis challenges identification of obsessive–compulsive symptoms in schizophrenia. As noted earlier, Fenton and McGlashan (1986) suggested alternative OCD-related behavioral categories in schizophrenia, while questioning the typical presentation of obsessive–compulsive symptoms in schizophrenia:

- repeated behaviors that interfere with daily activities, such as touching rituals so pervasive that they consume hours each day;
- indecision/stuckness, i.e., obsessional hesitancy so severe as to interfere with daily activities;
- repeated behaviors performed before some goal-directed activity, such as inspecting hands and feet before entering any doorway or arranging and rearranging shoes for an hour before bedtime;
- repeated behaviors aimed at magically avoiding harm to self or others, such as washing after contact with anything that might have touched the floor;
- obsessive and pedantic speech, described as dominating verbal communication and controlling others;
- verbal rituals, such as repetition of phrases, anecdotes, or minutiae, or reversing syllables;
- compulsive repetition of acts the patient finds repulsive, such as searching through trash cans;
- complaints of recurrent, persistent ideas experienced as senseless or repugnant – classic obsessions.

The authors unexpectedly found that the majority of patients had *typical* obsessions and compulsions (e.g., washing, cleaning, checking). Indeed, in a majority of the study patients, obsessive–compulsive symptoms were independent of psychotic symptoms, and the transformation of obsessions into delusions was revealed only in two of 21 schizo-obsessive patients (Fenton and McGlashan, 1986).

Modern research of obsessive–compulsive phenomena in schizophrenia is characterized by the use of rigorous DSM diagnostic criteria for both schizophrenia and OCD and structured clinical assessments, supplemented by relevant rating scales for symptom detection and their severity. The OCD module of the Structured Clinical Interview for DSM-IV (SCID) (First *et al.*, 1996), the Yale–Brown Obsessive–Compulsive Scale (Y-BOCS) (Goodman *et al.*, 1989), and the symptom checklist incorporated into the Y-BOCS were frequently used in current studies and contributed to a more comprehensive clinical characterization of obsessive–compulsive symptoms in schizophrenia. The Y-BOCS has been shown to be a valid and reliable instrument in patients with OCD and OCD-related disorders (Goodman *et al.*, 1989). de Haan *et al.* (2006) examined the psychometric properties of Y-BOCS for assessing severity of obsessive–compulsive symptoms in patients with schizophrenia, and found good internal consistency and inter-rater reliability of the scale, which further supports its usefulness in schizophrenia patients as well.

The Y-BOCS is a semistructured interview developed to measure a severity of obsessive–compulsive symptoms in OCD. The scale is divided into two parts: the obsessions subscale and the compulsions subscale. On each subscale five aspects of pathology are rated on scales ranging from 0 (no symptoms) to 4 (extreme symptoms): time spent, degree of interference, distress, resistance, and perceived control over symptoms. Scores obtained from the subscales are summed to yield a Y-BOCS total score. The Y-BOCS includes 15 major symptom domains of OCD: obsessions – aggressive, contamination, sexual, hoarding/saving; religious (scrupulosity), symmetry or exactness, somatic, miscellaneous (e.g., need to ask, fear of saying certain things, intrusive nonsense sounds); compulsions – cleaning/washing, checking, repeating, counting, ordering/arranging, hoarding/collecting, miscellaneous (e.g., mental rituals, need to ask, need to touch).

We now know that similar to their OCD counterparts, a majority of schizo-obsessive patients have both obsessions and compulsions (Eisen *et al.*, 1997; Tibbo *et al.*, 2000; Byerly *et al.*, 2005; Rajkumar *et al.*, 2008). The mean number of obsessions and compulsions per patient is considerable (range 3.8–7.3), with a few patients exhibiting only monosymptomatic OCD (Eisen *et al.*, 1997; Tibbo *et al.*, 2000; Ongür and Goff, 2005). There is also substantial consistency across studies as to the most frequently observed obsessive–compulsive symptoms, as well as a striking similarity of primary obsessive–compulsive symptoms in schizo-obsessive individuals and those reported in "pure" OCD (Foa *et al.*, 1995). The obsessions that were most often reported in the first smaller studies of schizo-obsessive patients were aggressive, contamination, somatic, and symmetry; the most prevalent compulsions were checking, cleaning/washing, ordering/arranging and counting (Porto *et al.*, 1997; Tibbo *et al.*, 2000; Ohta *et al.*, 2003; Rajkumar *et al.*, 2008). Two recent reports with large sample sizes (110 and 186 schizo-obsessive patients, respectively) (Faragian *et al.*, 2009; de Haan *et al.*, 2011) substantiated these preliminary findings. There is a remarkable similarity in the revealed frequencies of obsessions and compulsions (Table 4.4). Roughly half of all schizo-obsessive patients present with aggressive obsessions and checking and washing compulsions, a third with contamination, somatic, and symmetry obsessions and ordering and counting compulsions, and approximately 20% with sexual and religious obsessions. In addition, the

Table 4.4 Frequencies of obsessions and compulsions in schizophrenia patients[a]

	Obsessions			Compulsions	
	Faragian et al.	De Haan et al.		Faragian et al.	De Haan et al.
Aggressive	44%	42%	Checking	56%	53%
Contamination	33%	30%	Washing	52%	35%
Somatic	31%	27%	Ordering/arranging	40%	33%
Symmetry/exactness	26%	39%	Counting	28%	39%
Sexual	22%	30%	Hoarding/collecting	22%	6%
Religious	20%	25%			
Hoarding	10%	–			

[a] Symptoms from more than one obsessive–compulsive symptom category may be present in a patient. *Source*: Data extracted from Faragian *et al.* (2009) and de Haan *et al.* (2011). Data based on the symptom checklist incorporated into the Yale–Brown Obsessive–Compulsive Scale (Goodman *et al.*, 1989).

mean severity of obsessive–compulsive symptoms in schizo-obsessive patients, as measured by Y-BOCS, ranges from moderate to severe (total Y-BOCS = 16–40) (Byerly *et al.*, 2005). The severity of obsessive–compulsive symptoms seems to progress during the course of schizophrenia. There was a positive correlation between duration of schizophrenia and severity of obsessive–compulsive symptoms, and significantly higher Y-BOCS scores were revealed in recurrent episodes compared to first-episode schizophrenia patients (Poyurovsky *et al.*, 2003). Based on the above, it is apparent that obsessive–compulsive symptoms in schizophrenia contribute to significant patient distress and disability.

Notably, the relationship between obsessive–compulsive symptoms and specific subtypes of schizophrenia is unclear. Although there is some indication of more frequent occurrences of obsessive–compulsive symptoms in patients with paranoid-hallucinatory (Rosen, 1956), schizo-affective (Eisen *et al.*, 1997), or undifferentiated (Hwang *et al.*, 2000) subtypes of schizophrenia, a majority of recent reports failed to reveal predominance of any specific subtypes of schizophrenia (Krüger *et al.*, 2000; Tibbo *et al.*, 2000; Fabisch *et al.*, 2001; Ohta *et al.*, 2003).

Obsessive–compulsive symptom dimensions

OCD without symptoms of schizophrenia is a clinically heterogeneous disorder. Two patients with a clear OCD diagnosis can display completely different symptom patterns. It becomes increasingly clear that symptoms of OCD assemble within several potentially overlapping symptom dimensions (Mataix-Cols *et al.*, 2005). In view of the above notable similarities in phenomenological expression, symptom severity, and the most prevalently experienced symptoms between obsessive–compulsive phenomena in schizophrenia and "pure" OCD, it was conceivable to assume that symptom dimensions similar to those in OCD may be present also in schizophrenia.

An exploratory factor analytic study was conducted to determine whether the revealed factor structure in symptoms of OCD also exists in schizophrenia patients with obsessive-compulsive symptoms (Faragian *et al.*, 2009). Each of the 13 symptom categories on the Y-BOCS checklist (seven obsessions, six compulsions) except for miscellaneous obsessions and compulsions, was scored as 0 = absent or 1 = present, and only current symptoms were included in the factor analysis. Principal components analysis with Varimax rotation was conducted on the Y-BOCS checklist categories in accordance with the original method (Baer, 1994). In the principal component analysis, criteria for retention of factors were eigenvalue greater than 1 (Kaiser's criterion), interpretability of the factors and Cattell's Scree Test. The initial factor solutions were followed with a Varimax rotation in order to facilitate interpretation. To evaluate the structural integrity of these factors, Pearson correlations were used for each symptom category.

The principal component analysis of 13 Y-BOCS checklist categories yielded a five-factor solution and accounted for 58.7% of the total variance (Table 4.5). The first factor *(forbidden thoughts)* accounted for 15.9% of the variance and included aggressive, sexual, and religious obsessions and counting compulsions; loadings ranged from 0.52 to 0.67. The second factor *(symmetry)* (13.6% of the variance) included symmetry obsessions and ordering and hoarding compulsions; loadings ranged from 0.54 to 0.86. The third factor *(cleaning)* (11.2% of the variance) included contamination obsession and cleaning compulsion; loadings 0.79 and 0.82, respectively. The fourth factor *(somatic)* (9.8% of the variance) included somatic obsession and repeating compulsion; loadings 0.70 and 0.81, respectively. The fifth factor *(hoarding)* (8.2% of the variance) included hoarding obsession and checking and repeating compulsions; loadings ranged from 0.72 to 0.74. Pearson correlations demonstrated significant associations between some of the major Y-BOCS symptom categories. The most significant correlations (r values = 0.4–0.5, $p < 0.001$) were between contamination obsession and cleaning compulsion, symmetry obsession and ordering compulsion. In addition, significant but less robust correlations (r values = 0.2–0.4, $p < 0.01$) were found between aggressive and sexual obsessions and counting compulsions, somatic obsessions and counting and repeating compulsions, symmetry obsessions and hoarding compulsions.

In general, the five symptom dimensions resulting from the analysis are similar to a large extent to those revealed in factor- and cluster-analysis studies conducted in patients with "pure" OCD. Indeed, a meta-analysis of 21 factor analytic studies involving 5124 participants, generated four major symptom dimensions explaining a substantial proportion of the heterogeneity of the clinical symptoms in OCD: (1) *symmetry*: symmetry obsessions and repeating, ordering, and counting compulsions; (2) *forbidden thoughts*: aggression, sexual, religious, and somatic obsessions and checking compulsions; (3) *cleaning*: cleaning and contamination; and (4) *hoarding*: hoarding obsessions and compulsions (Bloch *et al.*, 2008). Interestingly, contrary to most factor-analysis studies of OCD, hoarding obsessions and compulsions in schizo-obsessive patients were not loaded on the same factor (Faragian *et al.*, 2009). Since hoarding obsessions and compulsions were the least frequent symptoms in the sample (10% and 11%, respectively), it is possible that the total number of hoarders was too small to be a separate group. Noteworthy, hoarding compulsions were linked to symmetry obsessions and ordering compulsion, supporting the view that hoarding and symmetry factors are closely related (Bloch *et al.*, 2008).

Boyette *et al.* (2011) went on to explore the underlying factor structure using principal components analysis and the severity items of the Y-BOCS in a large group of 217 patients

Table 4.5 Varimax rotated factor structure and loadings for Yale–Brown Obsessive–Compulsive Scale symptom category scores[a]

Yale-Brown Obsessive Compulsive Scale symptom category	Factor loading				
	Factor 1: Aggressive, sexual, religious/ counting[b]	Factor 2: Symmetry/ ordering, hoarding[c]	Factor 3: Cleanliness/ washing[d]	Factor 4: Somatic/ repeating[e]	Factor 5: Hoarding/ checking[f]
Aggressive	**0.67**	−0.07	−0.04	−0.03	−0.04
Contamination	0.05	−0.00	**0.82**	0.25	0.07
Sexual	**0.52**	−0.15	−0.05	0.29	−0.14
Hoarding	0.18	0.05	−0.06	0.25	**0.72**
Religious	**0.55**	0.05	0.27	−0.12	0.08
Symmetry	0.05	**0.86**	0.06	−0.02	0.05
Somatic	−0.01	−0.05	0.13	**0.81**	−0.17
Cleaning	0.13	0.06	**0.79**	−0.05	0.05
Checking	−0.13	0.06	0.18	−0.18	**0.74**
Repeating rituals	0.02	0.10	0.03	**0.70**	0.31
Counting	**0.65**	0.07	0.10	0.02	0.12
Ordering	−0.25	**0.78**	0.11	−0.01	−0.01
Hoarding	0.37	**0.54**	−0.29	0.11	0.19

[a] Total percent of variance = 58.7%. Factor loadings > 0.5 are considered robust.
[b] Percent of variance = 15.9%.
[c] Percent of variance = 13.6%.
[d] Percent of variance = 11.2%.
[e] Percent of variance = 9.8%.
[f] Percent of variance = 8.2%.
Source: Faragian S, Pashinian A, Fuchs C, Poyurovsky M (2009) Obsessive–compulsive symptom dimensions in schizophrenia patients with comorbid obsessive–compulsive disorder. *Progress in Neuropsychopharmacology and Biological Psychiatry* **33**, 1009–1012. Reprinted with permission.

with schizophrenia or related disorders and comorbid obsessive–compulsive symptoms (Table 4.6). A two-factor solution consistent with the originally proposed scoring structure of the Y-BOCS provided the optimal fit. The produced two factors related to severity of obsessions and compulsions and showed good reliability and strong correlation with the Y-BOCS total score. This highlighted the suitability of the Y-BOCS to assess the severity of obsessive–compulsive symptoms in patients with schizophrenia.

One substantial limitation of these studies is worth mentioning. A cross-sectional design precludes conclusions regarding the temporal stability of the OCD symptom structure in schizo-obsessive patients. Notably, symptom stability in patients with "pure" OCD has yet

Table 4.6 Principal component analysis two-factor solution model of the Y-BOCS

Item	Factor I	Factor II
1. Time spent on obsession	**0.85**	−0.09
2. Interference from obsession	**0.84**	−0.11
3. Distress from obsession	**0.88**	−0.19
4. Resistance to obsession	**0.61**	0.11
5. Control over obsession	**0.80**	0.10
6. Time spent on compulsion	−0.06	**0.78**
7. Interference from compulsion	0.17	**0.69**
8. Distress from compulsion	−0.02	**0.86**
9. Resistance to compulsion	−0.22	**0.65**
10. Control over compulsion	−0.01	**0.84**

Note: Factor loadings ≥ 0.50 are set in bold type.
Source: From Boyette L, Swets M, Meijer C, Wouters L, *et al.* (2011) Factor structure of the Yale–Brown Obsessive. *Psychiatry Research* **186**, 409–413. Reprinted with permission.

to be clarified. Initial reports point toward a lack of stability across time (Baer, 1994), and the latest reports indicate that temporal symptom changes emerged primarily within rather than between OCD symptom dimensions (Mataix-Cols *et al.*, 2002).

The following vignettes illustrate some of the obsessive–compulsive symptom dimensions in patients with schizophrenia.

*Case 4.3. **Forbidden thoughts:** aggressive obsessions and counting/checking compulsions in a schizophrenia patient.*

Ms. B, a 27-year-old housekeeper, mother of three children. Her mother suffered from OCD, and her brother had schizophrenic disorder. B's first obsessive–compulsive symptoms emerged at age 20, 2 years after she gave birth to her first child. She began complaining of repetitive, intrusive, and extremely distressful thoughts that she might kill her child. She had an urge to put a "suffocating bag" over his head, or to stab the child. She described repetitive, intrusive, and distressful images of a knife "in front of her eyes." In order to deal with severe anxiety induced by these "unbearable" aggressive thoughts she felt compelled to count to 33 in a certain order to neutralize her intrusive thoughts. The counting rituals lasted for hours, "paralyzing her" and making it impossible to take care of her son. She also felt an irresistible urge to touch the child "to ensure his safety." Additional rituals included repetitive checks of faucets and electrical appliances. She was completely aware of the excessive and unrealistic character of her fears and actions. B noted that all thoughts and actions were the product of "her brain," understood their pathological character, and asked for a professional explanation and help. She was diagnosed with DSM-IV OCD. Six months later after continuous treatment with an SSRI B developed an acute psychotic episode unrelated to the content of OCD. She presented with auditory imperative hallucinations, delusions of persecution, thought control, and gross disorganization of thoughts. Her obsessive–compulsive symptoms were not evident during the acute psychosis, but resurfaced after its resolution. She later experienced two additional psychotic episodes with a similar clinical picture and was diagnosed with DSM-IV schizophrenic disorder, undifferentiated type. Independent patterns of OCD and schizophrenia course were preserved.

Case 4.4. Cleaning: *contamination obsession and cleaning/washing compulsions in a schizophrenia patient.*

Mr. V, a 32-year-old unmarried man. Since his first hospitalization at age 20, he was diagnosed with DSM-IV schizophrenic disorder, paranoid type. The course of illness was characterized by episodes of psychosis followed by remissions associated with negative symptoms and progressive cognitive and functional decline. He was hospitalized four times due to psychotic exacerbations. V reported hearing voices commenting on his behavior and delusions of reference ("People are making remarks about me") and grandeur ("I am a king of Judea") that predominated his thought content. There was substantial disorganization of thought processes with parallel thoughts, tangentiality, and perseveration among the most prominent features. Treatment with typical antipsychotic agents was only partially successful, leaving residual psychotic symptoms during the remitted state. Initial clinically significant obsessive–compulsive symptoms were detected 3 years after his first admission, at age 23. After resolution of the first psychotic episode, V exhibited a new behavioral pattern of repeatedly washing his hands and showering for hours. He reported constant concern about the possibility of being contaminated by germs, insects, and bacteria, and bodily secretions. In addition, he constantly checked whether faucets were cleaned and properly turned off to ensure a "sterile environment." A diagnosis of DSM-IV OCD was suspected due to repetitive intrusive thoughts and ritualistic behaviors typical to OCD. Obsessive–compulsive symptoms were partially masked by psychotic symptoms during acute exacerbations but were evident during the remitted states accounting for distress and a substantial portion of his general functional impairment. A diagnosis of DSM-IV OCD was confirmed. Remarkably, despite marked thought disorders, chronic psychotic symptoms, and cognitive impairment, V revealed fair insight into his obsessive worries and compulsive rituals. He considered them excessive and distressful, and attempted to resist them. He recalled the occurrence of similar worries and rituals when he was 14, which at that time were transient and did not affect his daily routine.

Case 4.5. Symmetry: *symmetry obsessions and repeating, ordering, and counting compulsion in a schizophrenia patient.*

Mr. L, a 23-year-old man, was adopted as a child. His initial obsessive–compulsive symptoms were identified at age 13 when L was first seen arranging and rearranging things. He placed audio cassettes in a certain order and kept them in symmetry in order "to prevent his parents from being harmed in a car accident," "to prevent his favorite soccer team from losing a game," and "to prevent himself from getting bad grades in school." At first, his parents considered this behavior a game; however, later attempts to prevent him from conducting rituals ended in irritable responses and angry outbursts. He was seen by a psychiatrist at age 16 and when questioned reported additional obsessions and compulsions: an urge to keep his clothes, shoes, books, and internet files in a specific order that had a special meaning for him. L described an irresistible urge to keep the "whole world around" according to the "rule of symmetry." He admitted that intrusive thoughts and repeated actions were excessive but expressed certainty that symmetry was essential to prevent harm to himself and his family. Although a formal diagnosis of OCD was not established, it was strongly suspected. Attenuated psychotic symptoms, functional decline, and social withdrawal were followed by a full-blown psychotic episode 2 years later at age 18. The clinical picture then included *delusions of control, thought broadcasting, and withdrawal, with grossly disorganized thought process, affect, and behavior. He was diagnosed with a DSM-IV schizophrenic disorder, disorganized type. Notably, during a psychotic episode L exhibited additional behavioral patterns apparently not related to the delusional content. He counted and repeatedly arranged his bedding, explaining that he had to do it "just right." Symmetry obsessions accompanied by ordering, repeating, and counting compulsions remained after the resolution of psychosis. A diagnosis of DSM-IV OCD was eventually established in addition to the diagnosis of schizophrenic disorder.*

In summary, factor-analytic studies exploring an underlying structure of obsessive–compulsive symptoms in schizophrenia point toward its substantial similarity to "typical" OCD. This fact and a lack of intercorrelation between the major OCD symptom categories and schizophrenia symptom dimensions substantiate the independent nature of OCD in schizo-obsessive patients. The validity of the revealed symptom dimensions in patients with a primary diagnosis of OCD is supported by their putative association with distinct patterns of brain activation as measured by functional magnetic resonance imaging (fMRI), psychiatric comorbidity, and treatment response (Mataix-Cols et al., 2004). Whether a similar interrelationship exists in schizo-obsessive disorder remains to be elucidated.

Effect of obsessive–compulsive symptoms on schizophrenia symptom severity

How do obsessive–compulsive symptoms affect the severity of schizophrenia symptoms? This information is crucial in order to appreciate the interrelationship between the two components of the disorder, to predict illness outcomes, and to plan appropriate management strategies.

Reports concerning the effect of obsessive–compulsive symptoms on the severity of schizophrenia symptoms are inconsistent. Some studies, primarily those investigating recent-onset psychosis, show lower severity of delusions, formal thought disorders, and anergia (Poyurovsky et al., 1999; Tibbo et al., 2000; de Haan et al., 2006; Rajkumar et al., 2008), and others have shown higher severity of schizophrenia symptoms predominantly in chronic schizo-obsessive patients (Lysaker et al., 2000; Ongür and Goff, 2005; Owashi et al., 2010; Tiryaki and Ozkorumak, 2010). Most reports, however, did not reveal any differences in the severity of schizophrenia symptoms between schizophrenia patients with and without OCD (Poyurovsky et al., 2001; Ohta et al., 2003; Byerly et al., 2005; de Haan et al., 2005; 2011). Differences in study design, sample sizes, assessment instruments, and the inclusion of diverse patient populations may at least in part account for these discrepancies.

Cunill et al. (2009) performed the first systematic review and a meta-analysis of studies (23 and 18, respectively) that were completed by 2006, and that aimed to clarify the effect of obsessive–compulsive symptoms/disorder on the severity of schizophrenia symptoms. The authors found that the presence of obsessive–compulsive symptoms in schizo-obsessive patients was associated with higher global (95% CI), positive and negative symptoms in comparison to schizophrenia patients without OCD. It is quite remarkable that when the categorical DSM-IV definition of OCD was used, there was no association with more severe schizophrenic symptoms. The authors suggest some methodological and statistical explanations for these contradictory results. Using the categorical definition of OCD may well account for the inclusion of some subjects with varying degrees of obsessive-compulsive symptoms in the comparative schizophrenia group, resulting in a "dilution" of the between-group differences. To the degree that global symptoms refer to overall psychopathology, including anxiety, tension, preoccupation, and depression, in addition to positive and negative symptoms, it may not be surprising that schizo-obsessive patients scored higher on global symptoms than those with non-OCD schizophrenia. However, schizo-obsessive patients also had higher positive and negative symptom scores, indicating that the presence of obsessive–compulsive symptoms is also associated with more severe schizophrenic symptoms per se. This finding apparently contradicts earlier studies that suggested that the presence of obsessive–compulsive phenomena had a protective role and was an indicator of good prognosis in schizophrenia. It has been shown that the presence of OCD in the first stages of schizophrenia may be associated with fewer formal thought disorders and less affective flattening (Poyurovsky et al., 1999), rendering a "protective" effect against some, but not all, positive or negative symptoms. Nevertheless, the Cunill et al. (2009) meta-analysis did not aim to assess specific types of schizophrenia symptoms thus such a possibility cannot be ruled out and needs to be replicated.

How can the link between obsessive–compulsive symptoms and greater severity of psychotic symptoms be conceptualized? One possible explanation is that it is an artifact of the previously discussed phenomenological overlap of OCD and schizophrenia. Perhaps schizo-obsessive patients showed higher psychotic symptom severity because the obsessive–compulsive symptoms that resembled psychotic symptoms contributed to the quantification of psychosis. However, since most studies attempted to exclude patients with obsessions and compulsions that were exclusively related to schizophrenic symptoms from the schizo-obsessive group, and based upon the evidence that obsessions and compulsions can be reliably identified by instruments valid for OCD, this explanation of symptom overlap seems unlikely. It is also unlikely that the potential of atypical antipsychotics to induce or exacerbate obsessive–compulsive symptoms in schizophrenia patients accounted for the higher severity of psychotic symptoms. Subjects with more severe psychotic symptoms were treated with atypicals and consequently were at a higher risk of developing drug-induced obsessive–compulsive symptoms. However, most of the studies included in the meta-analysis that reported data on antipsychotic drug administration found no differences in the exposure to atypical antipsychotic agents between the schizo-obsessive and non-OCD schizophrenia groups. In fact, the finding of a greater severity of psychosis in schizophrenia patients with obsessive–compulsive symptoms is in line with a majority of reports that projected a graver general clinical picture for these patients associated with poorer social and vocational functioning and poorer prognosis.

Psychotic-related obsessive–compulsive symptoms in schizophrenia

Clinical experience shows that in addition to typical ego-dystonic obsessive–compulsive symptoms identified in a meaningful proportion of patients with schizophrenia, there is a subgroup which exhibits obsessions and/or compulsions that psychopathologically intertwine with psychotic symptoms. Schizophrenia patients with typical but poor insight to obsessions and/or compulsions are not included in this group. Noteworthy, Westphal, Kreapelin, and Schneider considered obsessive–compulsive and psychotic symptoms discrete non-overlapping psychopathological phenomena, and denied the possibility of a transition from an obsession to a delusion (Burgy, 2007). Accumulating evidence, indicates that obsessive–compulsive and psychotic symptoms are interconnected and represent a continuum of disturbances rather than discrete psychopathological phenomena.

Obsessive delusions

Bermanzohn and colleagues (1997) provide clinical descriptions and thorough psycho-pathological analysis of complex symptom profiles in which psychotic and obsessive–compulsive symptoms are interconnected. These persistent phenomena appear to be a "phenomenological hybrid," obsessional in form and psychotic or delusional in content. They might best be referred to as "obsessive delusions." The fact that roughly 20% of patients had obsessive delusions suggests that such an intertwining of delusional and obsessive features is relatively common in chronic schizophrenia patients. Viewing such phenomena as "just" obsessions or "just" delusions is apparently insufficient, as obsessive delusions have important features of both obsessions and delusions. Other than their psychotic content, obsessive delusions seem to be similar to ordinary obsessions experienced by patients without schizophrenia. Hence, obsessive delusions are intrusive, unwanted, repetitive, distressing phenomena that are often resisted by the patient. Compulsive-like behaviors generally arise out of these delusions. Another similarity with ordinary obsessions is that patients with obsessive delusions display variable insight. As noted previously, there is a range of conviction in the delusions in patients with schizophrenia, and the possibility of partial awareness of the falsity of a delusional idea has been described in some patients especially during clinical improvement (Spitzer, 1990). It seems that this is particularly relevant for schizo-obsessive patients. Emergence of "critical attitudes and doubt" towards delusions in the presence of obsessions was frequently found in schizo-obsessive patients (Mayer-Gross, 1924).

Two potential underlying mechanisms of "obsessive delusions" have been suggested: (1) obsessive delusions developed out of "simple" obsessions from which they lost insight; (2) obsessive delusions grew out of an obsessive preoccupation with a schizophrenic delusion (Bermanzohn et al., 1997). Both mechanisms may be at work and may have therapeutic implications: in patients with the former mechanism, obsessive delusions may respond to the addition of anti-obsessive agents, while patients with the latter mechanism may respond solely to monotherapy with an antipsychotic agent. Treatment aspects of these complex psychopathological phenomena are discussed in Chapter 9.

The following case vignettes depict obsessive delusions in schizophrenia patients as a "psychopathological hybrid," obsessional in form and delusional in content (Bermanzohn et al., 1997).

Case 4.6. Obsessive delusions developed out of "simple" obsessions.

Mr. H, a 26-year-old man, began having auditory hallucinations at age 21. He also developed a firm belief that he would cause harm to others if he ate certain foods. While he was "always convinced these thoughts are true," he often checked with clinical staff and family before eating. He also became preoccupied with the idea that if he wrote or drew with certain colors he would cause others to talk about him. Additionally, he believed others were following him and wanted to hurt him. His fear of eating certain foods preoccupied him for several hours every day, and caused him considerable distress, necessitating frequent reassurance from staff that it was all right for him to eat. Besides his preoccupation with eating certain foods, he developed other preoccupations, including the fear that he had cut off his toes with a fan, and fear of the letter K and the number 12. He constantly sought reassurance that he did not harm himself. H was maintained on neuroleptic medications which had no effect on these persistent thoughts, in particular his preoccupation with food and checking whether or not he could eat. A trial of an adjunctive anti-obsessive agent clomipramine was associated with a reduction in his preoccupations and checking behavior.

Case 4.7. Obsessive delusions developed out of an obsessive preoccupation with a schizophrenic delusion.

Mr. A, a 43-year-old man. At age 16 he began to be tormented by intrusive thoughts that people thought he was gay, and therefore talked about him, and made fun of him. He also believed that people wanted to hurt him and make his life miserable. He left school because of these intrusive and distressing thoughts, and became virtually housebound for about 7 years, during which time he spent hours each day monitoring his walking in front of a mirror to be sure he did not walk in a an "effeminate" manner that might confirm what he believed others thought about him. He heard a voice that kept a running commentary on his thoughts and actions and two or more voices conversing with each other. He also heard laughter, his name being called, and "noises that did not make sense." From age 17 to 20, A would repeatedly comb his hair until "I got the part exactly right," usually taking between 15 and 20 minutes daily, but sometimes hours. He became preoccupied with violent, sexually aggressive, and homosexual thoughts, which led him to see his neighborhood priest daily to confess. For several years these trips to confess were the only times he left his house. He also had to think in ritualistic ways, feeling that he had to synchronize his thinking with that of TV personalities. He said of these thoughts and actions: "I just could not stop" and recognized that they were excessive. During his long course of illness he was treated with a variety of typical neuroleptics and trials with adjunctive anti-obsessive agents that had no effect on A's preoccupation with thoughts that others believed he was gay and ridiculed him. Clozapine was initiated and slowly increased to 600 mg/day. During 4 weeks of this regimen, he experienced a definite reduction in the intrusiveness of these thoughts and in the distress they caused him.

Comparable to Bermanzohn *et al.*'s (1997) findings, our systematic clinical evaluation of patients who met DSM-IV criteria for both schizophrenia and OCD identified "atypical" psychotic-related, obsessive–compulsive phenomena in roughly 30% of schizoobsessive patients, and extended their psychopathological characterization (Poyurovsky *et al.*, 2003).

As noted above, delusional content and obsessional form come together to bring about this complex psychopathological phenomenon. Actually all schizophrenic delusions may be present: somatic, reference, persecution, grandeur, jealousy, and guilt. "Merging" with an obsessional form, the delusions become intrusive, repetitive, distressful, and often resisted. Both bizarre and non-bizarre delusions may become a focus of obsessive preoccupation. In some but not all patients obsessive delusions may be associated with compulsive rituals. Checking, washing, symmetry, arranging, hoarding, and other typical compulsions as well as mental rituals may accompany obsessive delusions. Obsessive delusions "growing out" of typical obsessions are generally detected during acute exacerbations of psychosis. In contrast to this transient psychopathological phenomenon, there are chronic persistent obsessive delusions observed in both acute and remitted phases of illness, putatively developed via a mechanism of "obsessive preoccupation" with a delusion. Once more, "obsessive delusions" phenomenologically differ from typical obsessions "with poor insight" in that they represent a combination of obsessive and delusional phenomena rather than merely a lack of awareness of the excessive and nonsensical nature of obsessions.

The following examples were drawn from the medical histories of patients with obsessive delusions.

Case 4.8. Mr. S, 32 years old, has a 10–year history of paranoid schizophrenia. Clinically significant contamination obsessions and washing and cleaning rituals preceded the occurrence of psychosis by a few years and warranted diagnosis of DSM-IV OCD. During psychotic exacerbations he exhibited delusions of grandeur, persecution, and influence, claiming that a TV broadcaster was talking about him and sending special messages. While in remission, S continued to report on these thoughts, but complained that they became intrusive, "annoying," unwanted, lasting for hours, and that they substantially restricted his daily functions. S now considered these thoughts as "his fantasy," and tried to resist them by "deliberately" watching TV and convincing himself that these thoughts are "ridiculous" and unrealistic.

Case 4.9. Mr. R, 24 years old, was diagnosed with DSM-IV OCD at age 17 due to the presence of typical ego-dystonic aggressive obsessions and checking and repeating compulsions. He was preoccupied with intrusive and distressful thoughts that he was homosexual and asked repeatedly for reassurance to the contrary. At age 20, R developed his first psychotic episode characterized by delusions of persecution and control and commentary auditory hallucinations, meeting criteria for DSM-IV schizophrenic disorder, paranoid type. He now claimed that his homosexuality was evident because he was sending special "thought fluids." People around him watched him, and laughed at him and his homosexuality. He expressed complete certainty about these experiences, but complained of their distressful and intrusive nature. To neutralize these intrusive thoughts he began to count in a certain order, touch the door frames, and repeat certain "magical phrases."

Case 4.10. Ms. S, a 40-year-old woman with DSM-IV schizoaffective disorder characterized by episodes of acute psychosis and major depressive disorder and typical OCD, presented with obsessive aggressive thoughts and images and compulsive checking behavior that preceded the emergence of psychosis. During psychotic exacerbations, she reported thoughts that her father transformed into a dog and that her grandmother became a bird; both followed her and noticed her. She expressed guilt feelings because her special power had turned them into animals and for that she deserved punishment. Her guilt thoughts were of delusional proportion. Her bizarre thoughts concerning her relatives were also associated with full conviction of their reality but were intrusive and unwanted and caused substantial distress and a desire "to get rid of them." She intensified her checking rituals to convince herself of the human identity of her relatives.

Case 4.11. Mr. N, a 35-year-old man with paranoid schizophrenia, first developed somatic delusions at age 30. He claimed that blood vessels in his brain were interconnected in a way that predisposed him to cancer. Repeated medical examinations including CT and MRI were unremarkable, but failed to convince him otherwise. Despite the delusional intensity of these thoughts, they were obsessional in form, namely intrusive, distressful, and unwanted. Moreover, N developed complex ritualistic behaviors to "prevent a cancer spread," including repetitive questions and phrases and compulsive touching. This behavior was perceived by N as excessive and distressful but he felt compelled to perform rituals.

Obsessive hallucinations

In addition to delusions that may acquire obsessional form, hallucinations may also become intertwined with obsessions. Notably, the French term *hallucination obsédante*, which translates as obsessional hallucination, was introduced by the French psychiatrist Jules Seglas in 1895 to denote a "hallucination proper accompanied by all the symptoms characteristic of an obsession, including anxiety, distress, and discomfort" (cited by Fuentenebro and Berrios, 2000). Karl Jaspers also raised the possibility of hallucinations becoming the intrusive focus of a patient's attention, and called them "compulsive hallucinations" (Jaspers, 1972). Although these types of hallucination psychopathologically related to obsessive–compulsive phenomena have primarily been described in individuals with OCD and schizophrenia, they may also occur in association with other mental disorders, as well as in individuals without a psychiatric diagnosis (Fuentenebro and Berrios, 2000).

Similar to obsessive delusions, obsessive hallucinations represent an amalgam of ordinary hallucinatory content and obsessional form. It is of note that roughly 10% of our sample of schizo-obsessive patients exhibited auditory hallucinations with typical hallucinatory content (e.g., voices commenting), but repetitive, intrusive, and distressful, that is obsessional form (Bleich-Cohen *et al.*, 2011). In some patients obsessive hallucinations are associated with typical compulsive behavior.

The following examples were drawn from the medical histories of patients with obsessive hallucinations.

Case 4.12. Ms. E is a 28-year-old unemployed woman with a 10-year history of paranoid schizophrenia. Since age 18 she began to have auditory hallucinations with voices cursing her and repeating phrases such as "Yes, correct." She described these voices as real and coming from the outside world. At the same time she described them as intrusive and distressful. Moreover, she attempted to ignore or suppress these voices but her attempts were usually unsuccessful. Her first psychiatric disturbance began at age 12, when she became preoccupied with aggressive and sexual thoughts and fear of saying the wrong things. In response she engaged in compulsive checking, counting, and repetitive behaviors. For several years, she spent from 2 to 3 hours a day performing rituals: this had a substantial effect on her school performance and daily functioning. Typical obsessions and compulsions accompanied by distress and functional impairment were suggestive of OCD; however, formal diagnosis was not established. She experienced a full-blown psychotic episode at age 19 when in addition to "obsessive auditory hallucinations" she had delusions of reference and persecution and believed that others were following her and wanted to harm her. Later negative symptoms and cognitive decline became evident and diagnosis of DSM-IV schizophrenic disorder was established. She continued to experience auditory hallucinations associated with obsessive-compulsive components.

Case 4.13. Mr. R is a 20-year-old religious man who since age 18 has had persistent thoughts that people send him messages, always look at him, harass him, and want to harm him because they believe he is homosexual. He also experienced continuous derogatory voices repeating the same word "homosexual" numerous times a day. He described these voices as real, related to an unknown person, and coming from the outside world. These auditory hallucinations however had a typical obsessional quality, that is intrusive and distressful. Complaining of "sticking voices," R began asking repetitive questions, counting up to the "magic number 7," and ordering things in a certain order to neutralize "unwanted voices" and associated anxiety.

Obsessions and formal thought disorders

Schneiderian first-rank symptoms may also intertwine with obsessive–compulsive symptoms and form complex psychopathological phenomena, psychotic in content and obsessive–compulsive in form. First-rank symptoms include the following psychopathological phenomena: audible thoughts, voices arguing and commenting, delusional perception, passivity phenomena (e.g., made thoughts, impulses, acts), thought insertion, thought withdrawal, thought broadcasting (Schneider, 1939). Although these symptoms are not unique to schizophrenia and may be detected in patients with affective psychoses as well, they are highly prevalent in schizophrenia (Peralta and Cuesta, 1999). In their genuine form some of these symptoms bear a resemblance to obsessive–compulsive phenomena. Hence, *audible thoughts* represent a *repetition* in the form of auditory hallucinations, of thoughts that have occurred a short but perceptible time before; *made acts* may also resemble compulsive rituals (Mellor, 1970). Generally, distinction of obsessions and compulsions from first-rank symptoms is based on the evaluation of thought possession (own vs. alien), agency thinking (own vs. alien), ego-boundary (intact vs. permeated), and insight (present vs. absent) (Mullins and Spence, 2003) (Table 4.7). Moreover, a paranoid delusion may accompany first-rank symptoms in schizophrenia patients and contribute to a differential diagnosis. In schizo-obsessive patients, however, at least some may "acquire" obsessional form and might follow with typical compulsive behavior.

Table 4.7 Comparative characteristics of selective first-rank symptoms and obsessions

Symptom	Ego-boundary	Permeation	Agency (thinking)	Thought possession
Thought insertion	Permeated	Inwards	Alien	Alien
Influenced[a] thinking	Permeated	Inwards	Alien	Own
Thought withdrawal	Permeated	Outwards	Alien	Own
Activity experiences	Permeated	Outwards	Own	Own
Obsessions	Intact	N/A	Own	Own

[a] "Influenced," "made," and "passivity" thinking are taken as equivalent.
Source: Modified from Mullins S, Spence SA (2003) Re-examining thought insertion: semi-structured literature review and conceptual analysis. *British Journal of Psychiatry* **182**, 293–298. Reprinted with permission.

Case 4.14. Mr. B, a 26-year-old man, had had aggressive and sexual obsessions since age 19. He described them as unpleasant and distressful. He was aware of the excessive and senseless nature of his intrusive thoughts, trying to resist by performing mental rituals. His first psychotic episode at age 24 was characterized by paranoid delusions, auditory hallucinations, and disorganized behavior. Additionally, he claimed that people around him could read his mind and specifically, the content of his obsessions. This feeling of openness to everybody of his "secret" sexual and aggressive thoughts was particularly distressful for B. After resolution of major psychosis, he continued to complain of "mind reading," maintaining a fair insight into the nonsensical nature of this phenomenon.

Case 4.15. Ms. M, a 51-year-old woman, had had chronic schizophrenia since age 20. Persistent positive symptoms, delusions of reference, and auditory hallucinations, along with social withdrawal and low level of functioning characterized her mental condition for years. One of the prominent features was M's reports of thoughts inserted deliberately by people to confuse her. Although M expressed conviction regarding the reality of these "thought insertions," they were experienced as unwanted and distressful, and were associated with typical checking rituals to neutralize them. She was also engaged in repetitive behaviors like arranging and rearranging things and asking repetitive questions, expressing distress from these acts.

Compulsions, in contrast to obsessions, are secondary phenomena that can follow both obsessive thoughts, delusional ideas, and hallucinations (Burgy, 2007). The following cases highlight this point of view:

Case 4.16. Mr. P, a 29-year-old man, stated that he suffered from obsessions. At home he had to turn the light switch four times and to pull the handbrake in the car four times in order to make sure that nothing happened to his family of four. This was an absolute necessity, although he knew at the same time that it was all nonsense. He also pressed the TV button four times, so that when being switched off no violence from the films was left behind in the apartment. He says that actually all of this was nonsense, but given the situation it was all real to him . . . In a lengthy exploration of the phenomena underlying the compulsive acts, acoustic hallucinations were finally identified, particularly the voice of God that had ordered him to check four times. Hence, the repetitive compulsive acts originated from chronic hallucinations and delusional ideas.

Case 4.17. Mr. E is a 41-year-old man with chronic paranoid schizophrenia, and transient subclinical obsessive–compulsive symptoms. He currently exhibits delusional ideas of reference and persecution claiming that his neighbors follow him and try to harm him by poisoning his food. He claimed that his body and clothes were infected by dirt because of poisoning. He began to wash his clothes, brush his teeth, and shower in a special order to deal with contamination. This ritualistic behavior continued for as long as 8 hours daily and paralyzed any productive activity. In contrast to the lack of insight of the pathological nature of his concerns, E revealed fair insight to the excessiveness of rituals and complained that he was not able to stop them.

Guillem *et al.* (2009) employed a dimensional symptomatic approach and multiple regression analyses in 59 stable schizophrenia outpatients to clarify an interrelationship between schizophrenic and obsessive–compulsive symptoms. A strong positive correlation was shown between bizarre delusions and obsessions while controlling for a potentially confounding effect of illness duration and antipsychotic drug dosages. This association is consistent with the view that delusions and obsessions reflect manifestations of overlapping underlying mechanisms. Additional association was found between auditory hallucinations and compulsions. The authors speculate that in fact, compulsions are often conceived as a response to an anxiogenic environment, i.e., obsessions. Similarly, hallucination could be viewed as a perceptual response to anxiogenic thoughts, i.e., delusions. Thus hallucinations and compulsions may both reflect a decreased capacity to inhibit behaviors or thoughts. The revealed inverse relationship between hoarding/collecting compulsions and bizarre delusions and auditory hallucinations is noteworthy, since it would be consistent with the view that some obsessive–compulsive symptoms have a protective effect against certain psychotic symptoms. A temporal stability of these associations remains to be shown in longitudinal design studies.

Recommendations for identification of obsessive–compulsive symptoms in schizophrenia

It is becoming increasingly clear that the schizo-obsessive group of patients is phenomeno-logically heterogeneous. Both typical and psychotic-related obsessive–compulsive symptoms are present in accord with symptoms of schizophrenia. Clinicians may encounter several subgroups of schizo-obsessive patients based on the interrelationship between obsessive–compulsive and schizophrenic symptoms. The subgroup that most frequently emerges is characterized by typical ego-dystonic obsessions and/or compulsions unrelated to the content of delusions and hallucinations. A less frequently observed subgroup includes patients who, in addition to "typical" ego-dystonic OCD symptoms, also have obsessive–compulsive symptoms that are related to the content of their delusions and hallucinations. These patients meet full DSM-IV criteria for OCD in addition to the diagnosis of schizophrenia. At least at some point during the course of schizophrenia all had readily detectable obsessive–compulsive symptoms with "typical" content, insight into the nature of obsessive–compulsive symptoms, and marked functional impairment due to the obsessive–compulsive component. Thorough clinical evaluation and assessment using instruments valid and reliable for targeting typical OCD (e.g., SCID, Y-BOCS) are useful in diagnosing obsessive–compulsive phenomena in these subgroups of schizo-obsessive individuals. There is also an alternative schizo-obsessive phenotype characterized by complete interference of obsessive–compulsive symptoms with delusions/hallucinations. In this schizo-obsessive subgroup a complex obsessive–compulsive–delusion/hallucination symptom profile appears to be obsessional in form and psychotic in content. Development of valid and reliable diagnostic instruments is warranted to identify these "atypical" obsessive–compulsive phenomena in schizophrenia.

Considering the substantial overlap between obsessive–compulsive and schizophrenic symptoms and diagnostic pitfalls in identification of obsessive–compulsive symptoms in schizophrenia, the following guidelines may assist in their identification in the presence of psychosis (Bottas *et al.*, 2005; Poyurovsky *et al.*, 2012):

- in general, obsessive–compulsive symptoms in schizophrenia are phenomenologically similar to typical OCD symptoms;
- recurrent intrusive ego-dystonic thoughts should not be considered obsessions if they are related exclusively to delusional themes; reassessment of these "questionable obsessions" may be necessary after resolution of acute psychotic symptoms;

- primary obsessional slowness may be mistaken for prodromal schizophrenia or a thought disorder; such patients may be unable to articulate any obsessions and may exhibit no compulsions;
- obsessional doubt may be mistaken for schizophrenic ambivalence; in rare cases of schizo-obsessive disorder both phenomena may coexist. Identification of additional symptoms of either disorder in interest may assist in differential diagnosis.

Overall, from the phenomenological perspective, a schizo-obsessive phenotype most likely represents a heterogeneous group of psychopathological expressions with a complex inter-relationship between obsessive–compulsive and schizophrenic symptoms. Differences in symptom profiles with distinct "proximity" of obsessive–compulsive to psychotic dimension may imply differences in pathophysiology; they could reflect differences between OCD as a comorbid disorder or as an additional psychopathological dimension of schizophrenia.

References

Amador XF, Strauss DH, Yale SA, et al. (1993) Assessment of insight in psychosis. American Journal of Psychiatry 150, 873–879.

Amador XF, Flaum M, Andreasen NC, (1994) Awareness of illness in schizophrenia and schizoaffective and mood disorders. Archives of General Psychiatry 51, 826–836.

American Psychiatric Association (1994) Diagnostic and Statistical Mannual of Mental Disorders, 4th edn. American Psychiatric Association, Washington, DC.

American Psychiatric Association (2000). Diagnostic and Statistical Manual of Mental Disorders 4th edn, text revn. American Psychiatric Association, Washington, DC.

Andreasen NC (1983) The Scale for the Assessment of Negative Symptoms (SANS). University of Iowa, Iowa City, IA.

Andreasen NC (1984) The Scale for the Assessment of Positive Symptoms (SAPS). University of Iowa, Iowa City, IA.

Appelbaum PS, Robbins PC, Roth LH (1999) Dimensional approach to delusions: comparison across types and diagnoses. American Journal of Psychiatry 156, 1938–1943.

Baer L (1994) Factor analysis of symptom subtypes of obsessive compulsive disorder and their relation to personality and tic disorders. Journal of Clinical Psychiatry 55 (Suppl.), 18–23.

Bermanzohn PC, Porto L, Arlow PB, et al. (1997) Are some neuroleptic refractory symptoms of schizophrenia really obsessions? CNS Spectrums 2, 51–57.

Berrios GE (1996) The History of Mental Symptoms: Descriptive Psychopathology since the Nineteenth Century. Cambridge University Press, Cambridge, UK.

Bleich-Cohen M, Hendler T, Pashinian A, Faragian S, Poyurovsky M (2011) Obsessive musical hallucinations in a schizophrenia patient: psychopathological and fMRI characteristics. CNS Spectrums 16, 579–582.

Bloch MH, Landeros-Weisenberger A, Rosario MC, Pittenger C, Leckman JF (2008) Meta-analysis of the symptom structure of obsessive-compulsive disorder. American Journal of Psychiatry 165, 1532–1542.

Bottas A, Cooke RG, Richter MA (2005) Comorbidity and pathophysiology of obsessive-compulsive disorder in schizophrenia: is there evidence for a schizo-obsessive subtype of schizophrenia? Journal of Psychiatry and Neuroscience 30, 187–193.

Boyette L, Swets M, Meijer C, Wouters L, G R O U P Authors (2011) Factor structure of the Yale-Brown Obsessive. Psychiatry Research 186, 409–413.

Burgy M (2007) Obsession in the strict sense: a helpful psychopathological phenomenon in the differential diagnosis between obsessive-compulsive disorder and schizophrenia. Psychopathology 40, 102–110.

Byerly M, Goodman W, Acholonu W, Bugno R, Rush AJ (2005) Obsessive–compulsive symptoms in schizophrenia: frequency and clinical features. *Schizophrenia Research* **76**, 309–316.

Catapano F, Sperandeo R, Perris F, Lanzaro M, Maj M (2001) Insight and resistance in patients with obsessive-compulsive disorder. *Psychopathology* **34**, 62–68.

Cunill R, Castells X, Simeon D (2009) Relationships between obsessive-compulsive symptomatology and severity of psychosis in schizophrenia: a systematic review and meta-analysis. *Journal of Clinical Psychiatry* **70**, 70–82.

de Haan L, Hoogenboom B, Beuk N, van Amelsvoort T, Linszen D (2005) Obsessive-compulsive symptoms and positive, negative, and depressive symptoms in patients with recent-onset schizophrenic disorders. *Canadian Journal of Psychiatry* **50**, 519–524.

de Haan L, Hoogeboom B, Beuk N, *et al.* (2006) Reliability and validity of the Yale–Brown Obsessive-Compulsive Scale in schizophrenia patients. *Psychopharmacology Bulletin* **39**, 25–30.

de Haan L, Sterk B, Wouters L, Linszen DH (2011) The 5-year course of obsessive-compulsive symptoms and obsessive-compulsive disorder in first-episode schizophrenia and related disorders. *Schizophrenia Bulletin* Jul 28. Epub ahead of print.

Eisen JL, Rasmussen SA (1993) Obsessive compulsive disorder with psychotic features. *Journal of Clinical Psychiatry* **54**, 373–379.

Eisen JL, Beer DA, Pato MT, Venditto TA, Rasmussen SA (1997) Obsessive-compulsive disorder in patients with schizophrenia or schizoaffective disorder. *American Journal of Psychiatry* **154**, 271–273.

Eisen JL, Phillips KA, Baer L, *et al.* (1998) The Brown Assessment of Beliefs Scale: reliability and validity. *American Journal of Psychiatry* **155**, 102–108.

Esquirol JE (1838) *Des Maladies Mentales*. Baillière, Paris.

Fabisch K, Fabisch H, Langs G, Huber HP, Zapotoczky HG (2001) Incidence of obsessive-compulsive phenomena in the course of acute schizophrenia and schizoaffective disorder. *European Psychiatry* **16**, 336–341.

Faragian S, Pashinian A, Fuchs C, Poyurovsky M (2009) Obsessive-compulsive symptom dimensions in schizophrenia patients with comorbid obsessive-compulsive disorder. *Progress in Neuro psychopharmacology and Biological Psychiatry* **33**, 1009–1012.

Fenton WS, McGlashan TH (1986) The prognostic significance of obsessive-compulsive symptoms in schizophrenia. *American Journal of Psychiatry* **43**, 437–441.

First MB, Spitzer RL, Gibbon M, Williams JBW (1996) *Structured Clinical Interview for DSM-IV Axis I Disorders, Clinician Version (SCID-CV)*. American Psychiatric Press, Washington, DC.

Fish F (1967) *Clinical Psychopathology: Signs and Symptoms in Psychiatry*. John Wright and Sons, Bristol, UK.

Foa EB, Kozak MJ, Goodman WK, *et al.* (1995) DSM-IV field trial: obsessive-compulsive disorder. *American Journal of Psychiatry* **152**, 90–96.

Fuentenebro F, Berrios GE (2000) Introduction: Jules Seglas and "hallucinatory obsessions." *History of Psychiatry* **11**, 109–112.

Goodman WK, Price LH, Rasmussen SA, *et al.* (1989) The Yale–Brown Obsessive-Compulsive Scale: I. Development, use, and reliability. *Archives of General Psychiatry* **46**, 1006–1011.

Gordon A (1950) Transition of obsession into delusions: evaluation of obsessional phenomenon from the prognostic standpoint. *American Journal of Psychiatry* **107**, 455–458.

Guillem F, Satterthwaite J, Pampoulova T, Stip E (2009) Relationship between psychotic and obsessive compulsive symptoms in schizophrenia. *Schizophrenia Research* **115**, 358–362.

Hwang MY, Morgan JE, Losconzcy MF (2000) Clinical and neuropsychological profiles of obsessive-compulsive schizophrenia: a pilot study. *Journal of Neuropsychiatry and Clinical Neurosciences* **12**, 91–94.

Insel TR, Akiskal HS (1986) Obsessive compulsive disorder with psychotic feature: a phenomenological analysis. *American Journal of Psychiatry* **143**, 1527–1533.

Jaspers K (1923) *General Psychopathology*. (Transl. Hoenig J., Hamilton, MW, Manchester University Press, Manchester, UK, 1972.) *Allgemeine Psychopathologie* Springer, Berlin.

Jaspers K (1972) Compulsion phenomena. In: *General Psychopathology*, transl. Hoenig J, Hamilton MW. University of Chicago Press, Chicago, pp.123–137.

Kendler KS, Glazer WM, Morgenstern H (1983) Dimensions of delusional experience. *American Journal of Psychiatry* **140**, 466–469.

Kozak MJ, Foa EB (1994) Obsessions, overvalued ideas, and delusions in obsessive-compulsive disorder. *Behaviour and Research Therapy* **32**, 343–353.

Krüger S, Bräunig P, Höffler J, *et al.* (2000) Prevalence of obsessive-compulsive disorder in schizophrenia and significance of motor symptoms. *Journal of Neuropsychiatry and Clinical Neurosciences* **12**, 16–24.

Lelliott P, Noshirvani HF, Başoğlu M, Marks IM, Monteiro WO (1988) Obsessive-compulsive beliefs and treatment outcome. *Psychological Medicine* **18**, 697–702.

Lysaker PH, Marks KA, Picone JB, *et al.* (2000) Obsessive and compulsive symptoms in schizophrenia: clinical and neurocognitive correlates. *Journal of Nervous and Mental Disease* **188**, 78–83.

Lysaker PH, Whitney KA, Davis LW (2006) Awareness of illness in schizophrenia: associations with multiple assessments of executive function. *Journal of Neuropsychiatry and Clinical Neurosciences* **18**, 516–520.

Mataix-Cols D, Marks IM, Greist JH, Kobak KA, Baer L (2002) Obsessive-compulsive symptom dimensions as predictors of compliance with and response to behavior therapy: results from a controlled trial. *Psychotherapy and Psychosomatics* **71**, 255–262.

Mataix-Cols D, Wooderson S, Lawrence N, *et al.* (2004) Distinct neural correlates of washing, checking, and hoarding symptom dimensions in obsessive-compulsive disorder. *Archives of General Psychiatry* **61**, 564–576.

Mataix-Cols D, Rosario-Campos MC, Leckman JF (2005) A multidimensional model of obsessive-compulsive disorder. *American Journal of Psychiatry* **162**, 228–238.

Matsunaga H, Kiriike N, Matsui T, *et al.* (2002) Obsessive-compulsive disorder with poor insight. *Comprehensive Psychiatry* **43**, 150–157.

Mayer-Gross W (1924) *Selbstschilderungen der Verwirrtheit die Oneiroide Erlebnisforme: Psychopathologische-Klinische Untersuchungen*. Springer, Berlin.

Mellor CS (1970) First-rank symptoms in schizophrenia. *British Journal of Psychiatry* **117**, 15–23.

Mullen P (1979) Phenomenology of disordered mental function. In: Hill P, Murray R, Thorley A (eds.) *Essentials of Postgraduate Psychiatry*. Academic Press, London, pp.24–54.

Mullins S, Spence SA (2003) Re-examining thought insertion: semistructured literature review and conceptual analysis. *British Journal of Psychiatry* **182**, 293–298.

Ohta M, Kokai M, Morita Y (2003) Features of obsessive-compulsive disorder in patients primarily diagnosed with schizophrenia. *Psychiatry and Clinical Neurosciences* **57**, 67–74.

Ongür D, Goff DC (2005) Obsessive-compulsive symptoms in schizophrenia: associated clinical features, cognitive function and medication status. *Schizophrenia Research* **75**, 349–362.

Owashi T, Ota A, Otsubo T, Susa Y, Kamijima K (2010) Obsessive-compulsive disorder and obsessive-compulsive symptoms in Japanese inpatients with chronic schizophrenia: a possible schizophrenic subtype. *Psychiatry Research* **179**, 241–246.

Peralta V, Cuesta MJ (1999) Diagnostic significance of Schneider's first-rank symptoms in schizophrenia: comparative study between schizophrenic and non-schizophrenic psychotic disorders. *British Journal of Psychiatry* **174**, 243–248.

Pinto A, Mancebo MC, Eisen JL, Pagano ME, Rasmussen SA (2006) The Brown

Longitudinal Obsessive Compulsive Study: clinical features and symptoms of the sample at intake. *Journal of Clinical Psychiatry* **67**, 703–711.

Pollitt J (1956) Discussion: obsessive compulsive states (abridged). *Proceedings of the Royal Society of Medicine* **49**, 842–845.

Porto L, Bermanzohn PC, Pollack S, Morrissey R, Siris SG (1997) A profile of obsessive-compulsive symptoms in schizophrenia. *CNS Spectrums* **2**, 21–25.

Poyurovsky M, Fuchs C, Weizman A (1999) obsessive-compulsive disorder in patients with first-episode schizophrenia. *American Journal of Psychiatry* **156**, 1998–2000.

Poyurovsky M, Hramenkov S, Isakov V, *et al.* (2001) Obsessive-compulsive disorder in hospitalized patients with chronic schizophrenia. *Psychiatry Research* **102**, 49–57.

Poyurovsky M, Kriss V, Weisman G, *et al.* (2003) Comparison of clinical characteristics and comorbidity in schizophrenia patients with and without obsessive-compulsive disorder: schizophrenic and OC symptoms in schizophrenia. *Journal of Clinical Psychiatry* **64**, 1300–1307.

Poyurovsky M, Faragian S, Kleinman-Balush V, *et al.* (2007) Awareness of illness and insight into obsessive-compulsive symptoms in schizophrenia patients with obsessive-compulsive disorder. *Journal of Nervous and Mental Disease* **195**, 765–768.

Poyurovsky M, Zohar J, Glick I, *et al.* (2012) obsessive-compulsive symptoms in schizophrenia: implications for future psychiatric classifications. *Comprehensive Psychiatry* **53**, 480–483.

Rajkumar RP, Reddy YC, Kandavel T (2008) Clinical profile of "schizo-obsessive" disorder: a comparative study. *Comprehensive Psychiatry* **49**, 262–268.

Rosen I (1957) The clinical significance of obsessions in schizophrenia. *British Journal of Psychiatry* **103**, 773–785. (Thesis for the degree of M.D. submitted to the University of Witwatersrand in 1954; abridged.)

Schneider K (1939) *Psychischer Befund und psychiatrische Diagnose.* Georg Thieme, Leipzig, Germany.

Solyom L, DiNicola VF, Phil M, Sookman D, Luchins D (1985) Is there an obsessive psychosis? Aetiological and prognostic factors of an atypical form of obsessive-compulsive neurosis. *Canadian Journal of Psychiatry* **30**, 372–380.

Spitzer M (1990) On defining delusions. *Comprehensive Psychiatry* **31**, 377–397.

Strauss JS (1969) Hallucinations and delusions as points on continua function. *Archives of General Psychiatry* **21**, 581–586.

Tibbo P, Kroetsch M, Chue P, Warneke L (2000) Obsessive-compulsive disorder in schizophrenia. *Journal of Psychiatric Research* **34**, 139–146.

Tiryaki A, Ozkorumak E (2010) Do the obsessive-compulsive symptoms have an effect in schizophrenia? *Comprehensive Psychiatry* **51**, 357–362.

Westphal C (1878) Über Zwangsvorstellungen. *Archiv für Psychiatrie und Nervenkrankheiten* **8**, 734–750.

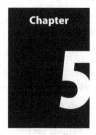

Obsessive–compulsive symptoms in schizophrenia: prodrome

The term "prodrome" derives from the Greek word *prodromos*, the forerunner of an event. In clinical medicine, a prodrome refers to the early symptoms and signs of an illness that precede the characteristic manifestations of the acute, full-blown disorder. Similarly, prodrome in psychotic disorders is defined as the period from the first noticeable signs to the first prominent psychotic symptoms. Prodrome refers to pre-psychotic disturbances, the period of deviation from one's previous experience and behavior. By definition, prodrome is the nascent stage of a disorder; however, it can be diagnosed only after the disorder has declared itself (Heckers, 2009). The course of symptoms that emerges during the prodromal phase of schizophrenia is of interest because (1) there is a temporal and possible nosological association between the prodromal phase and the full-blown disorder; (2) knowledge of the presence and duration of prodromal symptoms may contribute to a better understanding of the etiology, psychopathology, and outcome of schizophrenia; (3) the variability and multidimensionality of the clinical phenomenology of the prodromal phase might help clarify the heterogeneity of schizophrenia (Gourzis *et al.*, 2002; Woods *et al.*, 2009).

Prodromal phase of schizophrenia

The clinical staging model of psychosis places prodrome along a continuum of at least four identified phases of the progression to schizophrenia (Maier *et al.*, 2003).

First, a premorbid phase with no gross psychosocial impairment, but detectable endophenotypic vulnerability traits and risk factors. *Second*, an early prodromal phase, mainly anomalous subjective experiences (e.g., transient feelings of depersonalization, distortions of the stream of consciousness, self-perceived disturbances of thought, concentration, and attention), initial psychosocial impairment, and deterioration of quality of life and inter-peer performance. *Third*, a late prodromal phase of subthreshold, attenuated psychotic symptoms such as pre-delusional feelings of irrevocable change in the sense of self and the world, increasing suspiciousness, subthreshold transitory auditory hallucinations, and/or brief, limited, intermittent psychosis (i.e., frank psychotic symptoms that did not last longer than a week and spontaneously abated). *Fourth*, an overt psychotic phase of full-blown prolonged symptoms of psychosis, with potential to develop into schizophrenia. Such staging indicates a continuum of increasing risk, in which unspecific conditions phenotypically overlap with the initial stages of other disorders and gradually progress to a more clearly defined clinical–diagnostic profile of schizophrenia (Raballo and Laroi, 2009).

Initially prodromal research relied on retrospective reconstruction of changes from premorbid personality, through the first prodromal symptoms, to frank psychosis. Thus, Hafner and colleagues (1992) used the Interview for the Retrospective Assessment of the

Onset of Schizophrenia (IRAOS), a standardized structured instrument for the retrospective characterization of the prodrome, to describe four subgroups of prodromal psychopathological phenomena: non-specific signs, schizophrenic psychotic symptoms, non-schizophrenic psychotic symptoms, and neurotic symptoms, *including obsessions*. Huber and colleagues drew attention to the "basic symptoms," which are subjectively experienced abnormalities in the realms of attention, cognition, and perception, as precursors of the psychotic phase of schizophrenia (Gross, 1989; Huber and Gross, 1989). According to this school of thought, the subjectively experienced basic symptoms, elicited by the descriptive–phenomenological method of Jaspers (1972) and Schneider (1939), constitute the primary symptoms of schizophrenia, which are "nearer" to the substrate of the disorder than the psychotic phenomena that are formed and modified by secondary processes. Negative symptoms ("direct dynamic deficiencies") and cognitive thought disorders are fundamental to the concept of basic symptoms. They in turn may provoke "indirect dynamic deficiencies," such as *obsessional thought patterns*, coenesthesias, and sleep and vegetative disturbances. For example, a patient may present with an obsessive-like repetition of insignificant thoughts or mental images (*"I always have to mull over what I just said. I can't stop thinking about what I might have said wrong or what I could have added although I really don't think that anything was wrong with what I said."*) (Schultze-Lutter, 2009). The development of the Bonn Scale for Assessment of Basic Symptoms (BSABS) (Klosterkötter et al., 1997), and more recently, the Schizophrenia Proneness Instrument–Adult Version (SPI-A) (Schultze-Lutter et al., 2007) made it possible to operationalize the assessment of these subjective experiences and prodromal symptoms.

Yung and McGorry (1996) summarized subjective symptoms and observable behavioral changes described in the early retrospective studies as occurring during the prodromal phase of schizophrenia (Table 5.1). Among non-specific neurotic-type symptoms identified during the prodrome, *obsessive–compulsive phenomena* have consistently been reported (Bleuler, 1911/1950; Pious, 1961; Chapman, 1966; Docherty et al., 1978; Hafner et al., 1992; Hambrecht et al., 1994).

The prodrome was seen as a process that involved changes in experiences and behavior over time, "a moment to moment march of psychological changes" rather than a simple symptom inventory at any one point (Docherty et al., 1978). Regarding the sequence of changes that leads to psychosis, many authors suggest that the prodrome consists primarily of non-specific neurotic-type symptoms (e.g., anxiety, obsessions, phobias), followed by attenuated psychotic experiences, eventually leading to frank psychosis (Docherty et al., 1978; Heinrichs and Carpenter, 1985). On the contrary, neurotic symptoms were thought to be a reaction to early specific pre-psychotic symptoms (e.g., disturbances in attention, perception, speech, motility), followed by overt psychosis (Chapman, 1966). A "hybrid" interactive model incorporating the two patterns in conjunction with basic symptoms was also suggested (Yung and McGorry, 1996). Regardless of the theoretical model, frequent occurrence and clinical significance of non-specific neurotic-like symptoms, particularly *obsessive–compulsive phenomena*, co-occurring with attenuated psychotic symptoms, negative symptoms, social isolation, and academic dysfunction, during the prodromal phase of schizophrenia have consistently been underscored.

According to current conceptualizations, psychotic prodrome confers a heightened *vulnerability* to developing schizophrenia, instead of considering it to be inevitably followed by psychosis. This model implies that an individual who presents with certain disturbances of attention and perception commonly accompanied by anxiety and depressive symptoms,

Table 5.1 Prodromal features of schizophrenia

	Obsessive–Compulsive Phenomena
(1) "Neurotic" symptoms	Anxiety Restlessness Anger, irritability
(2) Mood-related symptoms	Depression Anhedonia Guilt Suicidal ideas Mood swings
(3) Changes in volition	Apathy, loss of drive Boredom, loss of interest Fatigue, reduced energy
(4) Cognitive changes	Disturbance of attention and concentration Preoccupation, daydreaming Thought-blocking Reduced abstraction
(5) Physical symptoms	Somatic complaints Loss of weight Poor appetite Sleep disturbances
(6) Behavioral changes	Deterioration in role functioning Social withdrawal Impulsivity Odd behavior Aggressive, disruptive behavior
(7) Other symptoms	Dissociative phenomena Increased interpersonal sensitivity
(8) Attenuated or subthreshold versions of psychotic symptoms	Perceptual abnormalities Change in sense of self, others, or the world Suspiciousness

Source: Modified from Yung AR, McGorry PD (1996) The prodromal phase of first, episode psychosis: past and current conceptualizations. *Schizophrenia Bulletin* **22**, 353–370. Reprinted with permission.

may or *may not* develop a psychotic disorder. The concept "at-risk mental state" was introduced, criteria of the prodromal phase were articulated, and three prodromal subgroups at high risk of developing psychosis were identified (McGorry and Singh, 1995; Yung and McGorry, 1996).[1] The criteria are a combination of (1) recent-onset functional decline plus genetic risk, (2) recent onset of subthreshold or (3) brief threshold psychotic symptoms (Table 5.2). Using the framework of an "at-risk mental state," several groups sought to prospectively determine the risk of conversion to full-blown psychosis and

---

[1] Terminology in the study of risk for schizophrenia has been the subject of considerable debate. Here the terms prodromal, at-risk, ultra-high risk (UHR), and clinical high-risk (CHR) are used interchangeably to denote subjects meeting criteria for at-risk mental state (Yung and McGorry, 1996).

Table 5.2 High-risk prodromal subgroups

Subgroup	Characteristics
Brief intermittent psychotic state	Psychotic symptoms emerged in the recent past but occurred too briefly to meet official criteria for a diagnosis of psychosis
Attenuated positive symptoms state	Non-psychotic, pre-delusional unusual thoughts; pre-hallucinatory perceptual abnormalities; or pre-thought-disordered speech disorganization
Genetic risk deterioration state	Genetic risk for psychosis (first-degree relative with schizophrenia spectrum disorder or schizotypal personality disorder in proband) plus a recent loss of social or work capacity, or both amounting to a 30% decline on the Global Assessment of Functioning (GAF) scale in the past 12 months

Source: Data extrapolated from Yung *et al.* (1996); Miller *et al.* (1999); McGlashan *et al.* (2001b).

develop algorithms for prediction. Some explicitly focused on the rate of occurrence and clinical presentation of OCD, and its potential role in the prediction of conversion to psychosis in high-risk individuals (Table 5.3).

Prevalence and clinical significance of obsessive–compulsive symptoms in prodromal phase of schizophrenia

Niendam and colleagues (2009) from the UCLA Center for the Assessment and Prevention of Prodromal States (CAPPS) investigated the presentation and effects of the presence of obsessions and compulsions on the clinical course in youth who were putatively prodromal for psychosis. Both categorical SCID-related definitions of OCD and a dimensional measure derived from the self-report Padua Inventory (Sanavio, 1988) were employed. Participants were screened with the Structured Interview for Prodromal Syndromes (SIPS) (McGlashan *et al.*, 2001a) for the presence of prodromal syndromes. The study revealed that 14% (9 of 64 ultra-high risk [UHR] individuals) met DSM-IV criteria for OCD, and an additional 6% (4 of 64) were considered subthreshold OCD. Of particular interest, none of the UHR youth with a DSM-IV diagnosis of OCD converted to full-blown psychotic illness over the mean 11-month follow-up period (conversion rate: 0% in OCD+ group vs. 22% in the OCD− group; $\chi^2 = 3.39$, $p = 0.06$). The UHR youth in this study endorsed significantly more obsessive–compulsive symptoms on the Padua Inventory compared to the control group of normal youth. Moreover, there was a significant association between obsessive–compulsive symptom severity with severity of SIPS positive symptoms, as well as self-reported symptoms of distress, depression, and suicidality ($r = 0.32$–0.63, $p = 0.04$–0.005). Again, while severity of self-reported obsessive–compulsive symptoms was associated with increased clinical severity, it was not associated with an increased rate of subsequent conversion to psychosis. Interestingly, corroborating clinical studies of schizophrenia patients with OCD, a qualitative analysis revealed that obsessive–compulsive symptoms in adolescents with a clinically high risk for psychosis manifest in two ways. Hence, a subset of UHR youth reported "typical" obsessions and compulsions, such as fears of contamination associated with repetitive hand-washing. In contrast, a separate small set of UHR youth described obsessive–compulsive symptoms related to their subpsychotic beliefs; for example, compulsive checking behavior that was associated with paranoid fears, such as a need to check the house for cameras or recording devices; or

Table 5.3 Prevalence of OCD in prodromal phase of schizophrenia

Reference	Study center; country	Study sample	Study design	Prevalence of OCD	Comments
Lencz et al. (2004)	The Zucker Hillside Hospital Recognition and Prevention (RAP) Program, NY, USA	82 help-seeking UHR referrals	Prospective, SOPS and SIPS for prodromal state, K-SADS-E for Axis I disorders	11%	Highlights significance of negative and non-specific symptoms in prodromal phase of schizophrenia
Rosen et al. (2006)	The Prevention through Risk Identification, Management, and Education (PRIME) Clinic, New Haven, USA	29 help-seeking UHR referrals	Prospective, SIPS for prodromal state, SCID-I/P for Axis I and Axis II disorders	4%	Mood disorders, cannabis dependence, and OCD are among common prodromal symptoms
Shioiri et al (2007)	Japan	219 inpatients with DSM-IV schizophrenia	Retrospective analysis of patients' records	9.2%	50% with prodromal obsessive–compulsive symptoms received initial diagnosis of OCD
Niendam et al. (2009)	UCLA Center for the Assessment and Prevention of Prodromal States, USA	64 help-seeking UHR adolescent referrals	Prospective, SIPS for prodromal state, SCID-I/P for Axis I disorders	14%	6% subthreshold OCD. Clinical diagnosis of OCD was not associated with a risk of conversion to psychosis
Sterk et al. (2010)	Specialized Clinic for UHR, Amsterdam, Netherlands	29 help-seeking UHR referrals	Prospective, SIPS for prodromal state, SCID-I/P for Axis I disorders	3.4%	20.7% subthreshold OCD
Fontenelle et al. (2011)	The PACE Clinic at Orygen Youth Health, Melbourne, Australia	312 help-seeking UHR referrals	Prospective, CAARMS for prodromal state and OCD, SCID for Axis I disorders	8.1%	Clinical diagnosis of OCD was not associated with a risk of conversion to psychosis

SIPS, the Structured Interview for Prodromal Syndromes; SOPS, the Scale of Prodromal Symptomatology; CAARMS, Comprehensive Assessment of At-Risk Mental States; SCID-I/P, Structured Clinical Interview for DSM-IV, Patient Edition; UHR, ultra-high risk for psychosis.

compulsive behavior associated with delusional beliefs of guilt and a need to inflict pain. These examples illustrate the symptomatic complexity of obsessive–compulsive features that is present in youth who demonstrate early clinical risk indicators for psychosis.

Lencz et al. (2004) focused on negative and non-specific symptoms in a clinically high-risk (CHR) population of treatment-seeking adolescents and young adults in the Zucker Hillside Hospital Recognition and Prevention (RAP) Program (New York, USA). Using the Scale of Prodromal Symptoms (SOPS) (McGlashan et al., 2001a) for the assessment of prodromal symptoms in CHR youth, the authors developed a prodromal classification algorithm and divided their study group ($N = 82$) into three subgroups; mild negative symptoms, attenuated positive symptoms, and schizophrenia-like psychosis. The most commonly reported symptoms among all three subgroups were social isolation/withdrawal and decline in school performance. Major depressive disorder (MDD), attention deficit hyperactivity disorder, and OCD were the most common non-specific syndromes (31%, 28%, and 11%, respectively). A similar rate of OCD was identified in all three subgroups. This study highlights the importance of negative and non-specific pre-psychotic symptoms, echoing earlier retrospective accounts of the schizophrenia prodrome that repeatedly reported social isolation and academic distress, as well as depression, anxiety, and obsessive–compulsive phenomena to mark the prodromal phase in adolescence (Yung and McGorry, 1996). Remarkably, Lysaker et al. (2009) also identified a subgroup of schizo-obsessive patients with predominant negative symptoms and an especially low level of functioning. It is critical to address whether a constellation of negative and non-specific, primary obsessive–compulsive symptoms represents an independent development with a different etiology, biochemistry, and underlying brain pathophysiology. Alternatively, it is inevitable that a prodromal state with negative and obsessive–compulsive symptoms produces more false-positive cases for schizophrenia than other groups with predominantly positive symptoms. Even so, careful evaluation of this group can provide an important glimpse of the potential pathophysiologic substrates of impairment in schizophrenia, without the confounding factor of overlapping psychosis (Lencz et al., 2004). Notably, a substantial proportion of the subsample meets criteria for schizotypal personality in addition to OCD.

Rosen and colleagues (2006) from the Prevention through Risk Identification, Management and Education (PRIME) Research Clinic (Yale University, USA) investigated the presence of comorbid psychiatric conditions in individuals identified with at-risk prodromal syndrome compared with help-seeking controls. Similar to their schizophrenia counterparts, roughly half of the sample of prodromal individuals (48%, 14 of 29) qualified for Axis I psychiatric disorders, with MDD and cannabis dependence the most common comorbidities. Nearly 30% of the prodromal sample experienced one or more anxiety disorders with OCD diagnosed in one (4%) of the prodromal individuals. The presence of psychiatric comorbidity, however, did not distinguish prodromal patients from help-seeking controls, raising the question of its role (specific vs. associated feature) in the development of psychosis.

Fontenelle et al. (2011) went on to clarify the effect of different OCD trajectories on transition to psychosis. The authors consecutively recruited a large cohort of 312 UHR individuals on admission to the Personal Assessment and Crises Evaluation (PACE) clinic (Australia), and followed them for a mean of 7.4 years. At baseline all were assessed with the Comprehensive Assessment of At-Risk Mental States (CAARMS) (Yung et al., 2005) and met criteria for UHR for psychosis. The CAARMS also includes a screening section for OCD symptoms, including questions on whether patients have distressing or intrusive thoughts, forced repetitive behaviors, rituals/superstitions, need to do things a certain way, or checking compulsions, rated on a six-point severity scale. There were three study groups based on the history of OCD: (1) Baseline OCD, all individuals who had a lifetime history of OCD, persistent or remitted; (2) Incident OCD, individuals who did not have a lifetime history of OCD at the first assessment, but displayed OCD during the follow-up; (3) Non-OCD group. The authors found that 8% (32 of 396) UHR subjects had a diagnosis of OCD at baseline and at follow-up. No differences were found between UHR individuals with and without OCD in terms of psychopathology. Moreover, a diagnosis of OCD at baseline did not predict conversion to DSM-IV psychotic disorders. Nevertheless, two (40%) out of six cases with early-onset persistent OCD had developed schizophrenia at follow-up. Notably, incident OCD was associated with an increased rate of non-schizophrenic psychoses and mood disorders. These findings are consistent with early observations suggesting that delusions can arise in the course of OCD but do not necessarily signify a diagnosis of schizophrenia (Insel and Akiskal, 1986).

An interrelationship between schizophrenic and obsessive–compulsive symptoms at both subclinical and clinical levels was convincingly demonstrated in the Netherlands Mental Health Survey and Incidence Study (NEMESIS) (Van Dael *et al.*, 2011). A representative population sample of 7076 participants was assessed using the Composite International Diagnostic Interview (CIDI) at baseline, and 1 and 2 years later for the presence of both subclinical and clinical forms of the two disorders. There are two important findings in this study. First, the association between obsessive–compulsive and psychosis phenotypes became progressively stronger when increasingly more stringent definitions were used. Thus, OCD was present in 0.5% (28 of 5838) of the subjects with no history of psychotic experiences, in 1.2% (11 of 930) of the subjects who had a psychotic experience but had no evidence for psychotic symptoms or disorder, in 3.9% (8 of 203) of the subjects with a psychotic symptom, and in 13.1% (14 of 107) of those with a psychotic disorder. Second, the risk-increasing effect of "comorbid" obsessive–compulsive and psychotic symptoms on a future psychosis was considerably stronger than the risk-increasing effect of comorbid obsessive–compulsive and psychotic symptoms on a future OCD outcome. This suggests a specific impact of obsessive–compulsive symptoms on psychotic symptoms in increasing the risk for progression to psychosis.

To summarize current knowledge of obsessive–compulsive phenomena in schizophrenia prodrome:

- OCD is prevalent in individuals at high risk for developing psychosis. The prevalence of prodromal obsessive–compulsive phenomena is even higher when subthreshold OCD is considered in addition to a full-scale DSM-IV OCD. Moreover, the rate of occurrence of OCD in the prodromal phase is comparable to that revealed in first-episode and chronic schizophrenia patients. It is plausible that OCD is *prevalent* and *persistent* during the entire course of schizophrenia. Nevertheless, longitudinal studies covering prodromal, acute, and remitted phases of schizophrenia have not yet been conducted to substantiate this assumption.
- The clinical significance of prodromal obsessive–compulsive symptoms is emphasized by their potential association with higher severity of prodromal positive symptoms, distress, depression, and suicidality.

- Similar to active phases of illness, the prodromal phase of schizophrenia seems to be associated with both typical ego-dystonic and "atypical" psychotic-related, obsessive–compulsive symptoms. Clinical complexity is also underscored by the putative existence of distinct prodromal subgroups, based on the co-occurrence of obsessive–compulsive symptoms with predominant positive or negative symptoms. The association of obsessive–compulsive and negative symptoms is particularly challenging in terms of differential diagnosis from severe OCD, treatment, and prognosis.

- Whether prodromal OCD predicts further transition to psychosis remains unclear. Notably, a meta-analysis has shown that the risk of development of a psychotic episode in high-risk cohorts was 18% at 6 months after onset of symptoms, 22% at 1 year, 29% at 2 years, and 32% at 3 years of follow-up (Fusar-Poli *et al.*, 2012).

The following clinical vignettes illustrate the co-occurrence of obsessive–compulsive phenomena with each of the (Figure 5.1) high-risk putative subgroups

Case 5.1. Obsessive–compulsive symptoms in an individual with attenuated positive symptoms.

Mr. D, a 23-year-old student, was referred for psychiatric evaluation due to depressed mood, anxiety, social isolation, and reduced academic performance. His family history included subthreshold OCD in a maternal relative. D's developmental milestones were achieved as expected. He was a good student throughout grade school, successfully completed military service, and was admitted to the faculty of computer engineering in the local university. However, during his sophomore year and roughly 6 months prior to the psychiatric evaluation, it became difficult for him to focus and he often daydreamed in class. He also became socially isolated, broke up with his girlfriend of 5 years, and felt increasingly anxious and tense.

On examination, he appeared anxious and complained of inability to concentrate on his studies. He became increasingly self-conscious and suspicious. Although he thought that classmates thought negatively of him, and on several occasions heard his name being called in a crowd, there was no evidence of clear-cut delusions and hallucinations. He denied

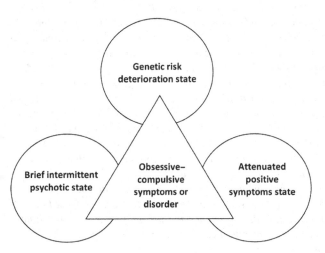

Figure 5.1 Schematic representation of a putative association between obsessive–compulsive phenomena and high-risk prodromal subgoups.

mind-reading, thought broadcasting, or other Schneiderian symptoms. When asked about possible obsessions or compulsions, he admitted recent emergence of intrusive thoughts that he might run over a pedestrian while driving. These thoughts were intense and distressful, and were associated with an irresistible urge to drive back and check whether anybody was hurt. He reported that a week before the assessment, a new intrusive and distressful theme emerged: that he might rape his female classmates. He stated that these thoughts were the product of his mind, were inappropriate, and caused anxiety and guilt feelings. D also recalled that when he was about 10 years old, he repeatedly washed his hands due to contamination fears that spontaneously remitted a few years later. Additional symptoms included decreased mood and lack of motivation.

D presented with a wide range of affective, perceptual, and thought abnormalities; however, he did not meet full criteria for any DSM-IV psychotic or mood diagnoses. He met research criteria for "an attenuated psychosis state" (Yung and McGorry, 1996). Although D exhibited typical obsessions and compulsions that were among the central presenting features, he did not meet a DSM-IV diagnosis of OCD since they lasted less than 1 hour a day and did not significantly interfere with his routine. D consented to a therapeutic trial with the atypical antipsychotic olanzapine (5 mg/day) and within 2 weeks there was a parallel amelioration of both attenuated psychotic and subthreshold obsessive–compulsive symptoms. The medication was discontinued after 3 months. Follow-up during 12 months revealed no progression to psychosis.

Case 5.2. Obsessive–compulsive disorder in an individual with genetic risk – schizotypal personality disorder – deterioration state.

Mr. S, a 25-year-old man, exhibited typical OCD symptoms, including intrusive distressful, aggressive thoughts of stabbing his younger brother, and checking and touching rituals to neutralize anxiety associated with obsessions, since the age of 13. At age 17, he was seen by a psychiatrist and diagnosed with DSM-IV OCD. Cognitive–behavior therapy was recommended, but he refused to cooperate. Family history was remarkable. His father was recognized as an odd and eccentric personality, although no formal diagnosis was established, and a maternal aunt had OCD. S was described as having been a shy and strange child. His social functioning and emotional reactions were always stilted. He preferred solitary activity to group games with peers, and had difficulties making friends. His discoordinated walk and gestures were cause for mockery. S was uncompromising in his thinking and began to articulate strong beliefs about morality at a young age. He developed his own theory about justice and equality, and scrupulously analyzed people according to his own moral standards. He was a good student in elementary school; however, by the 12th grade he started to have problems with concentration and complained that he was distracted by "external sounds and visual stimuli." He failed his matriculation exams. He was not recruited to military service due to low performance on cognitive tests and suspected schizophrenia-spectrum disorder. Between ages 18 and 24, S worked at several jobs, but was fired because he could not get along with his co-workers. His most recent job as a telephone company operator lasted for 2.5 years, until he was fired because of absenteeism. S's parents expressed concern that during the last year he lost his job, and increasingly avoided social interactions. About 3 months before the psychiatric examination S was completely socially isolated, locked himself in his room, and stopped taking care of his appearance and personal hygiene. S sometimes became verbally aggressive when family members confronted him regarding his behavior or asked him to help with household chores.

On examination, S's primary complaints were intrusive distressful thoughts of stabbing his brother, intensified whenever he was near a sharp object. He also reported rituals lasting for hours, including checking, touching, and ordering objects to "control the environment" and decreased fear associated with intrusive aggressive thoughts. He was aware of the excessive and baseless nature of his obsessive–compulsive symptoms. S also exhibited constricted affect, circumstantial, and metaphoric speech, naïve and odd beliefs about justice and punishment, and constantly quoted Dostoevsky's book Crime and Punishment. His appearance was peculiar, his long hair covered his face. S reported that he occasionally heard his thoughts spoken in his head, but he denied full-blown auditory hallucinations, thought insertion, or broadcasting. He also denied that others could hear his thoughts. He expressed skepticism and suspiciousness about people's attitudes toward him; however, there was no evidence of persecutory or other types of delusions. S said that he had periods of low moods lasting no more than a day, but no sadness, anhedonia, or somatic symptoms of depression were reported. His sleep cycle had shifted in the past 6 months: he remained awake until the early morning hours and slept until the late afternoon.

S's diagnosis of typical DSM-IV OCD was confirmed on examination. He also met criteria for schizotypal personality disorder owing to a pervasive and enduring pattern of social and interpersonal deficits, as well as affective and cognitive distortions and behavioral eccentricities. With regard to psychotic symptoms, the revealed perceptual abnormalities and unusual thought content did not reach the intensity of hallucinations or delusions, and thus did not merit a formal diagnosis of a psychotic disorder. He also did not meet criteria for major depressive disorder, despite brief periods of decreased mood. At this juncture, owing to the presence of schizotypal personality disorder and a substantial decline in social and work functioning during the past year, S met research criteria for "genetic risk deterioration state" (Yung and McGorry, 1996) in addition to a DSM-IV diagnosis of OCD. He consented to a therapeutic trial with the selective serotonin reuptake inhibitor escitalopram (up to 40 mg/day for 12 weeks), and showed meaningful improvement in the severity of OCD and general funtioning. No progression to psychosis was noted during the 12-month follow-up.

Case 5.3. Obsessive–compulsive disorder in an individual with brief intermittent psychotic state.

Mr. M, 16 years old, pleasant, and well-groomed. His father was an aloof, detached person, with a probable schizoid personality. M had a 22-year-old brother, hospitalized with schizophrenia and comorbid OCD. His 32-year-old sister also suffered from OCD and was the person that first detected M's obsessive worries and referred him for psychiatric evaluation. At his initial examination at age 14, M was well oriented, and asked for help and advice. He openly described his troubles. At age 9 he began to worry about his parents' health, constantly inquiring about their well-being and phoning for reassurance. He was also concerned with his own health. If a small object entered his eye he would repeatedly check to single out serious health consequences. He also reported aggressive thoughts about his parents, and a compulsive urge to "hate" them. He reported intrusive thoughts about spoiled food and compulsive checking to see if his food was ready to eat. He was fully aware of the unreasonable nature of his thoughts and ritualistic behavior that were distressful, intrusive, and time-consuming. His scholastic achievements were affected by the occurrence of obsessive thoughts that distracted him and prevented him from being a good pupil. At that point M met DSM-IV criteria for

OCD. There was no evidence of tic disorders, conduct disorders, attention deficit hyperactivity disorder (ADHD), or other developmental impairments.

At the 2-year follow-up, there was a gradual deterioration in scholastic achievements, social isolation, and brief emergence of paranoid transformation of obsessive thoughts concerning food poisoning. He now claimed that his parents intentionally poisoned his food. These delusional thoughts were accompanied by irritability, suspiciousness, and verbal aggression. There were two such brief intermittent psychotic episodes that lasted for no more than several days and spontaneously abated. At that point M met research criteria for a brief intermittent psychotic state (Yung and McGorry, 1996) in addition to DSM-IV OCD.

M's first psychiatric admission was at age 16 due to an acute psychotic episode reflected in clear-cut paranoid delusions of reference and persecution, as well as imperative auditory hallucinations, "voices of the parents who ordered him to check food for the presence of poison." As a result, he performed bizarre stereotypic movements to prevent food from "entering his body." He was also certain that a TV broadcaster sent him messages to direct his body movements. Patient M met DSM-IV criteria for schizophrenic disorder, paranoid type, and was successfully treated with risperidone (3 mg/day).

The presented cases highlight the clinical complexity of obsessive–compulsive phenomena in suggested schizophrenia prodrome: both full-scale OCD (Cases 5.2 and 5.3) and subthreshold OCD (Case 5.1), as well as typical (Cases 5.1 and 5.2) and "atypical" psychotic-related (Case 5.3) obsessive–compulsive symptoms may be detected in prodromal individuals. Moreover, obsessive–compulsive symptoms can be transient and emerge only in the context of a prodromal state along with attenuated positive symptoms (Case 5.1). However, this clinical situation represents only a minority of cases, since in a vast majority of schizophrenia patients, obsessive–compulsive symptoms are seen beyond the prodromal phase of schizophrenia. Detection of obsessive–compulsive symptoms in a prodromal phase impacts treatment strategies. A brief trial with an antipsychotic agent to target worsening subsyndromal psychotic symptoms is sometimes necessary and may be sufficient to address the associated obsessive–compulsive symptoms (Case 5.1). Alternatively, full-scale OCD that occurs in the context of a putative genetic risk deterioration state (e.g., schizotypal personality disorder) may be treated as though it existed alone, although the attenuated positive symptoms should be closely monitored (Case 5.2).

Recommendations for diagnosis and management of obsessive–compulsive symptoms in prodromal phase of schizophrenia

Guidelines have not yet been formulated for the identification and management of obsessive–compulsive phenomena in high-risk individuals or patients in a prodromal stage of schizophrenia. Clinical experience provides the basis for the following recommendations that may be considered:

- Individuals who are at high risk or in a prodromal stage of psychosis should be screened for OCD and its subthreshold forms owing to their high prevalence and clinical significance.
- Conversely, it is important to inquire about subpsychotic experiences in patients who present with OCD and have a family history of psychotic disorders, schizotypal personality disorder, and/or a precipitous decline in functioning.

- Metabolic, endocrine, or neurological causes for co-occurring obsessive–compulsive and attenuated psychotic symptoms need to be ruled out. Disorders that particularly involve the basal ganglia (e.g., Sydenham's chorea, Huntington's disease, basal ganglia stroke) can present with both psychotic and obsessive–compulsive symptoms (Mittal et al., 2010).

- Differential diagnosis is essential given that presenting prodromal symptoms can in fact indicate an emerging affective, anxiety, or substance-use disorder that may have "masqueraded" as subsyndromal psychotic symptoms (Haroun et al., 2006).

- Active follow-up is recommended for both obsessive–compulsive and attenuated psychotic components. The validity of the original diagnosis of prodromal syndrome and risk is elucidated with time, when progression to psychosis or to another treatable disorder, continuing prodrome, or remission and reduction of risk occur (McGlashan et al., 2001b).

- Vis-à-vis treatment interventions, psychoeducation, stress reduction, ongoing support related to family, peer, or school/work problems are imperative (Haroun et al., 2006). If pharmacotherapy is considered, anti-obsessive medications for clinically significant OCD along with rigorous monitoring of attenuated positive symptoms may be appropriate. Some high-risk patients are given a trial with a low-dose antipsychotic agent, even though they are not currently recommended in treatment guidelines (International Early Psychosis Association Writing Group, 2005). Apparently, long-term use of antipsychotic agents should be reserved *only* for the established diagnoses of DSM-IV psychotic disorders. Alternative pharmacotherapeutic approaches based on increasing understanding of the pathophysiology of the prodromal stage of schizophrenia are urgently needed (Cannon, 2008). Thus, experimental treatment with long-chain omega-3 polyunsaturated fatty acids to reduce the risk for progression to psychosis (Amminger et al., 2010) and OCD (Fux et al., 2004) is noteworthy, but yet to be replicated. All treatment approaches require scrupulous risk–benefit evaluations.

References

Amminger GP, Schäfer MR, Papageorgiou K, et al. (2010) Long-chain omega-3 fatty acids for indicated prevention of psychotic disorders: a randomized, placebo-controlled trial. *Archives of General Psychiatry* 67, 146–154.

Bleuler E (1911/1990) *Dementia Praecox or the Group of Schizophrenias*, transl Zinkin J. International Universities Press, New York.

Bloch MH, Landeros-Weisenberger A, Kelmendi B, et al. (2006) A systematic review: antipsychotic augmentation with treatment refractory obsessive-compulsive disorder. *Molecular Psychiatry* 11, 622–632. Erratum *Molecular Psychiatry* 11, 795.

Cannon TD (2008) Neurodevelopment and the transition from schizophrenia prodrome to schizophrenia: research imperatives. *Biological Psychiatry* 64, 737–738.

Chapman J (1966) The early symptoms of schizophrenia. *British Journal of Psychiatry* 112, 225–251.

Docherty JP, van Kammen DP, Siris SG, Marder SR (1978) Stages of onset of schizophrenic psychosis. *American Journal of Psychiatry* 135, 420–426.

Fontenelle LF, Lin A, Pantelis C, et al. (2011) A longitudinal study of obsessive-compulsive disorder in individuals at ultra-high risk for psychosis. *Journal of Psychiatric Research* 45, 1140–1145.

Fusar-Poli P, Bonoldi I, Yung AR, et al. (2012) Predicting psychosis: a meta-analysis of evidence. *Archives of General Psychiatry* 69, 220–229.

Fux M, Benjamin J, Nemets B (2004) A placebo-controlled cross-over trial of adjunctive EPA in OCD. *Journal of Psychiatric Research* **38**, 323–325.

Gourzis P, Katrivanou A, Beratis S (2002) Symptomatology of the initial prodromal phase in schizophrenia. *Schizophrenia Bulletin* **28**, 415–429.

Gross G (1989) The "basic" symptoms in schizophrenia. *British Journal of Psychiatry* **155** (Suppl. 7), 21–25.

Hafner H, Riecher-Rossler A, Maurer K, *et al.* (1992) IRAOS: an instrument for the assessment of onset and early course of schizophrenia. *Schizophrenia Research* **6**, 209–223.

Hambrecht M, Hafner H, Loffler W (1994) Beginning schizophrenia observed by significant others. *Social Psychiatry and Psychiatric Epidemiology* **29**, 53–60.

Haroun N, Dunn L, Haroun A, Cadenhead KS (2006) Risk and protection in prodromal schizophrenia: ethical implications for clinical practice and future research. *Schizophrenia Bulletin* **32**, 166–178.

Heckers S (2009) Who is at risk for a psychotic disorder? *Schizophrenia Bulletin* **35**, 847–850.

Heinrichs DW, Carpenter WT (1985) Prospective study of prodromal symptoms in schizophrenic relapse. *American Journal of Psychiatry* **142**, 371–373.

Huber G, Gross G (1989) The concept of basic symptoms in schizophrenic and schizoaffective patients. *Schizophrenia Bulletin* **6**, 592–605.

Insel TR, Akiskal HS (1986) Obsessive-compulsive disorder with psychotic features: a phenomenologic analysis. *American Journal of Psychiatry* **143**, 1527–1533.

International Early Psychosis Association Writing Group (2005) International clinical practice guidelines for early psychosis. *British Journal of Psychiatry* **48** (Suppl.), s120–124.

Jaspers K (1972) Subjective phenomena of morbid psychic life. In: *General Psychopathology*, transl. Hoenig J., Hamilton MW. University of Chicago Press, Chicago.

Klosterkötter J, Gross G, Huber G, *et al.* (1997) Evaluation of the Bonn Scale for the Assessment of Basic Symptoms - BSABS as

an instrument for the assessment of schizophrenia proneness: a review of recent findings. *Neurology Psychiatry and Brain Research* **5**, 137–150.

Lencz T, Smith CW, Auther A, Correll CU, Cornblatt B (2004) Nonspecific and attenuated negative symptoms in patients at clinical high-risk for schizophrenia. *Schizophrenia Research* **68**, 37–48.

Lysaker PH, Whitney KA, Davis LW (2009) Associations of executive function with concurrent and prospective reports of obsessive-compulsive symptoms in schizophrenia. *Journal of Neuropsychiatry and Clinical Neurosciences* **21**, 38–42.

Maier W, Cornblatt BA, Merikangas KR (2003) Transition to schizophrenia and related disorders: toward a taxonomy of risk. *Schizophrenia Bulletin* **29**, 693–701.

McGlashan TH, Miller TJ, Woods SW, Hoffman RE, Davidson L (2001a) A scale for the assessment of prodromal symptoms and states. In: Miller TJ, Mednick SA, McGlashan TH, Liberger J Johannessen JO (eds.) *Early Intervention in Psychotic Disorders*. Kluwer Academic Publishers, Dordrecht, pp.135–149.

McGlashan TH, Miller TJ, Woods SW (2001b) Pre-onset detection and intervention research in schizophrenia psychoses: current estimates of benefit and risk. *Schizophrenia Bulletin* **27**, 563–570.

McGorry PD, Singh BS (1995) Schizophrenia: risk and possibility. In: Raphael B, Burrows CD (eds.) *Handbook of Studies on Preventive Psychiatry*. Elsevier Science Publishers, Amsterdam, pp.491–514.

Miller TJ, McGlashan TH, Woods SW, *et al.* (1999) Symptoms assessment in schizophrenic prodromal states. *Psychiatric Quarterly* **70**, 273–287.

Mittal VA, Karlsgodt K, Zinberg J, Cannon TD, Bearden CE (2010) Identification and treatment of a pineal region tumor in an adolescent with prodromal psychotic symptoms. *American Journal of Psychiatry* **167**, 1033–1037.

Niendam TA, Berzak J, Cannon TD, Bearden CE (2009) Obsessive compulsive symptoms in the psychosis prodrome:

correlates of clinical and functional outcome. *Schizophrenia Research* **108**, 170–175.

Pious WL (1961) A hypothesis about the nature of schizophrenic behavior. In: Burton A (ed.) *Psychotherapy of the Psychoses*. Basic Books, New York, pp.43–68.

Poyurovsky M, Weizman A, Weizman R (2004) Obsessive-compulsive disorder in schizophrenia: clinical characteristics and treatment. *CNS Drugs* **18**, 989–1010.

Raballo A, Laroi F (2009) Clinical staging: a new scenario for the treatment of psychosis. *Lancet* **374**, 365–366.

Rosen JL, Miller TJ, D'Andrea JT, McGlashan TH, Woods SW (2006) Comorbid diagnoses in patients meeting criteria for the schizophrenia prodrome. *Schizophrenia Research* **85**, 124–131.

Ruscio AM, Stein DJ, Chiu WT, Kessler RC (2010) The epidemiology of obsessive-compulsive disorder in the National Comorbidity Survey Replication. *Molecular Psychiatry* **15**, 53–63.

Sanavio E (1988) Obsessions and compulsions: the Padua Inventory. *Behaviour Research and Therapy* **26**, 169–177.

Schneider K (1939) *Psychischer Befund and psychiatrische Diagnose*. Georg Thieme, Leipzig, Germany.

Schultze-Lutter F, Ruhrmann S, Picker H, *et al.* (2007) Basic symptoms in early psychotic and depressive disorders. *British Journal of Psychiatry* **51** (Suppl.), S31–S37.

Shioiri T, Shinada K, Kuwabara H, Someya T (2007) Early prodromal symptoms and diagnoses before first psychotic episode in 219 inpatients with schizophrenia. *Psychiatry and Clinical Neurosciences* **61**, 348–354.

Sterk B, Lankreijer K, Linzen DH, de Haan L (2010) Obsessive-compulsive symptoms in first episode psychosis and in subjects at ultra high risk for developing psychosis: onset and relationship to psychotic symptoms. *Australian and New Zealand Journal of Psychiatry* **45**, 1–7.

Van Dael F, van Os J, de Graaf R, *et al.* (2011) Can obsessions drive you mad? Longitudinal evidence that obsessive-compulsive symptoms worsen the outcome of early psychotic experiences. *Acta Psychiatrica Scandinavica* **123**, 136–146.

Woods SW, Addington J, Cadenhead KS, *et al.* (2009) Validity of the prodromal risk syndrome for first psychosis: findings from the North American Prodrome Longitudinal Study. *Schizophrenia Bulletin* **35**, 894–908.

Yung AR, McGorry PD (1996) The prodromal phase of first-episode psychosis: past and current conceptualizations. *Schizophrenia Bulletin* **22**, 353–370

Yung AR, Yuen HP, McGorry PD, *et al.* (2005) Mapping the onset of psychosis: the Comprehensive Assessment of At-Risk Mental States. *Australian and New Zealand Journal of Psychiatry* **39**, 964–971.

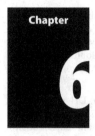

Obsessive–compulsive symptoms in schizophrenia: across lifespan

Early-onset forms of disorders often help elucidate the underlying mechanisms of disease. Illness that emerges at an early age is generally more homogeneous and severe, tends to have more salient genetic causes, and is less susceptible to environmental influence and effects of treatment (Childs and Scriver, 1986). The National Comorbidity Survey Replication study, which included face to face assessments of over 9000 people in their homes, and is representative of the US population, indicated that the peak age of onset for mental health disorders is roughly 14 years (Kessler *et al.*, 2005b). Schizophrenia, OCD, anxiety disorders, affective disorders, eating disorders, and substance abuse all most commonly emerge during adolescence. The emergence of these psychopathologies is putatively related to anomalies or exaggerations of typical adolescent maturation processes together with psychosocial factors (e.g., school, relationships) and/or biological factors (e.g., pubertal hormonal changes) (Paus *et al.*, 2008).

Childhood-onset and adolescent schizophrenia

Many clinicians view schizophrenia in childhood and adolescence as relatively rare; however, this assumption is not fully substantiated. Although the prevalence of childhood-onset schizophrenia (onset of psychotic symptoms before 13 years of age) is indeed low (approximately 1/100 cases of schizophrenia), the incidence of schizophrenia rises sharply at about 12–14 years of age (Häfner and Nowotny, 1995). Prior to age 18, approximately 12–33% of individuals with schizophrenia experience signs of the onset of their illness and thus could be classified as having early-onset schizophrenia (Kumra *et al.*, 2008). Longitudinal studies have shown diagnostic stability to be high in this form of illness (Hollis, 2000). Early-onset schizophrenia affects approximately twice as many boys as girls; however, in adolescence the rate evens out between the sexes. Prospective evaluation of outcomes, such as length of remission, number and duration of hospitalization, and social disability, consistently indicate poorer prognosis for early-onset than adult-onset schizophrenia (Eggers and Bunk, 1997), with some evidence that onset before puberty is associated with the most detrimental clinical and psychosocial outcomes (Rabinowitz *et al.*, 2006).

There appears to be clinical and neurobiological continuity between early- and adult-onset schizophrenia with greater early childhood neurodevelopmental deviance in early-onset schizophrenia (Hollis, 2000; Nicolson *et al.*, 2000). Hence, delayed motor milestones, poor coordination, and repetitive movements, as well as delayed speech production and problems with receptive and expressive language, were widely reported in early-onset schizophrenia. Abnormal social behavior including introversion and social withdrawal are the most replicable features reported in pre-schizophrenic children and adolescents (Kinros *et al.*, 2010). Childhood and adolescent intellectual functioning in individuals later diagnosed with schizophrenia was consistently lower than in both healthy controls and psychiatric controls, suggesting that persistent low scores in premorbid cognitive testing have some specificity for schizophrenia. Notably, premorbid functioning and IQ scores have consistently been found to be the best predictors of outcome for children and adolescents with schizophrenia (Jones et al., 1994; Cannon et al., 2002). Aberrant development may be secondary to a higher level of familial loading for schizophrenia. Indeed, parents of patients with childhood-onset schizophrenia had a sizably higher morbid risk for schizophrenia spectrum disorder (24.7%) than parents of patients with adult-onset schizophrenia (11.3%), and both had a greater morbid risk for schizophrenia than did parents of control subjects (1.5%) (Nicolson et al., 2003).

Findings from structural and functional brain imaging studies offer a neurobiological foundation for continuity between early- and adult-onset disorders. Brain imaging studies of childhood-onset schizophrenia revealed gray matter reduction, reduced overall cerebral volume, and ventricular enlargement similar to adults (Gogtay et al., 2011; Rapoport and Gogtay, 2011). Childhood-onset schizophrenia may be associated with a greater reduction of gray matter brain volume that correlates with symptom severity and impairments in cognitive functioning over time (Rapoport and Gogtay, 2011). In contrast to adults, however, findings regarding temporal lobe structures are less consistent, suggesting that volume reduction in these critical brain areas may be moderated by age of onset and illness duration. An intriguing finding of early-onset schizophrenia research to date is an apparent impairment of parietal lobe integrity and connectivity in schizophrenia, since the earliest deficits were detected in parietal gray matter (Thompson et al., 2001). Notably, longitudinal data revealed that the gray matter loss in early-onset schizophrenia had a characteristic back-to-front (parieto-frontal-temporal) pattern of spread during adolescent years (Thompson et al., 2001). This back-to-front wave of cortical gray matter loss has recently been replicated in first-episode adult-onset patients, further supporting a commonality between early- and adult-onset disease (Thompson et al., 2009). In rare cases of very early childhood-onset schizophrenia the typical decrease in frontal gray matter volume that is seen in healthy subjects during adolescence was exaggerated fourfold (Sporn et al., 2003). Preliminary findings regarding abnormal white matter integrity as detected by diffusion tensor imaging (DTI) in childhood-onset schizophrenia patients also suggest that the involvement of the distributed brain regions is broadly consistent with that found in adults (Kyriakopoulos et al., 2008).

From the clinical perspective, early-onset schizophrenia in children and adolescents can be reliably diagnosed using the same criteria as those applied to adults (American Psychiatric Association, 2000). The incidence of schizophrenia subtypes, constellation of symptoms, and patterns of treatment response do not substantially differ from those in adult-onset disorder (Russell, 1994; Correll, 2010; Masi and Liboni, 2011). However, severity of symptoms, primarily negative and cognitive, and social impairment are more pronounced in early-onset schizophrenia (Häfner and Nowotny, 1995). Elementary auditory hallucinations appear to be the most frequent positive symptoms, while delusions are less complex than in adults and are usually related to childhood themes. The most frequent delusions are bizarre (i.e., "a monster took control of my voice"), persecutory, somatic, reference, grandiose, and religious (Russell, 1994). Negative symptoms are predominant. Formal thought disorders are also prevalent; though they may not be severe in the initial stages of the disorder, they tend to become more evident as the illness progresses. Insidious onset of illness in most cases of childhood schizophrenia, non-specific character of premorbid disturbances, and the hesitancy of clinicians to diagnose schizophrenia in a child often delay identification of the disorder.

Early-onset OCD

OCD is characterized as childhood onset if symptoms present before puberty. Early-onset OCD was found in about 20% of all affected persons, suffering from manifestations of OCD at age 10 or even earlier (Kessler et al., 2005a). Delorme et al. (2005) consider the disorder to have a bimodal age distribution, with the first peak at age 11 and the second in early adulthood. Akin to schizophrenia, there is generally a clinical and neurobiological continuity between childhood- and adult-onset OCD. DSM-IV defines OCD in both adults and children similarly as recurrent obsessions and compulsions that are time-consuming or cause marked distress or significant impairment in daily functions (American Psychiatric Association, 2000). Common obsessions in children include pre-occupations with contamination, harm to self or others, and symmetry, as well as fear that bad things will happen if a ritual is not completed in just the right way. Common compulsions in children include compulsive questioning, washing, ordering, and repetitive rituals with magical thinking. The Yale–Brown Obsessive–Compulsive Scale (Y-BOCS) and the children's Y-BOCS (CY-BOCS) are very similar rating scales that further categorize the symptoms in adults and children, respectively, by providing specific measures of severity that are not influenced by the various types of obsessions and compulsions present (Goodman et al., 1989). DSM-IV criteria allow for the diagnosis of OCD to be made even for patients with poor insight, who do not recognize that their obsessions or compulsions are excessive or unreasonable (American Psychiatric Association, 2000). This is particularly relevant in the diagnosis of childhood-onset OCD, since young children often lack insight into the irrationality of their actions (Storch et al., 2008), and obsessions are not always associated with increased anxiety (Leckman et al., 1994). In addition, more than one-third of adults and roughly 40% of children diagnosed with OCD deny that their compulsions are driven by obsessive thoughts (Swedo et al., 1989).

Together with the evident similarities, there are some important differences between early- and adult-onset OCD in gender distribution, patterns of comorbidity, and symptom presentation. Thus, boys are more often affected by childhood-onset OCD than girls; however, at puberty, the sex ratio of affected individuals changes from predominantly boys to predominantly girls. When compared with girls, boys with childhood-onset OCD have a higher rate of comorbid tic disorders, a higher frequency of compulsions not preceded by obsessions, and a greater genetic contribution to the disease (Swedo et al., 1989). Children are more likely than adults to have comorbid attention deficit hyperactivity disorder (ADHD) and tic disorders, while comorbid major depressive disorder (MDD) and anxiety disorders are more typical for those who develop OCD during or after puberty (Kalra and Swedo, 2009). Family studies strongly suggest that of these comorbid conditions, only tic disorders share genetic etiology with OCD (Pauls, 2008).

Early-onset OCD is associated with a more persistent course, poorer prognosis, and an adverse impact on various aspects of personality and social integration (Sobin et al., 2000). In fact, OCD assumes chronic and disabling features in at least half of all early-onset cases; especially when OCD emerges between ages 5 and 8 years, as it can disrupt functioning across many domains and derail normal development (Swedo et al., 1989). The similar prevalence rates of childhood- and adult-onset OCD (roughly 2%) despite new emergent cases in adults, suggest that some patients with early-onset OCD may remit with treatment (Kalra and Swedo, 2009).

Similar to early-onset schizophrenia, early-onset OCD exhibits greater familial loading, indicating a stronger genetic contribution. The rate of OCD among relatives of children and adolescents with OCD was about ten times that found among controls. In contrast, when the probands were adults, the rate of OCD among relatives was about two times that among controls (Pauls, 2008). Twin studies also show somewhat greater heritability of obsessive–compulsive symptoms in children than in adults (van Grootheest et al., 2005).

Neuroimaging findings suggest the involvement of similar anatomical structures linked by well-described neuroanatomical circuits, namely the orbitofrontal cortex, anterior cingulated gyrus, caudate, and thalamus, in both pediatric and adult-onset OCD (Maia et al., 2008). Examination of the brain with MRI using voxel-based morphometry has shown increased regional gray matter volume in orbital frontal cortex (Szeszko et al., 2008), the caudate nucleus bilaterally, and right putamen (Zarei et al., 2011) in patients with childhood-onset OCD compared to healthy volunteers. In addition, more total gray matter in the anterior cingulated gyrus was found in patients with drug-naïve pediatric OCD (Szeszko et al., 2004). Increased gray matter in brain regions comprising cortical–striatal–thalamic–cortical circuits are consistent with structural and functional neuroimaging studies reporting increased regional gray matter volumes and increased metabolism or activation in striatal, anterior cingulated, and orbital frontal regions among adult OCD patients (Whiteside et al., 2004; Rotge et al., 2010). Adolescent patients with OCD also showed widespread white matter abnormalities, as indicated by increased fractional anisotropy in multiple brain areas that is broadly consistent with findings from adult DTI studies in OCD (Zarei et al., 2011). Notably, in the search for an explanation for striatal dysfunction, a link between streptococcal infections and the development of OCD and tic disorders in children has been suggested (Garvey et al., 1998). It was hypothesized that OCD in some individuals may be caused by an autoimmune response to streptococcal infections, with the diagnostic criteria described by Swedo et al. (1998) as Pediatric Autoimmune Neuropsychiatric Diseases Associated to Streptococcal Infections (PANDAS). Overall, patients with early-onset OCD have a wide range of gray matter and white matter changes compared to healthy individuals. Though apparently more extensive, these changes are broadly consistent with those identified in adult OCD.

Early-onset schizophrenia and OCD are relatively rare in the very young; however, when present they are stable and severe forms of the disorders. Early-onset schizophrenia and OCD share male preponderance, higher levels of familial loading and genetic predisposition, clinical and neurobiological continuity with the adult forms, poorer prognosis, and poorer treatment response (Table 6.1). An interface between early-onset schizophrenia and OCD represents a challenging clinical "hybrid" for which characteristics are currently being identified.

Table 6.1 Similarities between early-onset schizophrenia and early-onset OCD

Relatively rare

Onset before puberty

Male predominance

Greater familial inheritance

Psychopathological continuity with adult-onset disorder

Neurobiological continuity with adult-onset disorder

Stable course

Poorer treatment response

Poorer prognosis

Obsessive–compulsive symptoms in childhood-onset and adolescent schizophrenia

Prevalence

Data suggesting clinical continuity of early- and adult-onset schizo-obsessive disorder are emerging. The Colorado Childhood-Onset Schizophrenia Research Program focusing on genetic factors, physiological correlates, and treatment of children who develop schizophrenia prior to their 13th birthday examined the prevalence of comorbid disorders (Ross *et al.*, 2006). Using a structured clinical interview, the authors assessed 83 children (mean age 9.9 ± 2.5 years) and found that 99% of the sample had at least one lifetime comorbid Axis I diagnosis. The most common comorbid diagnoses were ADHD (84%), affective disorders (34%), and anxiety disorders (55%). OCD was identified in 13% (3 of 83) of the girls and 23% (14 of 83) of the boys, resulting in a total lifetime rate of 20%, a remarkably similar finding to that found in adult-onset schizophrenia. The fact that comorbid OCD was more prevalent among boys, than girls with schizophrenia is noteworthy, since it is conceivable that schizo-obsessive boys have an earlier age at onset of OCD similar to their counterparts with "pure" OCD. Notably, the rate of pharmacological treatment for comorbid syndromes in this study was low, less than 25%, suggesting that treatment focused on schizophrenia and tended to disregard comorbid conditions. This may be due to the lack of empirically supported guidelines for treatment of comorbid conditions, and may ultimately account for poor outcomes of schizophrenia patients with comorbid conditions.

Initial findings concerning the rate of occurrence of DSM-IV OCD in adolescent schizophrenia patients appears to be akin to that found in adult-onset patients. Nechmad *et al.* (2003) revealed that of 50 hospitalized adolescents with schizophrenia and schizoaffective disorder (32 boys, 18 girls; mean age 17.0 ± 2.1 years, age at schizophrenia onset 14.8 ± 2.2 years), 13 (26%) also met DSM-IV criteria for OCD. This rate of occurrence of OCD in adolescent schizophrenia patients echoes the prevalence of OCD in adult schizophrenia patients. Adolescent schizophrenia patients with and without OCD had similar demographic and clinical characteristics. However, schizo-obsessive adolescents had more severe affective flattening and blunting, as assessed by the corresponding subscale of the Scale for the Assessment of Negative Symptoms (SANS)

(Andreasen, 1983) ($p < 0.01$). Moreover, there was a positive correlation between the severity of obsessive–compulsive and negative ($p < 0.05$) but not positive ($p = 0.11$) schizophrenic symptoms. In addition, despite the similar ages at onset of schizophrenia, a higher percentage of schizo-obsessive patients than non-OCD schizophrenia patients required rehospitalization (53.8% vs. 37.8%). Taken together, these findings suggest that as with their adult counterparts, the interaction of OCD and schizophrenic symptoms creates a poorer prognosis for adolescent schizo-obsessive patients.

Case 6.1. An early-onset schizophrenia patient with obsessive–compulsive symptoms and a poor prognosis.

P, a 12-year-old boy, was continuously hospitalized in a long-stay psychiatric unit due to treatment-resistant schizophrenia with prominent obsessive–compulsive symptoms. Family history was significant; a maternal aunt had OCD and his father suffered from schizoaffective disorder. P's developmental, social, and school history was remarkable, with motor skills and language delay first noted in preschool. Substantial psychosocial adversities were primarily reflected in limited interactions with peers and lack of participation in age-appropriate social activities, as well as low academic performance, which were evident beginning in the first grade. Family members first noted P's repetitive behavior when he was 7 years old. He began asking repetitive questions expressing fears about his parents' health. He also went to the toilet again and again because he was afraid that he would not be able to control his bowel movements. At age 9 he began performing multiple time-consuming rituals such as tapping the door frames, counting floor tiles, and checking the mail box. P explained a necessity to perform rituals "just right" in order to prevent both his parents from developing cancer. P expressed a degree of insight regarding the excessive nature of his worries and behaviors but could not stop worrying about his parents and he continued to perform rituals. Gradually, P cut off all contacts with peers and stopped going to school. He had aggressive outbursts especially when his parents tried to persuade him to go back to school. He also said he was being watched and laughed at by his peers, and refused to eat until his parents checked his food because he was afraid of food poisoning. Marked deterioration in all areas of functioning and suspected psychosis led to hospitalization at age 11. During repeated examinations, P revealed hearing voices from time to time that commented on his ritualistic behavior. He also admitted that his thoughts were sometimes directed by outside sources that he assumed could be "people from Mars." Negative symptoms, blunted and restricted affect, poverty of content of speech, and asociality predominated the clinical picture. The diagnosis of DSM-IV schizophrenic disorder was established. In addition, he continued to perform rituals for at least 3–4 hours a day, repeatedly combing his hair, washing his hands, and counting floor tiles. He expressed no insight into the excessive nature of his behavior. Despite inability to explain his behaviors, P's repetitive acts that were seemingly performed according to elaborate rules were indicative of typical OCD rituals. Trials with antipsychotic monotherapy, including clozapine, combined with SRIs were ineffective. P remained in a long-stay unit due to the continuous presence of both schizophrenic and obsessive–compulsive symptoms and a very low level of daily functioning.

Clinical characteristics

A systematic phenomenological characterization of adolescent schizophrenia patients with OCD and their comparison to a carefully matched group of adolescent schizophrenia patients without OCD produced several valuable findings (Faragian *et al.*, 2008; Poyurovsky *et al.*, 2008). In general, noticeable similarities were found between clinical characteristics of adolescent schizo-obsessive patients and their adult counterparts. The small sample size, cross-sectional design, and lack of direct comparison of adolescent and adult schizophrenia populations, however, should be considered in the interpretation of the study results.

Thus, age at onset of schizophrenia, as determined by the emergence of first psychotic symptoms, is significantly earlier in the schizo-obsessive group (Table 6.2). Insidious onset is typical to a majority of the early-onset schizophrenia patients regardless of the presence of OCD. Obsessive–compulsive symptoms reveal key characteristics of "typical" OCD. Almost all patients have moderate-to-severe obsessions and compulsions, and the mean number of obsessions and compulsions per patient is around three. A few have only obsessions or only compulsions. The most prevalent obsessions are contamination, symmetry, and aggression; the most prevalent compulsions are checking, cleaning, and ordering/arranging. Unexpectedly, insight into obsessive–compulsive symptoms, as assessed by the Brown Assessment of Beliefs Scale, is quite good in the majority (86.3%, 19 of 22) of patients (Faragian *et al.*, 2008). These adolescents are aware of the excessive nature of their OCD-related beliefs and behaviors, admit that most people consider their behavior excessive, and usually try to "get rid" of these repetitive and intrusive thoughts and to control repetitive behaviors. They believe that these thoughts and behaviors are somehow illness-related and could be potentially corrected. Although sometimes their views are expressed in a naïve and childish way, it is clear that obsessive–compulsive symptoms in this subset of patients are ego-dystonic. Only a few patients reveal lack of insight, that is they express complete conviction that the rituals (e.g., checking, touching, washing) have to be performed to prevent a dreadful event. The effect size of the correlation between insight into OCD and awareness of schizophrenia, as assessed by the Schedule to Assess Mental Disorders (SUMD) (Amador *et al.*, 1994), in the schizo-obsessive group was negligible ($r = 0.15$, $p = 0.52$). In contrast to sufficient insight into OCD, a substantial proportion of patients showed poor or lack of awareness of having schizophrenia and of the need for treatment. Hence, similar to adults, obsessive–compulsive symptoms in adolescent schizo-obsessive patients appeared to be distinct psychopathological phenomena distinguishable from core schizophrenia symptoms.

In a majority of the patients OCD precedes the onset of schizophrenia, and only in a few does OCD emerge after the onset of schizophrenia symptoms. In roughly 75% of the adolescents obsessive–compulsive symptoms emerge as typical OCD prior to the develop-ment of the initial prodromal schizophrenic symptoms. Notably, half of the subgroup that had OCD prior to the onset of schizophrenia was initially diagnosed with "pure" OCD and treated with an anti-obsessive agent (Case 6.2). Among patients with an "alternating" course of the two disorders, obsessive–compulsive symptoms were usually not identifi-able during acute episodes of psychosis, and re-emerged after the resolution of psychotic symptoms. In others, obsessive–compulsive symptoms constituted an integral compon-ent of the prodromal phase of schizophrenia, along with behavioral problems, social withdrawal, and academic difficulties (Case 6.3). In this case scenario obsessive–compulsive symptoms seem to continue to accompany schizophrenic symptoms during the following acute and remitted stages of illness. This pattern of a temporal interrelationship between obsessive–compulsive and schizophrenic symptoms closely resembles that found in adults.

Table 6.2 Demographic and clinical characteristics and clinical rating scale scores of adolescent schizophrenia patients with and without obsessive–compulsive disorder (OCD)

Variable	Adolescent schizophrenia patients			
	With OCD ($N=22$)	Without OCD ($N=22$)	Statistics (df = 42)	P
Sex (M/F)	12/10	13/9	$\chi^2=0.09^a$	0.96
Age, years	16.3 (1.8)	17.0 (1.4)	$t=-1.38$	0.18
Age at onset of schizophrenia, years	12.4 (2.6)	14.9 (2.3)	$t=-3.37$	0.002
Age at onset of OCD, years	12.4 (2.9)	–		
Duration of schizophrenia, years	4.0 (2.0)	2.1 (1.9)	$t=3.11$	0.003
Number of hospitalizations	1.5 (0.7)	1.2 (0.4)	$t=1.60$	0.12
Education, years	8.7 (2.4)	9.8 (2.6)	$t=-1.38$	0.18
Rating scales:				
SAPS/SANS dimensions				
Positive	2.2 (2.3)	3.3 (1.6)	$t=-1.62$	0.11
Negative	10.4 (6.0)	9.1 (3.7)	$t=0.84$	0.41
Disorganized	4.4 (2.1)	4.5 (2.2)	$t=-0.43$	0.65
CGI	4.3 (0.7)	4.4 (0.7)	$t=-0.44$	0.66
HAM-D	3.8 (3.4)	4.5 (4.4)	$t=-0.58$	0.57
Y-BOCS				
Obsessions	9.5 (3.4)	–		
Compulsions	9.0 (4.0)	–		
Total	18.5 (6.7)	–		
BABS				
Conviction	1.4 (1.4)			
Perception of others' views	1.0 (1.1)			
Explanation of differing views	1.1 (1.1)			
Fixity of beliefs	0.8 (0.9)			
Attempts to disprove beliefs	1.3 (1.2)			
Insight	0.9 (0.9)			
Referential thinking	0.4 (0.8)			
Total	6.8 (6.1)			
SUMD				
Awareness of illness	2.8 (1.3)	3.1 (1.5)	$t=-0.71$	0.48
Awareness of treatment	2.7 (1.6)	2.5 (1.4)	$t=0.44$	0.66

SAPS, Schedule for the Assessment of Positive Symptoms; SANS, Schedule for the Assessment of Negative Symptoms; CGI, Clinical Global Impression scale for psychosis; HAM-D, Hamilton Rating Scale for Depression; Y-BOCS, Yale–Brown Obsessive–Compulsive Scale; BABS, Brown Assessment of Beliefs Scale; SUMD, Schedule to Assess Unawareness of Mental Disorder.
Figures in parentheses are standard deviations.
[a] df = 1.
Source: Modified from Poyurovsky M, Faragian S, Shabeta A, Kosov A (2008) Comparison of clinical characteristics, comorbidity and pharmacotherapy in adolescent schizophrenia patients with and without obsessive–compulsive disorder. *Psychiatry Research* **159**, 133–139. Faragian S, Kurs R, Poyurovsky M (2008) Insight into obsessive–compulsive symptoms and awareness of illness in adolescent schizophrenia patients with and without OCD. *Child Psychiatry and Human Development* **39**, 39–48. Reprinted with permission.

Case 6.2. Full-scale OCD that preceded schizophrenia in an adolescent patient.

S, a 16-year-old girl, was admitted to a psychiatric hospital following her first acute psychotic episode characterized by psychomotor agitation, delusions of reference and persecution, and auditory hallucinations. Twelve months prior to admission, she complained that her classmates were talking about her, reading her mind, and deliberately confusing her by sending "hypnotized messages." She also heard voices that made derogatory comments about her appearance. A gradual change in behavior that tended towards delinquency and a substantial decline in scholastic achievements accompanied these psychotic symptoms. A DSM-IV diagnosis of schizophrenic disorder, paranoid type was established. According to both the patient and her parents, since age 12, she constantly performed cleaning and washing rituals out of fear of contracting "a dirty disease." She also had an irresistible urge to check her school belongings and keep them in a special "magic" order. She had constant need for reassurance, and repeatedly asked her parents if she performed her rituals in 'just the right" order. She recognized that her worries and rituals were unreasonable and excessive, but was unable to control them. At age 14, 2 years prior to her first psychotic episode, DSM-IV OCD was diagnosed and treatment with an anti-obsessive agent, fluvoxamine (up to 200 mg/day), was initiated. Retrospective analysis of the course of illness revealed that initial psychotic symptoms developed during fluvoxamine administration that was discontinued when the psychotic symptoms became evident. Positive schizophrenia symptoms responded to monotherapy with the antipsychotic risperidone (3 mg/day). OCD symptoms were not noticed during the acute psychotic episode, and became identifiable again, after resolution of psychosis. After resolution of the acute psychosis, fluvoxamine (100 mg/day) was resumed as an adjunctive medication to an ongoing regimen of risperidone (2 mg/day). Six months of combined risperidone–fluvoxamine treatment was associated with a remission of positive schizophrenia symptoms and a gradual decline of OCD symptom severity.

Case 6.3. Obsessive–compulsive symptoms during prodromal and active phases of schizophrenia in an adolescent patient.

G, a 13-year-old boy, was hospitalized due to acute psychosis, characterized by delusions of reference and persecution, disorganized affect and behavior, and aggressiveness. His family history was significant; his older sister had OCD and his maternal aunt had schizophrenic disorder. The patient was born full term, normal birth with mild neonatal jaundice. G met developmental milestones with some delay in motor skills. He grew up as a shy boy, had very limited interactions with peers, and rarely participated in social activities. Academically he did relatively well until age 12, sixth grade, when his academic performance deteriorated due to gradual behavioral changes, characterized by previously uncharacteristic aggressive outbursts, impulsiveness, and cruelty toward peers. Due to increasingly inappropriate behavior G was expelled from school and remained at home for a year prior to his first hospital admission. While at home, G revealed increasing anxiety and suspiciousness. In parallel, new behavioral patterns became evident: G began to check repeatedly whether his belongings were kept in the proper order. This behavior lasted for hours. He also repeatedly washed his hands and constantly cleaned the things in his room. He explained this behavior by an urge "just" for order and cleanliness but could not articulate any obsessive thoughts to account for this ritualistic behavior. Later on he began to thoroughly clean objects including chairs, door handles, and every piece of furniture that his parents came in contact with. Any attempt to modify this behavior was associated with verbal and sometimes physical aggression. Finally, he began to claim that people around him, primarily his parents, followed him and implanted surveillance *devices in his room, to control his behavior. On the ward, G exhibited delusions of reference and persecution, auditory hallucinations, and disorganized speech. He met the DSM-IV criteria for schizophrenic disorder. Positive symptoms of schizophrenia responded beneficially to a trial with the antipsychotic perphenazine (up to 24 mg/day). His cleaning, washing, and ordering rituals typical to ordinary OCD intensified during the active phase of psychosis. This ritualistic behavior lasted for 6–8 hours a day and was as clinically significant as symptoms of schizophrenia. Notably, after the resolution of his psychotic symptoms, G began to express a degree of insight into the excessive and senseless nature of his ritualistic behavior, expressing frustration at his inability to control it. However he could not acknowledge any obsessive thoughts that accompanied his ritualistic behavior and claimed that he felt irresistible urges to "clean, wash, and order" in "just the right" way. The addition of the SSRI sertraline (150 mg/day) to his ongoing regimen of perphenazine (24 mg/day) gradually led to a reduction of the severity of his compulsive symptoms while maintaining his remission of psychosis.*

Additional comorbid disorders

Important similarities between early- and adult-onset schizo-obsessive disorder also emerged when additional comorbid disorders were evaluated (Poyurovsky *et al.*, 2008). There was a substantial aggregation of OCD-related disorders in adolescent schizo-obsessive patients, and their patterns were remarkably similar to those found in adult schizo-obsessive patients (Table 6.3). Fifty percent of patients in the schizo-obsessive group vs. only 5% in the schizophrenia group had at least one OCD-related disorder ($p < 0.01$).

Table 6.3 Comorbid Axis I psychiatric disorders in adolescent schizophrenia patients with and without obsessive–compulsive disorder (OCD)[a]

Comorbid diagnosis	Schizophrenia with OCD (N = 22)		Schizophrenia without OCD (N = 22)		Statistics	
	N	%	N	%	χ^2	P
OCD spectrum disorders						
Hypochondriasis	0	0.0%	0	0.0%	–	–
Anorexia nervosa	3	13.6%	1	4.5%	1.10	0.29
Bulimia nervosa	1	4.5%	0	0.0%	1.02	0.31
Body dysmorphic disorder	2	9.1%	0	0.0%	2.10	0.15
Tic disorder	6	27.3%	0	0.0%	6.95	0.008[b]
Major depressive disorder	9	40.9%	6	27.3%	0.91	0.34
Substance abuse	1	4.5%	4	18.1%	2.03	0.15
Anxiety disorders						
Panic disorder	2	9.1%	0	0.0%	2.10	0.15
Social phobia	1	4.5%	1	4.5%	0.0	1
Specific phobia	1	4.5%	2	9.0%	0.36	0.55

[a] Some patients had more than one comorbid disorder.
[b] Non-significant following Bonferroni post-hoc test (0.008 × 10 = 0.08).
Source: From Poyurovsky M, Faragian S, Shabeta A, Kosov A (2008) Comparison of clinical characteristics, comorbidity and pharmacotherapy in adolescent schizophrenia patients with and without obsessive–compulsive disorder. *Psychiatry Research* **159**, 133–139. Faragian S, Kurs R, Poyurovsky M (2008) Insight into obsessive–compulsive symptoms and awareness of illness in adolescent schizophrenia patients with and without OCD. *Child Psychiatry and Human Development* **39**, 39–48. Reprinted with permission.

The strongest association was found between a schizo-obsessive phenotype and tic disorders: almost 30% of the patients in the schizo-obsessive group and none in the non-OCD schizophrenia group reported the presence of tics. This association is not surprising owing to a pathophysiological linkage between OCD and tic disorders. There was an almost five-fold predominance of boys, compared to girls, with comorbid tics. In all cases tics preceded the emergence of schizophrenia, and preceded or emerged concurrently with symptoms of OCD. Chronic and transient tics were equally present. Simple motor tics, such as eye-blinking and facial grimacing, were the most prevalent. In a predominant majority of the cases, the severity of the tics was mild to moderate.

Importantly, a differential diagnosis between OCD and motor tics is not straightforward. Motor tics often have a premonitory urge similar to that seen with compulsive rituals, while the compulsions of early-onset OCD often lack obsessional triggers. Distinguishing between tics and compulsions is particularly difficult when the rituals are simple, repetitive movements such as tapping and touching. It is difficult to clearly differentiate the symptoms of OCD and Tourette's syndrome, but studies suggest that the compulsions associated with Tourette's syndrome may be less severe than those in children with "pure" OCD and without tics, and are more likely to involve symmetry, rubbing, touching, staring, or blinking rituals than washing or cleaning (Leckman *et al.*, 1997). Clinical experience shows that similar patterns may hold true for children and adolescents with schizo-obsessive disorder and comorbid tic disorders.

Differential diagnosis

Diagnosis of schizophrenia with or without OCD in children and adolescents is challenging. The following are some of the major psychiatric disorders that should be considered in differential diagnosis of early-onset schizophrenia, after medical conditions (e.g., seizure disorders, infectious, metabolic and endocrine disorders, central nervous system lesions) have been ruled out (Russell, 1994; Masi *et al.*, 2006; Correll, 2010).

- *Non-psychotic hallucinations and delusions.* Psychotic-like symptoms have been identified in children without mental disorders. According to a diagnostic interview at 11 years of age, roughly 8% in an epidemiological study reported experiencing hallucinatory phenomena at least some of the time (McGee *et al.*, 2000). These non-psychotic children who experience hallucinations usually have fewer premorbid language and motor disturbances characteristic of schizophrenia. They less frequently act on their misperceptions which are neither pervasive nor bizarre. Typically, hallucinations occur in a specific context or are triggered by environmental stressors. In addition, delusions and rare but appropriate social relationships are usually preserved. Nevertheless, a family history of psychosis is not uncommon, and at least in one follow-up study, 20% had experienced acute psychosis and almost one-third developed atypical psychosis (Del Beccaro *et al.*, 1988).

- *Depression.* Children with MDD may exhibit hallucinations (predominantly auditory) or, more rarely, delusions. Usually psychotic symptoms are mood-congruent and present mostly during depressive episodes. Grossly disorganized behavior or speech, as well as thought disorders and deterioration in functioning, are typically absent. Temporal stability of the diagnosis is high, and transition to schizophrenia is rare. Notably, the psychotic symptoms in major depression are associated with a higher frequency of bipolar disorder within the families of affected children and with a higher risk of developing bipolar disorder in probands.

- *Bipolar disorder.* From a phenomenological perspective, children with schizophrenia more frequently have an insidious onset of disease, more delusions and negative symptoms of flattened affect, and asociality than children with bipolar disorder. Children with bipolar disorder more frequently tend to have ADHD, while children with schizophrenia have more frequent premorbid personality abnormalities and developmental disabilities. The outcome is better in bipolar disorder. A family history of bipolar disorder can be a helpful indicator of an affective disorder.

- *Personality disorders.* Schizotypal personality disorder is characterized by marked abnormalities in social and interpersonal behavior, cognitive and perceptual distortions, and transient psychotic-like symptoms. Schizoid personality disorder in children and adolescents includes solitary activity, excessive interest in unusual topics (e.g., mystic), increased sensitivity, paranoid ideations, and a peculiar style of communication, which resembles that of the schizotypal personality disorder. A common clinical scenario for children and adolescents with both schizotypal and schizoid personality disorder is the general persistence of the disorders into adulthood. However, roughly 25% may develop a more severe schizophrenia-spectrum disorder, that is schizophrenia or schizoaffective disorder.

- *Pervasive developmental disorders* (PDD). A diagnosis of PDD is not rare among children with early-onset schizophrenia. In children who later develop schizophrenia, PDD symptoms are usually not as severe and pervasive as in autistic children, and they can progressively improve or, more rarely, can persist, albeit with a lesser severity, and with superimposition of psychotic symptoms.

- *Multidimensionally impaired disorder (MDI).* MDI has been proposed to describe a subgroup of children who cannot easily be considered to have any of the typical psychotic disorders. For instance, approximately one-fifth of children with putative very-early-onset schizophrenia in the National Institute of Mental Health study did not strictly meet the diagnostic criteria for this disorder (Kumra et al., 1998). Prevalent features of MDI are an impaired ability to distinguish reality from fantasy, mild psychotic symptoms (delusions of reference, perceptual disturbances), mood instability, impaired interpersonal relationships without clear isolation or withdrawal, deficits in information processing, and an absence of formal thought disorders. Psychotic symptoms are transitory, usually occur under stress, and are associated with emotional or behavioral outbursts. Negative symptoms such as blunted affect and poverty of speech are much rarer.

- *Obsessive–compulsive disorder.* As mentioned, younger children with OCD may not recognize that symptoms are the product of their mind, and the ego-dystonic quality of intrusive thoughts and repetitive behaviors may be lacking. Young children might describe their intrusive thoughts as internal or external "voices," and this report may lead to a misinterpretation resulting in the conclusion that the child is having auditory hallucinations. In these cases, diagnostic confusion may occur between severe OCD without insight and schizophrenic spectrum disorders with delusions and/or hallucinations.

Clearly there is an overlap between the observable behaviors in OCD and schizophrenia in children and adolescents. Moreover, there is also a substantial overlap between the symptoms of both disorders and age-related behaviors. Thus, while it is age-appropriate for a very young child (Piagetian preoperational stage) to believe that his/her action will prevent a bad outcome – i.e., not stepping on a crack will keep mommy and daddy safe – this type of thinking should not persist into later school-age years (Rodowski *et al.*, 2008). When it does, it is suggestive either of an obsession/ compulsion, i.e., this behavior is done to reduce the anxiety produced by an intrusive thought that one's parents will be harmed, or alternatively of psychotic symptoms, i.e., this behavior may be a direct consequence of formal thought disorders or auditory hallucinations. Sometimes this distinction is not clear-cut. Moreover, in rare cases, a psychopathological "hybrid," psychotic in content and obsessive–compulsive in form, may exist and further complicate differential diagnosis. Paraphrasing Aubrey Lewis (1935): "It must be a very short step... from feeling that one must struggle against thoughts that are not one's own (incongruous with self image), to believing that they are forced upon one by an external agency, the latter being the true projection of psychosis" (cited in Rodowski *et al.*, 2008).

Case 6.4. Childhood OCD presenting as schizophrenia (Rodowski et al.*, 2008).*

J is a 13-year-old girl with a long history of psychiatric treatment including multiple hospitalizations. Her working diagnosis was schizophrenia, undifferentiated type. Her outpatient psychiatrist described her behavior as almost catatonic. Although she denied auditory or visual hallucinations, she appeared to be preoccupied with "internal stimuli." She was fearful, was unable to function independently, and had not been able to attend school for months. Her presentation was notable owing to the recent development of abnormal repetitive movements, such as touching her eyes and face, and spells of stereotyped "stepping in place" that interrupted her normal walking pattern. There was a noticeable decline in her scholastic performance and intermittent refusal to eat, drink, bathe, or take medications. She also developed a fear that others were "out to get her." She had become more socially isolated and withdrawn from friends and family. Between the ages of 6 and 13, she had numerous episodes of aggressive and impulsive behaviors, mood swings, excessive anxiety, somatic complaints, and separation anxiety. By age 13, her functioning had declined further and she stopped attending school because she was very easily distracted and unable to complete simple tasks. Her developmental history was significant for mild "auditory processing" and expressive language delays. Her IQ scores dropped by age 13. Her family history included distant relatives with diagnoses of depression, bipolar disorder, and schizophrenia.

On examination, J had slowed movements and required one-on-one assistance with constant prompting to complete her basic activities of daily living. She even had difficulty efficiently completing tasks, such as raising a glass to drink. Although no "psychotic" symptoms were elicited, a schizophrenia-spectrum disorder could not be ruled out based on her history. In addition, because of J's paucity of movement and almost non-existent social interaction, a possibility of "catatonic" presentation of major mood disorder was also considered. Organic etiology was ruled out on the basis of her current routine laboratory screening and thorough prior medical work-up. Initial observations of J's behaviors noted a compulsive quality of her repetitive movements, most clearly her stepping on only the colored tiles of the floor. She also went back and forth in the doorway during transitions from one room to the next, but was not able to explain this hesitancy. She would also repetitively get up and down on her chair before finally rising. While she did not describe an "urge" in association with these behaviors, many of her movements had a purposeful quality. With further questioning, her parents endorsed a history of some counting behaviors, and minor rituals, as a younger child. Differential diagnosis included schizophrenia-spectrum disorder vs. OCD, while PDD was also considered because of her early history of developmental delays and social impairment. Targeting a working diagnosis of OCD, an anti-obsessive medication (sertraline) was initiated. In addition, behavioral interventions were implemented to limit the time she spent in transitions. This behavioral approach was designed to target the aggression that often developed when specific limits were set on her repetitive behaviors. Although it was not clear whether or not there was a specific "obsessive thought" that her compulsive repetitive behavior was attempting to relieve, it became quite apparent that interrupting these periods triggered a strong reaction. By the end of her third week in the hospital J was more independent; her repetitive movements diminished and did not interfere as much in her activities. She seemed less preoccupied and fearful. Her primary diagnosis was reconceptualized as OCD rather than a schizophrenia-spectrum disorder. Clozapine for symptoms of "schizophrenia" was gradually tapered off while the treatment with an SSRI was maintained. The patient was also referred for an intensive treatment program for OCD using a cognitive–behavioral approach for symptom reduction. A year later, J was functioning independently and had successfully returned to a full-time regular classroom setting and age-appropriate activities.

Past history and clinical presentation, the presence of insight into the connection between a thought and a behavior, and long-term follow-up to assess a natural course can help in establishing the differential diagnosis between OCD and schizophrenia-spectrum disorders in children and adolescents (Rodowski *et al.*, 2008). The authors also highlight that symptoms such as bizarre behaviors and atypical or disorganized thoughts should not lead the clinician to directly presume a schizophrenia-spectrum diagnosis. Childhood OCD obsessions may include unrealistic worry about contamination, catastrophic events, sexual thoughts, physical sensations, and excessive and recurrent worry, guilt, and morality. As mentioned earlier, studies of early-onset OCD have suggested that tapping, counting, repeating, ordering, checking, rubbing, and washing are common (Geller *et al.*, 1998; Miller, 2004). In the presented Case 6.4, checking behaviors and some repeating/tapping rituals around doorways and floor tiles led the clinicians to reconsider their diagnosis and seek other features of OCD. Despite an inability to explain her actions, J's stereotyped acts that were seemingly performed according to elaborate rules were suggestive of OCD. In contrast, psychosis was considered a less likely diagnosis due to the isolated nature of her repetitious behaviors. Positive response to combined psychopharmacological and cognitive–behavioral treatment that addressed OCD substantiated the author's diagnostic assumption.

Treatment

Schizophrenia patients with obsessive–compulsive symptoms, whether early- or adult-onset, is a difficult-to-treat subgroup. Unfortunately, there are presently no evidence-based data available to assist physicians in formulating treatment plans for youngsters with schizo-obsessive disorder. Recommendations for the treatment of adults with schizo-obsessive disorder might also be appropriate for the treatment of the disorder in children and adolescents. Findings from controlled pharmacological trials in pediatric patients with "pure" forms of schizophrenia and OCD should be considered as well.

Monotherapy with an antipsychotic agent is a reasonable first step in treating schizo-obsessive patients. Both typical and atypical antipsychotic agents have proven efficacy in children and adolescents for acute intervention in schizophrenia and as maintenance treatment to decrease the risk of relapse (Olfson et al., 2006; Sikich et al., 2008; Correll, 2010). However, the treatment of pediatric patients has unique developmental aspects. The specific maturational changes in the dopamine receptor system pertinent to antipsychotic drug action, such as decreases in dopamine cell density, peaking of basal dopamine levels, dopamine turnover and dopaminergic input in the prefrontal cortex, and changes in D_1 and D_2 receptor concentrations in the striatum (as well as other neurotransmitter systems) may be associated with increased basal dopamine neurotransmission in childhood and adolescence relative to adulthood (Kumra et al., 2008). This in turn can potentially have implications for clinical response as well as an increased susceptibility to side effects (e.g., extrapyramidal side effects [EPS], prolactin elevation, sedation, weight gain) observed in youth exposed to antipsychotic drugs. Antipsychotic agents have varying degrees of risk for these side effects, and a careful risk–benefit assessment is essential when choosing medications for young patients.

Typical antipsychotics should be administered with caution primarily due to their propensity to induce EPS and tardive dyskinesia. Moreover, since monotherapy with typical antipsychotics appears to be of minimal value in adult schizo-obsessive patients, their therapeutic utility in adolescents might also be limited. When considering treatment with atypical antipsychotics the following findings might influence the choice of medication. Olanzapine alone or in combination with an SRI revealed therapeutic efficacy in adult schizo-obsessive patients in small uncontrolled trials (Poyurovsky et al., 2000; Sasson et al., 2003). However, the magnitude of weight gain induced by olanzapine is substantially greater for adolescents than for adults and is alarming in comparison to other antipsychotic medications (Ratzoni et al., 2002). This might prompt clinicians to consider olanzapine as a "second-line" agent for children and adolescents with schizophrenia-spectrum disorders regardless of the presence of OCD (Kumra et al., 2008). Risperidone treatment in children and adolescents has been associated with galactorrhea, increased appetite, moderate weight gain, and dose-dependent EPS, suggesting that the overall risk–benefit profile of risperidone in schizophrenia youngsters with and without OCD appears to be optimal in lower dose ranges (1–4 mg) (Correll et al., 2006). Among children and adolescents with schizophrenia, aripiprazole was most commonly associated with akathisia, tremor, and somnolence, but weight gain was modest (Findling et al., 2008). A preliminary report indicates that aripiprazole exerts beneficial effect on both schizophrenia and obsessive–compulsive symptoms in some adult patients (Glick et al., 2008.). Therapeutic efficacy of aripiprazole, as well as quetiapine, amisulpiride, and ziprasidone, in children and adolescents with schizo-obsessive disorder merits investigation. Obsessive–compulsive symptoms in children and adolescents with schizophrenia should be considered the target for an anti-obsessive drug intervention only when severity of OCD reaches the threshold for clinical significance. In our study half of the patients from the adolescent schizo-obsessive group was treated with adjunctive SRIs (Poyurovsky et al., 2008). This finding indicates the tendency of treating psychiatrists to augment antipsychotic drug treatment with anti-obsessive medications to address the OCD component of schizo-obsessive disorder. Notably, the pattern of treatment response for pediatric OCD without schizophrenia appears quite similar to that seen in post-pubertal-onset OCD (Leckman et al., 2010). A meta-analysis that included controlled treatment trials in pediatric OCD reported that effective treatments for pediatric OCD were pharmacotherapy with SSRIs (effect size 0.48, 95% CI 0.36–0.61) or clomipramine (effect size 0.85, 95% CI 0.32–1.39), and cognitive–behavioral therapy (CBT) (effect size 1.45, 95% CI 0.68–2.22) (Watson and Rees, 2008).

SRIs should be administered only in stabilized antipsychotic-treated patients during remission of schizophrenia, since they may be deleterious in a psychotic phase. Adult schizo-obsessive patients with a history of impulsivity and aggressiveness are at higher risk of psychotic exacerbation during adjunctive SRI treatment. This observation may be pertinent to young patients as well. In addition, several adverse effects associated with SRIs are of particular concern when used in schizophrenia patients. Akathisia, activation syndrome, increased anxiety, and manic–like symptoms were consistently reported in both adults and adolescents with "pure" OCD (Lane, 1998). These SRI-induced adverse effects may be difficult to distinguish from symptoms of schizophrenia. Most activation occurs during the initial weeks of treatment and is frequently dose-dependent, and responds to dose reduction. In case of severe side effects discontinuation of an adjunctive SRI may be warranted. Pharmacokinetic interactions and potential side effects of an antipsychotic–SRI combination should be closely monitored. Anti-obsessive agents with minimal drug–drug interactions, (e.g., escitalopram, citalopram and sertraline) may be preferable as adjunctive agents.

Clozapine is generally reserved as a second-line intervention for pediatric patients with treatment-refractory schizophrenia due to its potential hematological side effects, weight gain, and seizures. When a trial of an adjunctive SSRI is considered to address the OCD component in schizo-obsessive patients, SSRIs should be added to clozapine with caution, and those that are devoid of clinically significant drug–drug interactions seem to be safer. A potential of some atypical antipsychotics, including clozapine, to induce *de novo* or exacerbate pre-existing obsessive–compulsive symptoms should be taken into consideration when treating adolescent schizo-obsessive patients.

In addition to pharmacotherapy, individual or group therapy and age-appropriate psychosocial interventions to address problem-solving, communication skills, and psychosocial functioning are also recommended for children and adolescents with schizophrenia. In addition, support and psychoeducation for the family are recommended. Considering that there is a sufficient degree of insight into obsessive–compulsive symptoms in a substantial proportion of adolescent schizo-obsessive patients, and a potential efficacy of CBT in pediatric OCD, CBT may potentially be incorporated in an integrative treatment approach in adolescent schizo-obsessive patients. However, its benefits and risks are yet to be evaluated.

Although far from being conclusive, the results of phenomenological characterization of schizophrenia with obsessive–compulsive symptoms in children and adolescents lend support to the notion that akin to "pure" schizophrenia and OCD, there is a clinical continuity between early- and adult-onset schizo-obsessive disorder. Elucidation of the neurobiological (genetic, imaging, neurocognitive) foundation for a phenomenological continuity between adolescent and adult forms of schizo-obsessive disorder merits further investigation.

Obsessive–compulsive symptoms in elderly schizophrenia patients

The clinical significance of obsessive–compulsive phenomena in adolescent and adult schizophrenia patients, along with evidence indicating that symptoms of both schizophrenia and OCD persist into old age in a substantial proportion of patients (Skoog and Skoog, 1999), prompted explicit evaluation of clinical characteristics of OCD in elderly schizophrenia patients.

Our group evaluated 50 elderly patients (63–83 years old; 14 men, 36 women) consecutively hospitalized in a psychogeriatric department for acute exacerbation of DSM-IV schizophrenia (23 paranoid type, 5 undifferentiated, 13 residual) or schizoaffective disorder (Poyurovsky *et al*, 2006). Diagnosis was based on the best-estimate approach including the Structured Clinical Interview for DSM-IV Axis I Disorders (SCID), medical records, caregivers, and treating psychiatrists. Exclusion criteria were: primary diagnosis of dementia, major affective disorders, or neurological disorders. Patients with severe cognitive impairment that interfered with the ability to complete rating scales were not included. Rating scales included the Schedule for the Assessment of Positive (SAPS) and Negative (SANS) Symptoms, Hamilton Rating Scale for Depression (HAM-D) (Hamilton, 1960), Mini Mental State Examination (MMSE) (Folstein *et al*, 1975). Clinically significant obsessive–compulsive symptoms were operationally determined using the Yale–Brown Obsessive–Compulsive Scale (Y-BOCS) as a minimum severity score of 16 and duration of at least 12 months.

Eight (16%) of the 50 patients with schizophrenia or schizoaffective disorder who participated in the study also met DSM-IV criteria for OCD. The two schizophrenia groups with and without OCD did not differ significantly in any of the demographic and clinical variables. Patients in both groups were in their seventies with mean age of schizophrenia onset approximately 35 years, mean duration of schizophrenia 30 years and an average of five hospitalizations. None had severe cognitive impairment, as revealed in the relatively high MMSE scores (schizo-obsessive, 26.4 ± 1.1; schizophrenia, 27.1 ± 1.4).

Within the schizo-obsessive group, the total Y-BOCS score was 22.2 ± 8.3, obsessions subscale 11.0 ± 5.1, and compulsion subscale 11.2 ± 6.4, indicating moderate-to-severe obsessive–compulsive symptoms. In half of the schizo-obsessive group, OCD first appeared in the third decade, preceded the onset of schizophrenia and persisted into old age (Case 6.5 below). In the remaining schizo-obsessive patients, OCD mean age of onset was 52.6 ± 5.2 years, roughly 15 years following the onset of schizophrenia. Since in all patients OCD preceded administration of atypical antipsychotic agents, their role in the occurrence of OCD in the study participants was negligible. Instead, the authors hypothesized that the late onset of OCD was related to a complex interaction of chronic course of schizophrenia, aging, and OCD-predisposing factors (e.g., parkinsonism), all putatively associated with basal ganglia pathology (Case 6.6 below). Obsessive–compulsive symptoms were typical and included contamination and aggressive obsessions, washing, checking, and hoarding compulsions. Remarkably, similar to elderly OCD patients without schizophrenia, certain symptom presentations, such as obsessions and compulsions related to scrupulosity and fear of forgetting names (Case 6.7 below), were quite common in the schizo-obsessive subgroup as well (Fallon *et al.*, 1990; Jenike, 1991). Significantly more patients in the schizo-obsessive group than in the non-OCD schizophrenia group were treated with adjunctive SSRIs (50% [4 of 8] vs. 2.4% [1 of 42]; $\chi^2 = 16.93$, $p < 0.001$), reflecting clinicians' tendencies to add anti-obsessive agents to antipsychotic therapy when obsessive–compulsive symptoms are identified.

Case 6.5. Obsessive–compulsive symptoms in an elderly schizophrenia patient.

Mr. A, a 62-year-old unmarried man, was diagnosed with schizophrenia at age 30, when he was first admitted to the hospital due to the deterioration of his mental condition associated with delusions of persecution, auditory hallucinations, and Schneiderian symptoms. This psychotic episode followed a period of roughly 2 years of prodromal symptoms and gradual functioning deterioration. According to hospital records, the patient and his family noted the occurrence of ritualistic behavior well before his first admission. He spent hours washing his hands and showering, owing to fear of contamination with germs. He also repeatedly cleaned objects around him to "protect himself from possible contamination and from contracting a dreadful disease." A's ritualistic behavior was not related to the content of delusions or hallucinations. Since his first admission, A was hospitalized twice at age 38 and 46 due to acute psychotic exacerbations following non-adherence to an antipsychotic medication. During the last 10 years A was under the supervision of a psychiatrist in an outpatient clinic, and remained in a good-quality remission. Moderate weight gain associated with olanzapine treatment was the only side effect. Otherwise A was in a good physical health. The course of his obsessive–compulsive symptoms was waxing and waning with periods of meaningful distress and functional impairment owing to increased symptom severity and periods of mild and manageable symptoms. The two disorders ran independent courses with symptoms of OCD undetectable during psychotic exacerbations and resurfacing during remission of schizophrenia. The adjunctive SSRI sertraline was quite efficious during remissions of schizophrenia in controlling clinically significant OCD symptoms.

Case 6.6. Late-onset obsessive–compulsive symptoms putatively following a basal ganglia lesion in a schizophrenia patient.

Mr. D, a 67-year-old man, was diagnosed with schizophrenic disorder, paranoid type, at age 37, and was hospitalized four times due to acute psychotic exacerbations during the 30-year history of his illness. After his last admission at age 59, D was treated with a typical antipsychotic, perphenazine (16 mg/day) and was in a stable remission. He was employed as a part-time clerk in a post office. Suspected obsessive–compulsive symptoms occurred approximately 12 months prior to the current psychiatric evaluation performed in an outpatient unit. D described recurrent obsessions of "needing to know" information associated with rituals that manifested as repeated questions for reassurance and repeated checking of his computer. This urge "to know" was related to the names, dates, events, and proper spellings of geographical regions, products, and people. He was reluctant to watch television or listen to the radio for fear of encountering new information that he would need "to decode." He also compulsively made and reorganized lists of a variety of informational facts in a diary that he never used. He telephoned family members, friends, and former colleagues following a compelling urge to ask questions, regardless of the expense or the time of day. D was fully aware of the excessive and unreasonable nature of his concerns and behaviors, but he could not control them. These typical repetitive, distressful, intrusive, and time-consuming (more than 5 hours daily) obsessive–compulsive symptoms were distinct from core symptoms of schizophrenia. Notably, D was never treated with atypical antipsychotic agents, ruling out the possibility of antipsychotic-induced OCD. There was no evidence of a family history of psychiatric illnesses, past history of OCD, affective disorder, or substance abuse. This patient's medical history was remarkable for type 2 diabetes mellitus and hypertension. At the time of evaluation, in addition to perphenazine (16 mg/day) and zopiclone (7.5 mg) at bedtime for insomnia, D's medication regimen included metformin (850 mg/day) and captopril (50 mg/day) for diabetes and hypertension, respectively. A recent MRI was significant for small lacunar infarct in the right basal ganglia. The location of the lesion and the recent and relatively abrupt onset of symptoms suggested a possible relationship to the patient's OCD. Treatment with adjunctive SSRI escitalopram (10 mg) was associated with a meaningful improvement in the severity of obsessive–compulsive symptoms, substantiating the diagnosis.

Case 6.7. Symptom presentation in a patient with late-onset OCD without schizophrenia (from Weiss and Jenike, 2000).

Mr. D, a 70-year-old married man, first developed obsessive–compulsive symptoms at the age of 62. He specifically recalled the exact date and time of symptom onset: it had occurred when *he recognized an actor in a television commercial but was unable to recall his name. He had become quite anxious and "needed to know;" eventually he called several acquaintances and the television network. This "need to know" worsened, and it became common for him to wake his wife or phone friends in the middle of the night to obtain answers to questions that plagued him. He memorized bumper stickers, newspaper headlines, names of songs and their composers, and even comic strip character names. He started to collect old newspapers to create a database to answer questions that might come up. With time, however, D was no longer able to read the newspaper because of a strong urge to memorize all of the headlines. He became unable to attend church because he felt compelled to look up all of the references during the sermon. Trials of nearly 35 medications from several different classes provided little to no relief. D had a history of hypertension, diabetes mellitus, and carotid artery disease (total occlusion of the right internal carotid artery with 30–40% stenosis on the left). This latter finding was discovered during a work-up of recurrent brief paresthesias involving the left arm and face, eventually thought to be due to sensory seizures. Neurological examination revealed rare paraphasic errors in spontaneous speech, and mild constructional apraxia, and mild difficulty with Luria sequencing bilaterally. There was generalized hyporeflexia, with absent ankle jerks bilaterally. There was also evidence of bilateral sensory loss in a stocking distribution. A CT scan of the head revealed a 3-by-4-cm wedge-shaped infarct in the posterior right frontal lobe, with extension to the deep subcortical white matter. A $[^{99m}Tc]$ HMPAO SPECT scan revealed hypoperfusion in the area of the infarct, but no other notable abnormalities.*

Recommendations for diagnosis and treatment of obsessive–compulsive symptoms in elderly schizophrenia patients

Research into OCD presented in elderly patients with or without schizophrenia is sparse. Putative clinical implications of obsessive–compulsive symptoms in elderly schizophrenia patients are as follows:

- Similar to youngsters and adults, obsessive–compulsive symptoms are present in elderly schizophrenia patients. The observed prevalence of obsessive–compulsive symptoms comparable to that found in younger schizophrenia patients needs to be replicated in larger independent clinical and community samples of elderly schizophrenia patients. This is particularly important owing to the clinical impact of obsessive–compulsive symptoms in elderly schizophrenia as reflected in an increased rate of readmissions (Prince *et al.*, 2008) and by a reduced quality of well-being (Wetherell *et al.*, 2003) in elderly schizo-obsessive patients compared to individuals with "pure" schizophrenia.

- There are several possible origins of obsessive–compulsive symptoms in elderly patients with schizophrenia. *First*, they may persist into old age running typical to the OCD waxing-and-waning course independent of schizophrenia (Case 6.5). *Second*, late-onset obsessive–compulsive symptoms can follow the age-related brain insults in elderly schizophrenia patients (Case 6.6). Late-onset OCD has been reported in association with stroke, traumatic brain injury, progressive supranuclear palsy, neoplasms, and dementias (Weiss and Jenike, 2000; Voon *et al.*, 2006; Pompanin *et al.*, 2012), which may be superimposed on schizophrenia in elderly individuals. Lesions to the basal ganglia and thalamus and their connected cortical sites (orbitofrontal cortex and anterior cingulate), the brain areas pertinent to the pathophysiology of OCD, most likely contribute to the late occurrence of the disorder (Chacko *et al.*, 2000; Graybiel and Rauch, 2000). *Third*, atypical antipsychotic agents have a potential to induce, exacerbate, or reactivate obsessive–compulsive symptoms in schizophrenia patients in early as well as in the advanced stages of treatment. An additional intriguing yet unresolved question is a possible interrelationship between parkinsonian symptoms induced by typical antipsychotic agents, to which elderly patients are particularly sensitive, and late development of obsessive–compulsive symptoms. Notably, obsessive–compulsive phenomena have consistently been identified in patients with Parkinson's disease (Alegret *et al.*, 2001; Maia *et al.*, 2003), and similar neurocognitive impairments were found in these two disorders with basal ganglia involvement (Hollander *et al.*, 1993).

- Because OCD is an illness that usually emerges in the second or third decade of life, onset after age 50 should alert the physician to possible age-related "organic" causes of obsessive–compulsive symptomatology. Thorough work-up, including laboratory tests, repeated brain imaging, and cognitive (e.g., Mini Mental State Examination) evaluations are essential in the differential diagnosis of late-onset OCD in elderly patients with or without schizophrenia.

- Obsessive–compulsive symptoms in elderly schizophrenia patients seem to be akin to ordinary OCD, echoing the impression that clinical expression of OCD symptoms in elderly patients without schizophrenia is almost identical to that observed in young patients (Jenike, 1991). The diagnosis of OCD in the elderly can be made by the same criteria used for younger patients (American Psychiatric Association, 2000). However, some putative age-related presentations of obsessive–compulsive symptoms were also noted. A few schizophrenia patients with late-onset obsessive–compulsive symptoms similar to their OCD counterparts had distressful intrusive thoughts that they needed to remember names, events, or words (Case 6.7). The emergence of repetitive engagement in memorizing daily events, naming objects, rereading paragraphs, and needing to know trivia may be the direct consequence of a lesion to complex and partially overlapping neural systems that serve to detect, appraise, and react to potential threats (Mataix-Cols *et al.*, 2004). These "new" mental compulsions could also be aimed at counterbalancing the negative consequences of age-related cognitive deficits and to prevent further deterioration (Weiss and Jenike, 2000). Thus, this ritualistic "cognitive" training seems to be adaptive and could reflect the other side of ritualistic "motor" acts, such as compulsive exercising, observed in patients with head-trauma-related OCD, who justify it as an effort to recover physical effectiveness and to neutralize anxiety-provoking OCD symptoms (Berthier *et al.*, 2001; Salinas *et al.*, 2009).

- Treatment of obsessive–compulsive symptoms in elderly schizophrenia patients, akin to their younger counterparts, is recommended when distress and/or functional impairment associated with OCD are clinically significant. Similar to younger patients, adjunctive SRIs for obsessive–compulsive symptoms can be administered only in remitted antipsychotic-treated patients. Because elderly patients frequently take multiple medications, and due to a decrease in cellular, organ, and systems reserves with age, adverse medication interactions are an important clinical concern. The clinical impact of drug–drug interactions varies considerably depending on the extent of the pharmacokinetic effects, genetic polymorphism of metabolic enzyme systems, and involvement of a single or multiple metabolic pathways. Both pharmacokinetic (the effects of one drug on absorption, distribution, metabolism, or excretion of another drug) and pharmacodynamic (the pharmacological activity of interacting drugs) interactions between SRIs and concurrently used medications in elderly patients should be considered (Schellander and Donnerer, 2010). For example, a life-threatening prolongation of the Q–T interval can occur as a result of pharmacokinetic interaction between the tricyclic agent anafranil and antipsychotics. Pharmacodynamic interactions between SSRIs and substances that influence serotonergic neurotransmission in the central nervous system, such as tramadol, the opioid for treatment of pain or anti-migraine triptans (e.g., sumatriptan), may account for an increased risk for serotonin syndrome. Increased bleeding risks when SSRIs are taken concurrently with anticoagulant drugs or cyclo-oxygenase (COX) inhibitors is another example of potentially harmful drug interactions.

In order to avoid drug–drug interactions as far as possible while treating elderly patients, the following general recommendations can be applied to elderly schizo-obsessive patients as well (Mallet et al., 2007):

- If possible, discontinue all the substances that interact strongly
- Review all currently administered drugs for appropriate indication and target the lowest possible effective dose
- Substitute the affected substance by another drug of similar efficacy but lower potential for interactions
- Order monitoring of drug concentration
- Be prepared to discontinue drugs rather than add new ones
- Once an optimal medication profile is selected, observe the patient long enough
- Exchange your experiences with other physicians and document the interaction management in order to promote a continuation of treatment.

Overall, obsessive–compulsive symptoms in adolescents, adults, and elderly patients with schizophrenia across the lifespan provides additional support for their clinical validity. Identification of this potentially treatable condition is imperative to provide adequate care of age-specific groups of schizophrenia patients.

References

Alegret M, Junqué C, Valldeoriola F, et al. (2001) Obsessive–compulsive symptoms in Parkinson's disease. Journal of Neurology, Neurosurgery and Psychiatry 70, 394–396.

Amador XF, Flaum M, Andreasen NC, et al. (1994) Awareness of illness in schizophrenia and schizoaffective and mood disorders. Archives of General Psychiatry 51, 826–836.

American Psychiatric Association (2000) Diagnostic and Statistical Manual of Mental Disorders, 4th edn, text revision. American Psychiatric Association, Washington, DC.

Andreasen NC (1983) The Scale for the Assessment of Negative Symptoms (SANS). University of Iowa, Iowa City, IA.

Berthier ML, Kulisevsky J, Gironell A, López OL (2001) Obsessive-compulsive disorder and traumatic brain injury: behavioral, cognitive, and neuroimaging findings. Neuropsychiatry, Neuropsychology, and Behavioral Neurology 14, 23–31.

Cannon M, Caspi A, Moffitt TE, et al. (2002) Evidence for early-childhood, pan-developmental impairment specific to schizophreniform disorder: results from a longitudinal birth cohort. Archives of General Psychiatry 59, 449–456.

Chacko RC, Corbin MA, Harper RG (2000)
Acquired obsessive-compulsive disorder
associated with basal ganglia lesions. *Journal
of Neuropsychiatry and Clinical Neurosciences*
12, 269–272.

Childs B, Scriver CR (1986) Age at onset and
causes of disease. *Perspectives in Biology and
Medicine* 29, 437–460.

Correll CU (2010) Symptomatic presentation
and initial treatment for schizophrenia in
children and adolescents. *Journal of Clinical
Psychiatry* 71(11), e29.

Correll C, Penzner J, Parikh U, et al. (2006)
Recognizing and monitoring adverse events
of second-generation antipsychotics in
children and adolescents. *Child and
Adolescent Psychiatric Clinics of North
America* 15, 177–206.

Del Beccaro MA, Burke P, McCauley E (1988)
Hallucinations in children: a follow-up study.
*Journal of the American Academy of Child
and Adolescent Psychiatry* 27, 462–465.

Delorme R, Golmard JL, Chabane N, et al.
(2005) Admixture analysis of age at onset in
obsessive-compulsive disorder. *Psychological
Medicine* 35, 237–243.

Eggers C, Bunk D (1997) The long-term course of
childhood-onset schizophrenia: a 42-year
follow-up. *Schizophrenia Bulletin,* 23, 105–117.

Fallon BA, Liebowitz MR, Hollander E, et al.
(1990) The pharmacotherapy of moral or
religious scrupulosity. *Journal of Clinical
Psychiatry* 51, 517–521.

Faragian S, Kurs R, Poyurovsky M (2008)
Insight into obsessive-compulsive symptoms
and awareness of illness in adolescent
schizophrenia patients with and without
OCD. *Child Psychiatry and Human
Development* 39, 39–48.

Findling RL, Kauffman RE, Sallee FR, et al.
(2008) Tolerability and pharmacokinetics of
aripiprazole in children and adolescents with
psychiatric disorders: an open-label, dose-
escalation study. *Journal of Clinical
Psychopharmacology* 28, 441–446.

Folstein MF, Folstein SE, McHugh PR (1975)
"Mini-mental state": a practical method for
grading the cognitive state of patients for the
clinician. *Journal of Psychiatric Research*
12, 189–198.

Garvey MA, Giedd J, Swedo SE (1998)
PANDAS: the search for environmental
triggers of pediatric neuropsychiatric
disorders – lessons from rheumatic fever.
Journal of Child Neurology
13, 413–423.

Geller DA, Biederman J, Jones J, et al. (1998)
Obsessive-compulsive disorder in children
and adolescents: a review. *Harvard Review of
Psychiatry* 5, 260–273.

Glick ID, Poyurovsky M, Ivanova O, Koran LM
(2008) Aripiprazole in schizophrenia patients
with comorbid obsessive-compulsive
symptoms: an open-label study of 15
patients. *Journal of Clinical Psychiatry* 69,
1856–1859.

Gogtay N, Vyas NS, Testa R, Wood SJ,
Pantelis C (2011) Age of onset of
schizophrenia: perspectives from structural
neuroimaging studies. *Schizophrenia
Bulletin* 37, 504–513.

Goodman WK, Price LH, Rasmussen SA, et al.
(1989) The Yale–Brown Obsessive–
Compulsive Scale: I. Development, use, and
reliability. *Archives of General Psychiatry* 46,
1006–1011.

Graybiel AM, Rauch SL (2000) Toward a
neurobiology of obsessive-compulsive
disorder. *Neuron* 28, 343–347.

Häfner H, Nowotny B (1995) Epidemiology of
early-onset schizophrenia. *European Archives
of Psychiatry and Clinical Neuroscience* 245,
80–92.

Hamilton M (1960) A rating scale for
depression. *Journal of Neurology,
Neurosurgery and Psychiatry* 23, 56–62.

Hollander E, Cohen L, Richards M, et al. (1993)
A pilot study of the neuropsychology of
obsessive-compulsive disorder and
Parkinson's disease: basal ganglia disorders.
*Journal of Neuropsychiatry and Clinical
Neurosciences* 5, 104–107.

Hollis C (2000) Adult outcomes of child-
and adolescent-onset schizophrenia:
diagnositc stability and predictive validity.
American Journal of Psychiatry 157,
1652–1659.

Jenike MA (1991) Geriatric obsessive-
compulsive disorder. *Journal of Geriatric
Psychiatry and Neurology* 4, 34–39.

Jones P, Rodgers B, Murray R, Marmot M (1994) Child development risk factors for adult schizophrenia in the British 1946 birth cohort. *Lancet* **344**, 1398–1402.

Kalra SK, Swedo SE (2009) Children with obsessive-compulsive disorder: are they just "little adults"? *Journal of Clinical Investigation* **119**, 737–746.

Kessler RC, Berglund P, Demler O, et al. (2005a) Lifetime prevalence and age-of-onset distributions of DSM-IV disorders in the National Comorbidity Survey Replication. *Archives of General Psychiatry* **62**, 593–602. Erratum *Archives of General Psychiatry* **62**, 768.

Kessler RC, Birnbaum H, Demler O, et al. (2005b) The prevalence and correlates of nonaffective psychosis in the National Comorbidity Survey Replication (NCS-R). *Biological Psychiatry* **58**, 668–676.

Kinros J, Reichenberg A, Frangou S (2010) The neurodevelopmental theory of schizophrenia: evidence from studies of early onset cases. *Israel Journal of Psychiatry and Related Sciences* **47**, 110–117.

Kumra S, Jacobsen LK, Lenane M, et al. (1998) Multidimensionally impaired disorder: is it a variant of very early onset schizophrenia? *Journal of the American Academy of Child and Adolescent Psychiatry* **37**, 91–99.

Kumra S, Oberstar JV, Sikich L, et al. (2008) Efficacy and tolerability of second-generation antipsychotics in children and adolescents with schizophrenia. *Schizophrenia Bulletin* **34**, 60–71.

Kyriakopoulos M, Vyas N, Barker G, Chitnis X, Frangou S (2008) A diffusion tensor imaging study of white matter in early-onset schizophrenia. *Biological Psychiatry* **63**, 519–523.

Lane RM (1998) SSRI-induced extrapyramidal side effects and akathisia: implications for treatment. *Journal of Psychopharmacology* **12**, 192–214.

Leckman JF, Goodman WK, North WG, et al. (1994) The role of central oxytocin in obsessive compulsive disorder and related normal behavior. *Psychoneuroendocrinology* **19**, 723–749.

Leckman JF, Grice DE, Barr LC, et al. (1995) Tic-related vs. non-tic-related obsessive compulsive disorder. *Anxiety* **1**, 208–215.

Leckman JF, Grice DE, Boardman J, et al. (1997) Symptoms of obsessive-compulsive disorder. *American Journal of Psychiatry* **154**, 911–917.

Leckman JF, Denys D, Simpson HB, et al. (2010) Obsessive-compulsive disorder: a review of the diagnostic criteria and possible subtypes and dimensional specifiers for DSM-IV. *Depression and Anxiety* **27**, 507–527.

Maia AF, Pinto AS, Barbosa ER, Menezes PR, Miguel EC (2003) Obsessive-compulsive symptoms, obsessive-compulsive disorder, and related disorders in Parkinson's disease. *Journal of Neuropsychiatry and Clinical Neurosciences* **15**, 371–374.

Maia TV, Cooney RE, Peterson BS (2008) The neural bases of obsessive-compulsive disorder in children and adults. *Development and Psychopathology* **20**, 1251–1283.

Mallet L, Spinewine A, Huang A (2007) The challenge of managing drug interactions in elderly people. *Lancet* **370**, 185–191.

Masi G, Liboni F (2011) Management of schizophrenia in children and adolescents: focus on pharmacotherapy. *Drugs* **71**, 179–208.

Masi G, Mucci M, Pari C (2006) Children with schizophrenia: clinical picture and pharmacological treatment. *CNS Drugs* **20**, 841–866.

Mataix-Cols D, Wooderson S, Lawrence N, et al. (2004) Distinct neural correlates of washing, checking, and hoarding symptom dimensions in obsessive-compulsive disorder. *Archives of General Psychiatry* **61**, 564–576.

McGee R, Williams S, Poulton R (2000) Hallucinations in nonpsychotic children. *Journal of the American Academy of Child and Adolescent Psychiatry* **39**, 12–13.

Miller MC (2004) Questions and answers: what is a repetition compulsion, and how can it be changed? *Harvard Mental Health Letters* **21**, 8.

Nechmad A, Ratzoni G, Poyurovsky M, et al. (2003) Obsessive-compulsive disorder in adolescent schizophrenia patients. American Journal of Psychiatry 160, 1002–1004.

Nicolson R, Lenane M, Hamburger SD, et al. (2000) Lessons from childhood-onset schizophrenia. Brain Research. Brain Research Reviews 31, 147–156.

Nicolson R, Brookner FB, Lenane M, et al. (2003) Parental schizophrenia spectrum disorders in childhood-onset and adult-onset schizophrenia. American Journal of Psychiatry 160, 490–495.

Olfson M, Blanco C, Liu L, Moreno C, Laje G (2006) National trends in the outpatient treatment of children and adolescents with antipsychotic drugs. Archives of General Psychiatry 63, 679–685.

Paus T, Keshavan M, Giedd JN (2008) Why do many psychiatric disorders emerge during adolescence? Nature Reviews Neuroscience 9, 947–957.

Pauls DL (2008) The genetics of obsessive compulsive disorder: a review of the evidence. American Journal of Medical Genetics Part C Seminars in Medical Genetics 148, 133–139.

Pompanin S, Perini G, Toffanin T, et al. (2012) Late-onset OCD as presenting manifestation of semantic dementia. General Hospital Psychiatry 34, 102.e1–4.

Poyurovsky M, Dorfman-Etrog P, Hermesh H, et al. (2000) Beneficial effect of olanzapine in schizophrenic patients with obsessive-compulsive symptoms. International Clinical Psychopharmacology 15, 169–173.

Poyurovsky M, Bergman J, Weizman R (2006) Obsessive-compulsive disorder in elderly schizophrenia patients. Journal of Psychiatric Research 40, 189–191.

Poyurovsky M, Faragian S, Shabeta A, Kosov A (2008) Comparison of clinical characteristics, comorbidity and pharmacotherapy in adolescent schizophrenia patients with and without obsessive-compulsive disorder. Psychiatry Research 159, 133–139.

Prince JD, Akincigil A, Kalay E, et al. (2008) Psychiatric rehospitalization among elderly persons in the United States. Psychiatric Services 59, 1038–1045.

Rabinowitz J, Levine SZ, Hafner H (2006) A population based elaboration of the role of age of onset on the course of schizophrenia. Schizophrenia Research 88, 96–101.

Rapoport JL, Gogtay N (2011) Childhood onset schizophrenia: support for a progressive neurodevelopmental disorder. International Journal of Developmental Neuroscience 29, 251–258.

Ratzoni G, Gothelf D, Brand-Gothelf A, et al. (2002) Weight gain associated with olanzapine and risperidone in adolescent patients: a comparative prospective study. Journal of the American Academy of Child and Adolescent Psychiatry 41, 337–343.

Rodowski MF, Cagande CC, Riddle MA (2008) Childhood obsessive-compulsive disorder presenting as schizophrenia spectrum disorders. Journal of Child and Adolescent Psychopharmacology 18, 395–401.

Ross RG, Heinlein S, Tregellas H (2006) High rates of comorbidity are found in childhood-onset schizophrenia. Schizophrenia Research 88, 90–95.

Rotge JY, Langbour N, Guehl D, et al. (2010) Gray matter alterations in obsessive-compulsive disorder: an anatomic likelihood estimation meta-analysis. Neuropsychopharmacology 35, 686–691.

Russell AT (1994) The clinical presentation of childhood onset schizophrenia. Schizophrenia Bulletin 20, 631–646.

Salinas C, Davila G, Berthier ML, Green C, Lara JP (2009) Late-life reactivation of obsessive-compulsive disorder associated with lesions in prefrontal-subcortical circuits. Journal of Neuropsychiatry and Clinical Neurosciences 21, 332–334.

Sasson Y, Chopra M, Harrari E, Amitai K, Zohar J (2003) Bipolar comorbidity: from diagnostic dilemmas to therapeutic challenge. International Journal of Neuropsychopharmacology 6, 139–144.

Schellander R, Donnerer J (2010) Antidepressants: clinically relevant drug interactions to be considered. *Pharmacology* **86**, 203–215.

Sikich L, Frazier JA, McClellan J, et al. (2008) Double-blind comparison of first- and second-generation antipsychotics in early-onset schizophrenia and schizo-affective disorder: findings from the Treatment of Early-Onset Schizophrenia Spectrum Disorders (TEOSS) Study. *American Journal of Psychiatry* **165**, 1420–1431.

Skoog G, Skoog I (1999) A 40-year follow-up of patients with obsessive-compulsive disorder. *Archives of General Psychiatry* **56**, 121–127.

Sobin C, Blundell ML, Karayiorgou M (2000) Phenotypic differences in early- and late-onset obsessive-compulsive disorder. *Comprehensive Psychiatry* **41**, 373–379.

Sporn AL, Greenstein DK, Gogtay N, et al. (2003) Progressive brain volume loss during adolescence in childhood-onset schizophrenia. *American Journal Psychiatry* **60**, 2181–2189.

Swedo SE, Rapoport JL, Leonard H, Lenane M, Cheslow D (1989) Obsessive-compulsive disorder in children and adolescents: clinical phenomenology of 70 consecutive cases. *Archives of General Psychiatry* **46**, 335–341.

Swedo SE, Leonard HL, Garvey M, et al. (1998) Pediatric autoimmune neuropsychiatric disorders associated with streptococcal infections: clinical description of the first 50 cases. *American Journal of Psychiatry* **155**, 264–271. Erratum *American Journal of Psychiatry* **155**, 578.

Szeszko PR, MacMillan S, McMeniman M, et al. (2004) Brain structural abnormalities in psychotropic drug-naive pediatric patients with obsessive-compulsive disorder. *American Journal of Psychiatry* **161**, 1049–1056.

Szeszko PR, Christian C, Macmaster F, et al. (2008) Gray matter structural alterations in psychotropic drug-naive pediatric obsessive-compulsive disorder: an optimized voxel-based morphometry study. *American Journal of Psychiatry* **165**, 1299–1307.

Thompson PM, Vidal C, Giedd JN, et al. (2001) Mapping adolescent brain change reveals dynamic wave of accelerated gray matter loss in very early-onset schizophrenia. *Proceedings of the National Academy of Sciences of the United States of America* **98**, 11 650–11 655.

Thompson PM Bartzokis G, Hayashi KM, et al. (2009) Time-lapse mapping of cortical changes in schizophrenia with different treatments. *Cerebral Cortex* **19**, 1107–1123.

van Grootheest DS, Cath DC, Beekman AT, Boomsma DI (2005) Twin studies on obsessive-compulsive disorder: a review. *Twin Research and Human Genetics* **8**, 450–458.

Voon V, Hassan K, Zurowski M, et al. (2006) Prevalence of repetitive and reward-seeking behaviors in Parkinson disease. *Neurology* **67**, 1254–1257.

Watson HI, Rees CS (2008) Meta-analysis of randomized, controlled treatment trials for pediatric obsessive-compulsive disorder. *Journal of Child Psychology and Psychiatry* **49**, 489–498.

Weiss AP, Jenike MA (2000) Late-onset obsessive-compulsive disorder: a case series. *Journal of Neuropsychiatry and Clinical Neurosciences* **12**, 265–268.

Wetherell JL, Palmer BW, Thorp SR, et al. (2003) Anxiety symptoms and quality of life in middle-aged and older outpatients with schizophrenia and schizoaffective disorder. *Journal of Clinical Psychiatry* **64**, 1476–1482.

Whiteside SP, Port JD, Abramowitz JS (2004) A meta-analysis of functional neuroimaging in obsessive-compulsive disorder. *Psychiatry Research* **132**, 69–79.

Zarei M, Mataix-Cols D, Heyman I, et al. (2011) Changes in gray matter volume and white matter microstructure in adolescents with obsessive-compulsive disorder. *Biological Psychiatry* **70**, 1083–1090.

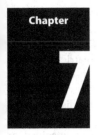

OCD-spectrum disorders in schizophrenia

As previously discussed, exclusion rules in the hierarchical design of the diagnostic system for psychiatric disorders prevent clinicians from "seeing" additional syndromes in schizophrenia and hamper the study of their clinical validity. Abandonment of hierarchical classification led to a proliferation of studies examining "non-schizophrenic" syndromes in schizophrenia patients that unequivocally determined that schizophrenia is a highly comorbid disorder with a substantial proportion of patients exhibiting one or more additional psychiatric syndromes during the lifespan. Substance-use disorders, major depressive disorder (MDD), and anxiety disorders (e.g., panic disorder, social phobia) are frequently diagnosed comorbidities in schizophrenia (Bermanzohn *et al.*, 2000). Similarly, OCD has also been strongly associated with MDD and anxiety disorders (Nestadt *et al.*, 2001; Diniz *et al.*, 2004), as well as body dysmorphic disorder (BDD), hypochondriasis, tic disorders, and eating disorders. It has been suggested that some comorbid psychiatric conditions, primarily BDD and tic disorders, may share common etiologic pathways with OCD, while others (e.g., MDD) may represent secondary syndromes (McElroy *et al.*, 1994; Nestadt *et al.*, 2001; Hollander *et al.*, 2008). Indeed, considerable overlap has been found in the clinical presentation, familial inheritance, basal ganglia dysfunction, and pharmacotherapy between BDD, tic disorders, and OCD, supporting the existence of a putative OCD-spectrum of disorders (Phillips *et al.*, 2010).

Studies that explicitly evaluate the co-occurrence of additional psychiatric syndromes in schizo-obsessive patients have begun to emerge. Hence, comorbid OCD in schizophrenia patients (de Haan *et al.*, 2011) was associated with more severe depressive symptoms as assessed by the Montgomery–Asberg Depression Scale (Montgomery and Asberg, 1979). Consistent with these findings, schizo-obsessive patients are more likely to experience greater levels of hopelessness, prefer avoidant coping strategies, and show more depressive symptoms (Lysaker *et al.*, 2000; 2006). Moreover, OCD appeared to be an independent risk factor for suicidal ideation and suicide attempts in schizophrenia patients (Sevincok *et al.*, 2007). A trend toward a higher rate of anxiety disorders (Rajkumar *et al.*, 2008) in schizo-obsessive patients has also been noted.

The question is whether there are generally more additional psychiatric syndromes in schizo-obsessive patients. Or alternatively, is the presence of obsessive–compulsive symptoms in schizophrenia associated with a specific aggregation of disorders considered to be related to the OCD-spectrum? Elucidation of this topic has clinical implications and may affect research into underlying mechanisms of a schizo-obsessive subgroup. One proposed hypothesis suggested that if obsessive–compulsive symptoms represent a separate psychopathological dimension, a preferential aggregation of OCD-spectrum disorders in schizo-obsessive patients akin to typical OCD would be plausible. Indeed, the results of such evaluation show that OCD-spectrum disorders do aggregate in schizo-obsessive patients but not in their non-OCD schizophrenia counterparts (Poyurovsky *et al.*, 2006).

In this study, psychiatric comorbid disorders, as evaluated using the SCID, were defined as the presence of additional lifetime or concurrent DSM-IV Axis I psychiatric diagnoses. Participants were screened for MDD, substance-use disorders, anxiety disorders (panic disorder with and without agoraphobia, social, and specific phobia), BDD, hypochondriasis, and eating disorders (anorexia nervosa, bulimia nervosa). Chronic tic disorders and Tourette's syndrome were diagnosed using additional modules based on DSM-IV criteria. For the diagnosis of BDD the presence of typical preoccupation with an imagined or exaggerated bodily defect associated with significant distress and/or functional impairment not related to schizophrenia symptoms was required. If preoccupation with bodily defect was exclusively restricted to patients' delusional or hallucinatory experience, such cases were not included. Similar requirements were applied to the diagnosis of hypochondriasis. The false belief regarding a serious illness despite the absence of pathological findings on medical examination had no delusional intensity and had to cause distress or functional impairment. OCD-spectrum disorders were defined as the sum of the rates of occurrence of BDD, hypochondriasis, eating disorders (anorexia nervosa, bulimia nervosa), and tic disorders (chronic tic disorder or Tourette's syndrome [TS]). Stepwise logistic regression was used to analyze differences in comorbid disorders between the study groups that included schizophrenia with and without OCD, OCD, and healthy controls.

As expected, more than half of the schizophrenia patients that participated in the study had at least one additional Axis I psychiatric disorder, substantiating the view that schizophrenia is a highly comorbid disorder (Table 7.1). Major depressive disorder was the most frequently co-occurring disorder, followed by anxiety disorders. Consistent with the hypothesis, there was a robust differentiation between the two schizophrenia groups with respect to combined OCD-spectrum disorders evaluated in the study. This difference was accounted for primarily by the substantially higher rate of tic disorders and BDD in the schizo-obsessive group compared to the non-OCD schizophrenia group. There was also a higher rate of comorbid eating disorders in the schizo-obsessive group; however, the difference was no longer significant after adjustment for age at onset of illness. Overall, combining OCD-spectrum disorders yielded a robust between-group difference in a number of patients with at least one OCD-spectrum disorder (schizo-obsessive 30/100 patients vs. schizophrenia 8/100 patients; odds ratio [OR] = 4.35, 95% CI = 2.13–11.41, $p < 0.001$, adjusted for onset of schizophrenia) (Table 7.2). Moreover, patients who had two comorbid OCD-spectrum disorders were found only in the schizo-obsessive group (8 vs. 0, $\chi^2 = 8.33$, $p = 0.0039$). In contrast, no significant between-group difference in the rate of MDD and anxiety disorders was revealed. These findings strongly suggest that there is a specific elevation in the rate of OCD-spectrum disorders in the schizo-obsessive group rather than an elevation of psychopathology in general. The revealed comparable rates of OCD-spectrum disorders in the schizo-obsessive and OCD groups that are both substantially higher than in the non-OCD schizophrenia group further substantiate a preferential aggregation of OCD-spectrum disorders in schizo-obsessive patients.

It is worth noting that the odds of having substance-use disorders, primarily cannabis and nicotine dependence, in the schizo-obsessive group were half those found in the non-OCD schizophrenia group, and comparable with the "pure" OCD group (Table 7.2). In accordance with this observation the findings from a large-scale study demonstrated inverse correlation between nicotine use and a severity of obsessive–compulsive symptoms in schizo-obsessive patients (de Haan *et al.*, 2011). The authors assumed that patients

Table 7.1 Comorbid Axis I psychiatric disorders in schizophrenia patients with and without obsessive–compulsive disorder (OCD), OCD, and healthy controls[a]

Comorbid diagnosis	Schizophrenia with OCD (N = 100)	Schizophrenia without OCD (N = 100)	OCD (N = 35)		Healthy controls (N = 161)	
	N (%)[b]	N (%)[b]	N	%	N	%
Any Axis I disorders	57	52	28	80.0	15	9.3
Any OCD-spectrum disorders	30	8	15	42.9	0	
Anorexia nervosa	9	2	1	2.9	0	
Bulimia nervosa	3	2	1	2.9	0	
Hypochondriasis	2	0	2	5.8	0	
Body dysmorphic disorder	8	0	3	8.6	0	
Tic disorders	16	4	12	34.3	0	
Major depressive disorder	28	32	23	65.7	7	4.3
Substance-use disorders	9	21	1	2.9	3	1.9
Any anxiety disorders	17	12	11	31.5	7	4.3
Panic disorder (with and without agoraphobia)	7	4	10	20.0	2	1.2
Social phobia	4	5	3	8.6	1	0.6
Specific phobia	6	3	1	2.9	5	3.1

[a] Some patients had more than one comorbid disorder.
[b] Since the sample size is 100, the number of patients equals percentage.
Source: From Poyurovsky M, Fuchs C, Faragian S, Kriss V, Weisman G, Pashinian A, Weizman R, Weizman A (2006) Preferential aggregation of obsessive–compulsive spectrum disorders in schizophrenia patients with obsessive–compulsive disorder. *Canadian Journal of Psychiatry* **51**, 746–754. Reprinted with permission.

with schizophrenia and OCD have a lower propensity to smoke or that, alternatively, smoking may diminish obsessive–compulsive symptoms. While the rate of smoking among schizophrenia patients is almost 80%, patients with OCD tend to smoke less than the general population (Bejerot and Humble, 2007). If confirmed, the presence of OCD in schizophrenia may serve as a "protective factor" against nicotine dependence, similar to ordinary OCD. This however may not hold true for alcohol-related and some other substance-use disorders. Notably, no significant differences were found in their prevalence between those with OCD and the general population (Murphy *et al.*, 2010).

Tic disorders in schizophrenia

Tics typically refer to sudden, rapid, recurrent, non-rhythmic motor movements, such as blinking or head-nodding, or vocalizations, such as sniffing or throat clearing, usually appearing in bouts while waxing and waning in frequency, intensity, and kind of tic. Tic disorders, including Tourette's syndrome (TS) which encompasses the combination of chronic (more than 1 year) motor and vocal tics, typically onset in childhood around the age of 5 years (Olson, 2004). Additional symptoms are echolalia (automatic repetition of vocalizations made by others), echopraxia (automatic repetitive mimicking of others),

Table 7.2 Results of stepwise logistic regression for the OCD-spectrum and the additional comorbid disorders between the schizophrenia with and without OCD groups and the OCD group

Comorbid diagnosis	Comparison between the two schizophrenia groups (with and without OCD)			Comparison between the schizo-obsessive and the OCD group		
	OR	95% CI	p	OR	95% CI	p
Any Axis I disorders	1.22	0.70 to 2.14	NS	0.33	0.13 to 0.83	0.027
Any OCD-spectrum disorders	4.35^a	2.13 to 11.41	0.001	0.57	0.23 to 1.26	NS
Eating disorders	3.27^a	1.02 to 10.52	NS	2.25	0.48 to 10.60	NS
Hypochondriasis^b			NS	0.34	0.05 to 2.49	NS
Body dysmorphic disorder^c			0.0039	0.93	0.23 to 3.71	NS
Tic disorders	4.57	1.47 to 14.21	0.018	0.37	0.15 to 0.88	0.044
Major depressive disorder	0.83	0.45 to 1.51	NS	0.20	0.09 to 0.46	0.0003
Substance-use disorders	0.40^b	0.16 to 0.96	NS	2.96	0.36 to 24.53	NS
Any anxiety disorders	1.32	0.57 to 3.06	NS	0.31	0.13 to 0.77	0.016

^{a} Adjusted for age at onset of schizophrenia.
^{b} Zero frequency in the non-OCD schizophrenia group.
^{c} Adjusted for the duration of schizophrenia.
NS, not significant.
Source: From Poyurovsky M, Fuchs C, Faragian S, Kriss V, Weisman G, Pashinian A, Weizman R, Weizman A (2006) Preferential aggregation of obsessive–compulsive spectrum disorders in schizophrenia patients with obsessive–compulsive disorder. *Canadian Journal of Psychiatry* **51**, 746–754. Reprinted with permission.

palilalia (repetition or echoing of one's own spoken words), and coprolalia (involuntary utterance of obscene words).

Studies of the pathophysiology of tic disorders and schizophrenia revealed similarities that suggest overlapping mechanisms. Alterations in brain areas within the cortical–striatal–thalamic–cortical circuits with reduced intracortical inhibition shown in studies using transcranial magnetic stimulation (TMS) and a saccadic movements paradigm, has been proposed for tic disorders as well as schizophrenia (Ziemann et al., 1997; Muller et al., 2002; Albin and Mink, 2006; Bohlhalter et al., 2006; Wang et al., 2011). Both disorders also share hyperactivity of dopaminergic neurotransmission in the striatum, shown in positron-emission tomography (PET) raclopride studies using amphetamine challenge, altered metabolic activity in the frontal cortex, impaired executive cognitive functioning, and sensory and sensorimotor gating deficits (Eidelberg et al., 1997; Stern et al., 2000; Swerdlow et al., 2008; Wong et al., 2008). Exacerbation of symptoms after administration of dopamine receptor agonists (e.g., amphetamines) and therapeutic response to dopamine D_2 receptor antagonists are among the most salient features of the two disorders. Although evidence for deviances in the dopaminergic system is emerging, other imbalances, such as in the serotoninergic, noradrenergic, glutamatergic, gamma-aminobutyric acid (GABA)-ergic, cholinergic, and opioid metabolism in tic disorders and TS seem probable, akin to schizophrenia (Swain et al., 2007). Moreover, there is increasing evidence that those systems play interactively together, especially the dopaminergic and the serotoninergic system (Roessner et al., 2011). Additionally, comparable to schizophrenia, only a minority of tic disorder patients (roughly 12%) does not exhibit additional psychiatric disorders (Freeman *et al.*, 2000). OCD, anxiety, affective disorders, substance-use disorders, and attention deficit hyperactivity disorder (ADHD) are common co-occurring disorders in TS patients.

Owing to notable neurobiological and clinical similarities between schizophrenia and tic disorders, studies have examined a comorbidity of the two disorders. In a study of 666 TS patients only 0.5% had schizophrenic psychopathology (Shapiro *et al.*, 1972), while Takeuchi *et al.* (1986) estimated a 4% prevalence of schizophrenia in the TS patient population. Reviewing the charts of 399 TS patients consecutively seen in a specialized TS clinic over a 30-year time-span, Kerbeshian *et al.* (2009) identified only 10 patients who met DSM-IV criteria for both TS and schizophrenic disorder. Likewise, no TS cases and only two cases of tic disorder were identified in 62 schizophrenia inpatients in one of the few reports on the prevalence of tic disorders in schizophrenia and other psychiatric disorders (Eapen *et al.*, 2001). It seems that the rate of occurrence of full-blown schizophrenia in patients with tic disorders is not substantially higher than that in the general population (Robertson, 2000). None of the above studies, however, aimed to explicitly compare the rate of occurrence of tic disorders in schizophrenia patients with and without comorbid OCD.

When schizophrenia patients were stratified on subgroups based on an additional DSM-IV diagnosis of OCD, a striking difference in the rate of co-occurring tic disorders was indeed found (Poyurovsky *et al.*, 2006). *First*, there was a clinically meaningful rate of occurrence (16%) of tic disorders in a schizo-obsessive group. Second, the odds for having tic disorders in the schizo-obsessive group were four times higher than in the schizophrenia group (16% vs. 4%). Markedly, in the "pure" OCD group, the frequency of tic disorders was the typical 35% found in the literature (Phillips *et al.*, 2010). The intermediate frequency of tic disorders in the schizo-obsessive group suggests a continuum between OCD, schizo-obsessive disorder, and schizophrenia. Remarkably, only a few cases of TS were found among schizophrenia patients with tic disorders. It has been suggested that TS and chronic tic disorders are part of the same disease entity, with the former being a more complex form of tic disorders (Saccomani *et al.*, 2005). The underlying mechanism of this distinct association of TS with typical but not schizophrenia-related OCD is yet to be revealed.

Clinical characteristics of tic disorders in schizophrenia

As emerged from our systematic evaluation of tic disorders in schizophrenia, similar to "ordinary" tics, among schizo-obsessive patients there is a fourfold predominance of men and the mean age of onset of tic disorders was 7.1 ± 1.3 years. In all cases tics preceded the emergence of schizophrenia, and preceded or emerged concurrently with symptoms of OCD in schizo-obsessive patients. Thus, the sequence of disorders was characteristically tic disorder – OCD – schizophrenia. These findings are consistent with clinical descriptions of tic disorders in schizophrenia that showed a preponderance in men and the precedence of tic disorders to schizophrenia symptoms (Sandyk and Bamford, 1988; Escobar and Bernardo, 1993; Wagle and Staley, 1999; Muller *et al.*, 2002).

Chronic tics were more common than a transient form of the disorder. Simple motor tics – eye-blinking, neck-jerking, facial grimacing – were the most prevalent, while

Table 7.3 Differential diagnosis of tic disorders in schizophrenia

Catatonic signs; stereotypy, mannerisms

Extrapyramidal side effects (e.g., acute dystonia, akathisia, tardive dyskinesia)

Antipsychotic-induced tics

General medical conditions (e.g., Wilson's disease)

Substance-induced tics (e.g., stimulants)

Compulsions

complex motor tics were rare. Similar to patients with typical tic disorders, some schizophrenia patients with tic disorders experience the tics as intentional movements and can temporarily suppress them. Though a few patients had severe tics, in roughly 75% of the cases, the severity of the tics was mild to moderate. Finally, no demographic or other clinical differences were found between schizophrenia patients with and without tic disorders.

Differential diagnosis of tic disorders in schizophrenia

Differential diagnosis of tic disorders in schizophrenia is challenging (Table 7.3). Motor and vocal symptoms including echophenomena (echolalia, echopraxia), repetitive, stereotypic movements, or bizarre gestures and grimacing also often occur in schizophrenia, particularly in the catatonic subtype. Motor tics can be mistaken for mannerisms and stereotypic movements of schizophrenia or may be masked by the use of antipsychotic agents; both factors might lead to an underestimation of the true prevalence of tic disorders in schizophrenia. Additionally, clinical and population-based studies indicate that up to 80% of individuals with tic disorders experience a significant decrease in the tic during adolescence and by age 18 intensity and frequency of the tics decreases to a level that tic-related impairment is no longer exhibited, although objective ratings indicate mild tic severity (Pappert et al., 2003). The same might hold true for tic disorders comorbid to schizophrenia. Alternatively, it is possible that treatment of tic disorders with antipsychotic agents may mask or delay the onset of schizophrenic illness, further obscuring the links between the two disorders. Differentiation of simple tics (e.g., eye-blinking) from complex stereotypic movements is relatively easy. The distinction between complex motor tics and stereotypic movements is less clear-cut. In general, stereotyped movements appear to be more driven and intentional, and tics have a more involuntary quality and are not rhythmic. It is sometimes quite difficult to distinguish between tic disorders and antipsychotic-induced extrapyramidal side effects (acute dystonia, akathisia, tardive dyskinesia). Thorough assessment of clinical expressions of motor phenomena is essential. Dystonic movements are slower, twisting movements interspersed with prolonged states of muscular tension. Akathisia is characterized by a sense of leg restlessness accompanied by characteristic restless movements. Choreoathetoid movements of tardive dyskinesia are slow, irregular, writhing movements, most frequently in fingers and toes, but often involving the face and neck. Analysis of the temporal relationship between motor phenomena and antipsychotic treatment may assist in differential diagnosis. Additionally, a diagnosis may be

Table 7.4 Comparison between tic disorders, OCD and movement disorders in schizophrenia

Tic disorder	OCD	Schizophrenia
Sudden, short (jerking)	Ritualized	Mechanical repetition of speed or physical activities
Fragmented movements	Goal-directed behavior	Stereotypic behavior
Sensorimotor urges	Thoughts/imaginations	Delusions/hallucinations
Not related to anxiety	Mostly related to anxiety	Mostly related to psychosis
Ego-syntonic	Ego-dystonic	Ego-syntonic
Involuntary	Voluntary	Voluntary
Waxing and waning	Waxing and waning	Chronic
Also during sleep	Not during sleep	Not during sleep
Suppressible (short-term)	Suppressible (long-term)	Suppressible

Source: Modified from Cath DC, Hedderly T, Ludolph AG, *et al.* (2011) European clinical guidelines for Tourette syndrome and other tic disorders. Part I: Assessment. *European Child and Adolescent Psychiatry* **20**, 155–171. Reprinted with permission.

complicated by the potential of typical and atypical antipsychotics and clozapine to induce acute or tardive tics and TS in schizophrenia patients (Klawans *et al.*, 1978; Lindenmayer *et al.*, 1995; Reid, 2004). In schizo-obsessive patients, tics must be distinguished from compulsions. Compulsions are typically quite complex, more cognitively driven, and goal-directed, and are performed in response to an obsession or according to rules that the patients rigidly apply. In contrast to compulsions, tics are typically less complex and are not aimed at neutralizing anxiety that results in obsessions. At times, it may be difficult to distinguish apparent goal-directed complex motor tics from compulsions, which are not always preceded by obsessions. When tics and obsessive-compulsive symptoms co-occur in schizophrenia patients both diagnoses are warranted, as was the case in 16% of the schizo-obsessive patients in our study (Poyurovsky *et al.*, 2006). Complex motor tics, such as the repetitive touching of objects or people, repetitive mimicking others (echopraxia), repetitive obscene movements (copropraxia), are the most diagnostically challenging in schizophrenia. Finally, it is essential to perform a comprehensive medical work-up to rule out common medical causes of tic disorders (e.g., Huntington's disease, Wilson's disease, Sydenham's chorea) and substance-induced (e.g., stimulants) tics (Table 7.4).

Treatment of tic disorders in schizophrenia

Clinical experience and research findings show that in a majority of schizophrenia patients co-occurring tic disorders are of mild-to-moderate severity and do not require specific therapeutic intervention. However, some tic disorders are severe and need to be addressed. For many years, typical neuroleptics with their marked dopamine D_2 receptor antagonism were mainstream treatment for both schizophrenia and tic disorders (Shapiro and Shapiro, 1998). The two potent D_2 antagonists, haloperidol and pimozide, have consistently been shown to produce a beneficial therapeutic effect on tics in randomized controlled trials (Ross and Moldofsky, 1978). In daily clinical practice, doses such as 1–4 mg/day for haloperidol and 2–4 mg/day for pimozide, which are lower than dosages usually administered in schizophrenia, are typically used to treat tic disorders. There is a high correlation between D_2 receptor occupancy and unfavorable adverse reactions, such as prolactinemia and EPS (Kapur and Mamo, 2003). It has also been reported that akathisia frequently occurred with typical antipsychotics (Weiden and Bruun, 1987). Moreover, the risk of tardive dyskinesia, a potentially debilitating and treatment-persistent adverse reaction, also should be taken into account when choosing treatment. Atypical antipsychotics, that showed therapeutic efficacy in both tic disorders and schizophrenia, have a significantly lower risk of EPS and tardive dyskinesia. In a thorough review, Roessner et al. (2011) reported that among atypical antipsychotics, risperidone exhibited the best evidence for treatment of tic disorders without symptoms of schizophrenia. Hence, risperidone seems to be an adequate choice for treatment for clinically significant tic disorders in schizophrenia patients; however, its optimal dose range in this subgroup has not yet been defined. Besides, rare cases of exacerbation of both tics and obsessive–compulsive symptoms in risperidone-treated schizophrenia patients have also been reported (Su et al., 2008). Findings regarding the therapeutic efficacy of olanzapine, quetiapine, and ziprasidone in patients with tic disorders are less consistent and their clinical utility in schizophrenia patients with tics is not clear (Roessner et al., 2011). Aripiprazole, a partial dopamine agonist, with additional partial agonistic activity at 5HT-1A receptors and antagonism at 5HT-2A receptors, seems to be a promising option for patients with tic disorders especially in those who did not respond to or could not tolerate previous trials of medication for tics (Lyon et al., 2009). This is particularly noteworthy since aripiprazole in a flexible dose (10–30 mg/day) appeared to be efficacious in some schizophrenia patients with obsessive–compulsive symptoms during a 6-week open-label trial (Glick et al., 2008). Aripiprazole's relatively low cardio-metabolic and weight-gain potential, but meaningful risk for akathisia among the other side effects, need to be considered. Clozapine, an antipsychotic agent often used for patients with treatment-resistant schizophrenia, has not been found helpful in the treatment of tic disorders. Moreover, it has been reported that among schizophrenia patients clozapine administration may exacerbate tics, along with stuttering (Begum, 2005). The emergence of tics and obsessive–compulsive symptoms in schizophrenia patients during clozapine administration and withdrawal was also described (Poyurovsky et al., 1998). The role of non-antipsychotic medications effective in controlling tics, such as the α2-adrenergic agonist clonidine, in schizophrenia patients with tic disorders merits investigation (Roessner et al., 2011). Finally, since selective serotonin reuptake inhibitors (SSRIs) are frequently used in addition to antipsychotics to address obsessive–compulsive symptoms in schizo-obsessive patients, elucidation of their therapeutic benefits and risks in patients with triple comorbidity (schizophrenia, OCD, tic disorders) is imperative. The potential of SSRIs to induce tics should be acknowledged (Fennig et al., 1994). Evidence-based treatment for schizophrenia patients with comorbid tic disorders, and especially for the schizo-obsessive subgroup where tic disorders seem to aggregate, is to be determined.

Following are case vignettes portraying schizophrenia patients with comorbid tic disorders.

Case 7.1. A schizophrenia patient with Tourette's syndrome and OCD (Escobar and Bernardo, 1993).

Ms. D, a 26-year-old divorced woman, began to have involuntary, repetitive, recurrent, and stereotyped motor movements when she was 10 years old. These movements later changed from facial grimacing to head, neck, and superior-limb movement. She also made guttural sounds, coughed, and had dirty words episodes. Since adolescence she exhibited washing, voiding, and cleaning rituals. She was aware of the absurdity of her behavior. Almost 2 years before her first hospitalization, she started to hallucinate, hearing voices that told her how to act. Six months before admission she said that the TV newscaster spoke about her and that there were microphones in her bedroom. During this time her motor and vocal tics and her cleaning and voiding rituals worsened. She was then admitted to a hospital. On admission, she was agitated and had simple and complex cephalic and upper-limb motor tics and simple and complex vocal tics. She was distracted and emotionally labile. Her thought was circumstantial, with bizarre and persecutory delusions and ideas of reference. She also had auditory hallucinations. Serum chemistries were within normal limits. EEG was normal. CT brain scan was reported normal. Inpatient treatment consisted of haloperidol (10 mg/day) with a subsequent addition of clomipramine (225 mg/day). Tics disappeared after a few days of treatment. An improvement in delusions, hallucinations, and obsessive–compulsive symptoms was later noted.

Case 7.2. A schizophrenia patient with a chronic tic disorder.

Mr. D, a 21-year-old former student, had a history of chronic motor tic disorder involving face and neck since age 6. In addition his psychiatric history included symptoms of impulsiveness, hyperactivity, and distractibility. During the course of his illness he was consecutively treated with methylphenidate, pimozide, and haloperidol. His family history was remarkable in that his father suffered from schizophrenia and his aunt had a tic disorder. On examination, D had motor tics of his face and shoulder that were exacerbated by emotional stress. No vocal tics were present. In addition, D exhibited clear-cut psychotic symptoms. He reported hearing voices that were threatening in nature, and he also admitted to auditory hallucinations. His thought content and process were idiosyncratic and disorganized. An EEG, CT, blood and urine tests were normal. He met DSM-IV criteria for both schizophrenic disorder, undifferentiated type, and chronic tic disorder. Symptoms of schizophrenia responded beneficially to treatment with risperidone (3 mg/day) which led to almost complete disappearance of motor tics and continuous improvement of schizophrenic symptoms.

Case 7.3. A schizophrenia patient with a chronic tic disorder and OCD.

Mr. T, a 29-year-old single, unemployed man. His first motor tics, involving eyes, face, and shoulders, were detected at the age of 7. Approximately 3 years later, T exhibited typical ego-dystonic rituals including repeated counting before meals, brushing his teeth, and keeping his belongings in symmetry in response to aggressive and sexual obsessions. His first contact with a psychiatrist was at age 14, when the diagnoses of chronic tic disorders and OCD were established after organic causes were ruled out. At 17, he started complaining about voices that said derogatory things about him. Over the next 5 years, hallucinations became worse and he also developed Schneiderian first-rank symptoms (thought insertion, thought broadcast, passivity phenomena). DSM-IV schizophrenic disorder was added to his diagnoses. Schizophrenic symptoms responded *poorly to adequate trials of perphenazine (up to 32 mg/day) and olanzapine (15 mg/day). A substantial improvement in the intensity of positive schizophrenic symptoms was achieved 8 weeks after the initiation of clozapine. Subsequently, sertraline (up to 150 mg/day) was added to clozapine (200 mg/day) to treat obsessive–compulsive symptoms that exacerbated during clozapine treatment. The patient gave up some of his rituals (symmetry and brushing his teeth) but persisted with others (counting). His tic disorders also persisted, were of substantial severity and caused distress. Risperidone (1.5 mg/day) was then added to the ongoing combination of clozapine and sertraline and the tics decreased substantially in frequency and intensity. Additional improvement in obsessive–compulsive symptoms was also observed.*

Body dysmorphic disorder in schizophrenia

The term "dysmorphophobia" was coined by the Italian psychiatrist Morselli to describe "a subjective feeling of ugliness or physical defect that patients feel is noticeable to others, although their appearance is within normal limits" (Morselli, 1891).

Body dysmorphic disorder as a separate disorder

In DSM-III, dysmorphophobia applied to "individuals who are preoccupied with some imagined defect in physical appearance that is out of proportion to any actual physical abnormality that may exist," and was an example of an atypical somatoform disorder that had no specific diagnostic criteria (American Psychiatric Association, 1980). Dysmorphophobia was accorded separate diagnostic status in the somatoform section of DSM-III-R, and was called body dysmorphic disorder (BDD), because "dysmorphophobia" was a misnomer considering that the disorder does not involve phobic avoidance (American Psychiatric Association, 1987). In the current edition of DSM (DSM-IV-TR) (American Psychiatric Association, 2000), BDD is also classified as a somatoform disorder.

Although for decades dysmorphophobia has been referred to as a non-delusional syndrome, the term was also used, primarily by European psychiatrists, to describe a preoccupation of delusional intensity, and the disorder was seen as one of the mono-symptomatic hypochondriacal psychoses reflecting similarities with Kraepelin's concept of paranoia (Munro, 1988). These psychotic disorders consist of a single delusional belief of a somatic nature, usually in the absence of other prominent psychotic symptoms, and thus similar to delusional disorder, somatic type, in DSM-III-R (Munro, 1988). The other two monosymptomatic hypochondriacal syndromes are *delusions of parasitosis* (the belief that one is infected with parasites or other vermin), and *olfactory reference syndrome*, or delusions of bromosis (the belief that one emits an offensive body odor).

Body dysmorphic disorder is a relatively common psychiatric disorder with a point prevalence of 0.7–2.4% in the general population (Rief *et al.*, 2006; Koran *et al.*, 2008). Higher BDD prevalence rates are reported in non-clinical adult student samples, as well as in inpatient and outpatient settings (2–16%) (Bohne *et al.*, 2002; Cansever *et al.*, 2003). Notably, since many patients are embarrassed by their symptoms and reluctant to reveal them, BDD often goes undiagnosed. BDD has been reported to occur in children as young as 5 and in adults as old as 80, but usually begins during adolescence and predominates in adults. BDD may be somewhat more common in women, but it clearly affects men as well. Retrospective data indicate that BDD generally has a chronic course and a slim possibility for a full remission (Phillips, 2009). Risk behaviors such as suicidality, substance abuse, and violence are strikingly elevated among individuals with BDD (Bjornsson *et al.*, 2010). The disorder has significant negative consequences on patients' functioning; a majority of BDD patients do not marry and are unemployed, and more than 40% have psychiatric hospitalizations (Rief *et al.*, 2006; Didie *et al.*, 2008; Koran *et al.*, 2008).

The following case vignette illustrates major clinical features of a patient with BDD:

Case 7.4. A patient with BDD.

Ms. V, a 24-year-old single woman, exhibited preoccupations focused on her facial "acne," "baldness," and "long" nose. She was already preoccupied with her appearance at age 13, focusing at that time on her "short stature." V spent hours every day thinking about her perceived physical flaws. In addition, she compulsively checked her reflection in the mirror, picked her skin to remove tiny blemishes, combed her hair repeatedly to cover a spot of perceived baldness, and searched the internet for acne and hair-loss treatments. These behaviors lasted for at least 2–3 hours a day, made it difficult to concentrate on her studies as a medical nursing student, and often made her late to class. V described her preoccupation with her appearance as upsetting but was too embarrassed to reveal anything to family or friends. V was convinced that she was deformed. She even believed that strangers sometimes laughed at her "behind her back" because of her "ugliness." She had no other psychotic symptoms such as hallucinations or formal thought disorders. V was so ashamed of her appearance that she avoided social activities with family and friends. V received dermatological treatment for acne, but it did not diminish her preoccupations. She sought cosmetic surgery for a nose "defect," but surgical intervention was denied because of a lack of objective indication. V was referred to psychiatric evaluation following depressed mood, feelings of hopelessness, and suicidal ideations that were attributed to her concerns about her appearance.

In addition to *appearance preoccupations* (e.g., mirror checking, excessive grooming), patients with BDD like Ms. V also exhibit *safety behaviors*, such as camouflaging disliked body parts, and *avoidance behavior* because they are afraid that others will consider them "ugly." Any parts of the body can be the focus of preoccupation, though the most frequent areas are the skin, hair, and nose. Some patients are preoccupied with their overall appearance, as in the case of *muscle dysmorphia* which is the belief that one's body is too small and not sufficiently muscular (Pope *et al.*, 2005).

The degree of insight into the erroneousness of presumed defective appearance is a key issue in the psychiatric classification of BDD. Studies have consistently found that patients with BDD exhibit poor insight and roughly 40% of BDD patients evaluated using the Brown Assessment of Belief Scale (Eisen *et al.*, 1998) were found to be delusional, that is completely certain that their beliefs about how they look were accurate (Eisen *et al.*, 2004). A delusional variant of BDD in which patients are completely convinced that they appear ugly or abnormal is classified in DSM-IV as a delusional disorder, somatic type, in the psychosis section of the manual. ICD-10 classifies BDD, along with hypochondriasis, as a type of "hypochondriacal disorder," also in the somatoform section (World Health Organization, 1992). It is becoming increasingly evident that BDD patients may have varying degrees of insight ranging from fair to poor insight or delusional beliefs. Moreover, fluctuations of insight during the course of illness have also been described in BDD patients

(Phillips, 2009). Studies comparing delusional and non-delusional BDD patients revealed more similarities in terms of demographic features, psychopathology, and course of illness than between group differences, and that the primary difference seems to be symptom severity (Phillips *et al.*, 1994; Eisen *et al.*, 2008). These findings and the fact that patients with delusional BDD appear to respond to SSRI monotherapy and may not respond to an antipsychotic agent suggest that the delusional form of BDD is not a typical psychotic disorder. Hence, it may be more accurate to view insight as existing on a continuum and to consider BDD a single disorder which encompasses both delusional and non-delusional variants (Phillips *et al.*, 2010). In addition, about two-thirds of BDD patients also have past or current delusions of reference, believing that others notice them negatively or mock or ridicule them because of how they look (Phillips *et al.*, 1994). Although overlap with delusional thinking might seem to imply a link with psychosis, lack of other psychotic symptoms such as auditory hallucinations, formal thought disorders, alternative delusional themes along with a lack of negative symptoms, and characteristic course and outcome clearly indicate that BDD is a separate disorder distinct from schizophrenia or other typical psychotic disorders. In fact, Phillips and colleagues (1993) found no personal or family history of schizophrenia as defined by DSM-III-R in BDD patients. Moreover, though direct comparisons between BDD and schizophrenia were not performed, emerging preliminary findings from neuropsychological and neuroimaging research in BDD also hint at the existence of distinct and selective neurocognitive impairments rather than a generalized deficit characteristic of schizophrenia (Bjornsson *et al.*, 2010). For instance, a neuropsychological paradigm revealed that BDD patients over-focused on details of visual stimuli rather than on their global aspects (Deckersbach *et al.*, 2000). A similar bias among BDD patients for using strategies to encode details of stimuli rather than use of holistic visual processing strategies was found in a functional magnetic resonance imaging (fMRI) study of facial strategies (Feusner *et al.*, 2007). Additional information-processing abnormalities such as threatening interpretations for non-threatening scenarios and overestimation of the attractiveness of others, alongside clinical expressions of the disorder, were also detected in BDD patients (Buhlmann *et al.*, 2006).

Overall, there is increasing evidence indicating that BDD is a separate disorder associated with distinct psychopathological features, course, treatment response, and prognosis. Although BDD is sometimes misidentified as schizophrenia because it often involves symptoms attributed to psychosis (e.g., delusional beliefs about appearance "abnormalities," referential thinking), BDD is clearly not a typical psychotic disorder. Nevertheless, BDD may *co-occur* with psychotic disorders, particularly schizophrenia. The comorbidity of schizophrenia and BDD may well be mediated, at least in some cases, by the presence of OCD, owing to a likely relatedness between BDD and OCD (Poyurovsky *et al.*, 2006; Phillips *et al.*, 2010).

Body dysmorphic disorder as a disorder related to OCD-spectrum

A possible link between dysmorphophobia and obsessive–compulsive phenomena was initially noted by Morselli, Kraepelin, and Janet, who provided a clinical description of the disorder. Morselli attempted to capture the clinical phenomenon of dysmorphobobia as follows: (a) obsessionality, impulsivity, and irresistibility; (b) awareness of disease and concomitant anxiety; (c) tendency to act upon the idea (cited in Berrios and Kan Chung-Sing, 1996). Kraepelin believed that the persistent, ego-dystonic nature of dysmorphophobic symptoms warranted its classification as a compulsive neurosis (Kraepelin, 1915).

Similarly, Janet called dismorphophobia "an obsession of shame of the body," and classified it within a large class of syndromes similar to obsessive–compulsive disorder (Janet, 1903). Contemporary studies substantiate the relatedness of BDD and OCD. Indeed, according to a survey of 187 OCD experts around the world BDD received the greatest support (72%) for its inclusion to a putative OCD-spectrum of disorders (Mataix-Cols et al., 2007). Both BDD and OCD are chronic disorders with age at onset in mid adolescence. The relationship between thoughts and behaviors in BDD appears akin to the relationship between obsessions and compulsions in OCD. The compulsive behaviors such as mirror-checking arise in response to the obsessive preoccupations with abnormal appearance. As in OCD, compulsive behaviors are repetitive, time-consuming, and hard to resist, and are directed to reduce anxiety and distress. Most BDD patients perform multiple compulsive behaviors, which may include repeated mirror-checking, grooming (e.g., combing hair or washing skin repeatedly), tanning (to improve skin color), excessive shopping for beauty products, and excessive exercise (Phillips, 2009). As noted earlier, avoidance is a common behavior in BDD which may serve a purpose similar to compulsive behaviors in the short term – that is temporary relief of BDD-related anxiety and distress. However, compulsions and avoidance seldom improve anxiety or reduce intensity of BDD-related thoughts: rather these behaviors may contribute to the chronicity and severity of illness. One substantial difference between BDD and OCD is a substantially poorer insight in BDD patients, with 27–60% having delusional beliefs (Eisen et al., 2004).

The relatedness of BDD and OCD is also supported by a high rate of co-occurrence of the two disorders. Findings from comorbidity studies showed that roughly 30% of BDD patients have lifetime comorbid OCD; conversely, BDD's lifetime prevalence averages 15–20% in patients with OCD (Phillips et al., 2010). Noteworthy, comorbid lifetime rates for MDD and social phobia in BDD patients are even higher, contributing to a considerable morbidity and functional impairment of BDD patients.

In a large-scale family study using direct clinical interview, Bienvenu and colleagues (2000) convincingly demonstrated an aggregation of BDD cases in first-degree relatives of OCD probands compared to relatives of control probands, regardless of the presence of BDD, thus providing an additional argument for a close relationship between the two disorders. Using the family history method, Phillips et al. (1998) found that first-degree relatives ($N = 325$) of BDD and OCD probands did not significantly differ in terms of lifetime rates of OCD, social phobia, or MDD. Taken together, these findings suggest that BDD may be part of a familial OCD spectrum further supporting a likely relation between the two disorders.

A search for neurobiological correlates of BDD is still in its initial stages, although there is preliminary evidence of a possible similarity between BDD and OCD in functional neuroanatomy of orbitofrontal–subcortical circuits, which may be associated with obsessive thoughts and compulsive behaviors (Saxena and Feusner, 2006; Feusner et al., 2010). Nevertheless, a difference between the two disorders, such as exaggerated amygdala activation in response to face stimuli in BDD but not in OCD, has also been found, suggesting that BDD and OCD are close but distinct disorders on the OCD spectrum (Saxena and Feusner, 2006).

Both disorders share preferential response to monotherapy with serotonin reuptake inhibitors (SRIs) (Ipser et al., 2009). Preliminary evidence suggests that delusional insight in BDD may also improve with SRI treatment. Remarkably, though SRI augmentation with an antipsychotic agent has been shown to be beneficial in the treatment of OCD, it does not seem to be efficacious in BDD; however, evidence is limited (Phillips, 2005).

Body dysmorphic disorder in patients with schizophrenia

Before entering the official psychiatric nomenclature as a separate disorder in DSM-III-R, dysmorphophobia has long been considered by psychiatrists, primarily in Europe, Russia, and Japan, as a non-specific syndrome that can occur in several psychiatric disorders, such as depression, neuroses, and personality disorders. The relation between dysmorphophobia and schizophrenia has been strongly suggested. Mid-twentieth-century psychiatric literature included numerous vivid examples of the syndrome and its occurrence in schizophrenia. Hence, Bychowski (1943) gave detailed case histories of patients for whom changes in the body image appeared at the initial phase of a psychosis and the illness then seemed to crystallize around these complaints. Fenichel (1945) mentioned bodily complaints in incipient schizophrenia, interpreting this as a sign of regression to narcissism. Stekel (1950) described dysmorphophobia in the context of a possible transition of obsessions into delusions, mentioning that "there are people who occupy themselves continually with a specific part of the body, e.g., nose, ears, eyes, bald head, bosom, genitals, etc. Then thoughts can be very tormenting and are frequently connected with feelings of inferiority-they can be elaborated into a whole compulsive system." The author goes on to state his opinion that dysmorphophobic obsessions frequently occur in psychotic conditions. That is to say, "the initial diagnosis may be obsessive–compulsive neurosis but a few years later the patient is found to be suffering from schizophrenia."

Hay (1970) viewed dysmorphophobia as a symptom in a variety of disorders which could vary from "a sensitive personality development to an attenuated schizophrenic illness or to occasionally affective disorder." The author studied 17 patients (12 men, 5 women) who exhibited symptoms of dysmorphophobia. Five (29.4%) patients were diagnosed with schizophrenia, based on the presence of at least one of Schneider's (1959) first-rank symptoms.

Case 7.5. Dysmorphophobic symptoms in a schizophrenia patient (Hay, 1970).

Ms. I, aged 20, complained of lines under her eyes. At age 17, while combing her hair at a college dance, she noticed in the mirror that she had lines under her eyes. She became upset and self-conscious. However, the next day the lines seemed to have disappeared. After a few nights of not sleeping well she again noticed lines under her eyes. She became panicky, feeling that if she did not sleep well, she would soon look old and unattractive. She complained of continually thinking about the lines. "I make it worse by not sleeping and worrying. I don't feel comfortable or at ease any more." On close questioning, she admitted that some months before she had had "peculiar sensations" in which she appeared to get thoughts in her head that were not her own thoughts. She also admitted to auditory hallucinations, hearing her name called out when nobody was around while she was fully awake. She felt the lines under her eyes were different than the lines other people have under their eyes. "They are deeper and run at a different angle." The patient was thought to be suffering from a schizophrenic illness, but her presenting complaint appeared phenomenologically to be a phobia, not a delusion. She resisted thinking about the lines and agreed that her concern over them was "silly." It seemed therefore that her illness was "pathoplastically veiled."

Connoly and Gibson (1978) examined notes of patients who underwent cosmetic rhinoplasty at the Plastic and Jaw Unit in Sheffield (UK) between 1955 and 1960. Using Schneider's (1959) criteria for the diagnosis of schizophrenia they found that six (7%) of 86 individuals who sought rhinoplasty for aesthetic reasons were diagnosed with schizophrenia, compared to only one (1%) of 100 individuals in the control group who underwent surgery following disease or recent injury. It is interesting that in the case records of schizophrenia patients included in this study no mention was made of dysmorphophobia, and the illness was identified roughly 6 to 7 years after the rhinoplasty, highlighting that dysmorphophobia was generally an under-recognized disorder.

Marks and Mishan (1988) presented a case series of patients with primary diagnoses of depression, OCD, and schizophrenia, and an additional dysmorphophobic syndrome. Two aspects of the presented cases are noteworthy: first, a schizophrenia patient who had an olfactory reference syndrome that was considered to be intimately related to dysmorphophobia; second, efficacy of a psychotherapeutic approach of exposure and response prevention in the treatment of dysmorphophobic symptoms in a schizophrenia patient.

Case 7.6. A schizophrenia patient with olfactory reference syndrome (Marks and Mishan, 1988).

A 44-year-old decorator had for 16 years been convinced that he passed flatus and smelled so that others noticed. He carefully located toilets wherever he went and turned down jobs where toilets were not easily accessible. He visited toilets 19 times daily for 10–15 minutes at a time, used exactly 20 sheets of toilet paper at a time, and showered twice daily. He avoided proximity to others and sat away from them on buses lest he have an urge to go to the toilet. For 3 months he had heard a voice ("Tommy") commenting on his actions and telling neighbors he was dirty, believed Tommy watched him with a mirror, and on the street shouted at and searched for Tommy. He hallucinated the voices of neighbors (men, women, children) talking about his bowel noises. For a week he stayed in his room. He thought he could guess other people's thoughts. Over 10 years, extensive bowel investigations, X-rays, and barium enema were normal . . . On examination the patient sat far away, spoke quietly with good eye contact, was suspicious, and heard voices. When reassured that no smell could be detected he replied "You are just trying to encourage me." He wondered if he was going mad, thought others could hear his thoughts, and heard voices in the third person talking of his past. He was diagnosed as having schizophrenia and dysmorphophobia . . .

Japanese psychiatrists conceptualized that dysmorphophobia could exist either as a separate disorder or as a symptom of other psychiatric disorders, particularly schizophrenia. Thus, Yamada and colleagues (1978) distinguished the former variant by early age at onset during adolescence, male preponderance, and relatively positive prognosis; while the later was often transient and associated with worse prognosis. Additional distinction between the two forms of dysmorphophobia lies in the presence of referential thinking, but not ideas of persecution, in primary dysmorphophobia in contrast to the schizophrenia-related variant of the disorder. Following are two cases portraying a difference between the two variants of dysmorphophobia:

Case 7.7. A patient with "primary" dysmorphophobia (Yamada et al., 1978).

A 22-year-old university student. In his junior year of high school, he took a 1-hour daily nap while preparing for his university entrance examination, and was told by a friend that "Your eyes are bloodshot." When he looked at his face in the mirror, he saw that his eyes were bloodshot, and also noticed that his eyelids had become puffy, and that he had a single eyelid instead of the double eyelid he believed himself to have. He went to an ophthalmologist for medical treatment, and soon after an injection the discoloration disappeared, but swelling of the eyelids did not improve. He was satisfied with the ophthalmologist's explanation that "It is probably due to lack of sleep." After being accepted to his university of choice, he had a relatively routine daily life, but the swelling of his eyelids did not improve, and he began to believe that his vision in the left eye was diminishing rapidly. Unable to stand it any longer, he consulted his mother, and was told to his surprise that when he was about 2 years old he fell in the garden and hit his left eyelid on a stone. Afterwards, unless he looked at himself in the mirror many times a day and used an eye lotion, he became anxious. Concerned about his face, he would skip lectures, and spend most of his time looking in the mirror in his dormitory. As a result, he remained on the same courses for 2 years . . . He persistently complained that when he was emotionally strained, the left eyelid became swollen, and his doubled eyelid became single, creating a difference in the size of his eyelids. As a result, he refused to try to find a job. Later, his attitude changed, exemplified by his remark, "I've given up worrying about my face. It's not the face, but the heart that counts." He has since been doing relatively well.

Case 7.8. A dysmorphophobic syndrome in a schizophrenia patient (Yamada et al., 1978).

An 18-year-old senior high school girl, the eldest of two siblings. Her paternal uncle was once admitted to a mental hospital for treatment of schizophrenia, paranoid type. She had been gentle and shy since childhood. She could not clearly communicate her thoughts to other people. Her grades at school were good, but she was told by a teacher that her grades were not good enough for her to be accepted to the university she desired, so she reluctantly decided to take an entrance examination for a junior college. From around that time, she began to notice a strange smell like perfume, that she found offensive, and started taking baths several times a day. She was obsessed with the idea that she might be emitting the offensive odor. In college, she appeared to have had no psychiatric problems. Immediately after graduation, her family brought up the subject of marriage, and when she opposed the idea, her uncle slapped her across the face and her cheek swelled. From that time on, she became reluctant to leave the house. When visiting a beauty salon, she would make an appointment when there were no other customers. At the beauty shop she would giggle, or cry, without any reason, while looking in the mirror. On evaluation, she said her face swelled and returned to normal like a balloon, which she positively attributed to her being hit by her uncle. She also insisted that such a phenomenon would occur repeatedly while looking at her reflection in the mirror. At age 23, she got married, but immediately after the wedding, she started projecting delusions of persecution on her husband together with apathy and autism which led to the diagnosis of schizophrenia. At the same time, her complaint about dysmorphophobia began to vanish.

Russian psychiatrists focused on the occurrence of dysmorphophobia along with other "secondary" syndromes, such as hypochondriasis and OCD, in patients with schizophrenia. (Korkina, 1959; Vaghina, 1966). They considered these syndromes within the definitions of schizophrenia that are considered too broad by current nosological standards, including those suggested by Hoch and Polatin (1949) as a "pseudoneurotic" subtype. Pointing towards a lack of a phobic component in dysmorphophobia, in the strict sense, Korkina (1959) proposed an alternative term "dysmorphomania" to highlight a psychotic quality of a syndrome in a substantial proportion of patients.

A prospective evaluation of a large sample of 214 schizophrenia patients with dysmorphophobia conducted by Korkina (1984) facilitated clinical descriptions of the syndrome which may be relevant to present day psychiatrists as well. Hence, initial symptoms of dysmorphphobia emerge during adolescence, and there is a relatively long time lapse until characteristic symptoms of schizophrenia (e.g., auditory hallucinations, thought disorders) can be detected. During this period multiple psychiatric and non-psychiatric assessments and diagnoses other than schizophrenia are typically done. There are two major courses of illness: first, a dysmorphophobic syndrome retains its features during the entire course accompanied by typical schizophrenia symptoms; second, transient occurrence of dysmorphophobia during the initial stages of illness with further transformation into paranoid, hallucinatory, or other characteristic schizophrenia syndromes. Dysmorphophobia may co-occur with other "secondary" syndromes in patients with schizophrenia, particularly OCD, anorexia nervosa, and hypochondriasis, complicating even more its diagnosis and management. Finally, overall prognosis in schizophrenia patients with dysmorphophobia is unsatisfactory, since a particularly high suicidality, cognitive decline, and social disability have been observed in this patient population.

Early reports addressing the interrelation between the two disorders had notable limitations; they were primarily observational in nature and had fuzzy diagnostic boundaries. Contemporary reports aimed to overcome these drawbacks by using structured clinical interviews, stringent DSM-IV diagnostic criteria, and both epidemiological and clinical samples of participants. Surprisingly, consistently low rates of BDD in schizophrenia were noted, quite contrary to the sizable comorbidity rates of BDD and major depression, OCD, and social phobia (Phillips et al., 1993; Grant et al., 2001; Conroy et al., 2008). Remarkably small, absolute numbers of schizophrenia patients enrolled in these studies, making it difficult to determine the true rates of co-occurrence of the two disorders. Moreover, a majority of large-scale studies looking at additional "secondary" syndromes in schizophrenia did not include BDD.

Body dysmorphic disorder in patients with schizo-obsessive disorder

As noted above, our group conducted a study aimed to explicitly evaluate the rate of additional DSM-IV-defined disorders in schizophrenia patients with and without OCD, and to address the hypothesis of a differential aggregation of OCD-related disorders in schizo-obsessive patients (Poyurovsky et al., 2006). Indeed, there was a robust differentiation between the two schizophrenia groups primarily with respect to BDD with a substantially higher BDD rate in the schizo-obsessive group, compared with the non-OCD schizophrenia group. Since the publication of these findings, additional patients were enrolled, and the following figures emerged: 18 (12.7%) of 140 schizo-obsessive patients and 4 (3.5%) of 113 schizophrenia patients met DSM-IV criteria for BDD ($\chi^2 = 6.68$, $p < 0.01$). These latest results substantiate and extend initial findings and indicate that BDD may be detected in a meaningful proportion of schizophrenia patients, and that the presence of OCD moderates the co-occurrence of BDD and schizophrenia.

Following are two clinical vignettes portraying BDD in schizophrenia patients with and without OCD.

Case 7.9. Body dysmorphic disorder in a schizo-obsessive patient.

Mr. E, a 24-year-old college student, was admitted to a psychiatric hospital following his first acute psychotic episode characterized by imperative auditory hallucinations, persecutory delusions, and grossly impaired thought processes. He claimed that the mafia followed him, and affected his mental capacity by "inserting brain-destroying devices" in his apartment and neighborhood. Deterioration of his mental condition began about 12 months before he was hospitalized, with the emergence of initial prodromal symptoms of psychosis, such as emotional instability, social withdrawal, and transient paranoid ideation. He met DSM-IV criteria for schizophrenic disorder, undifferentiated type. When he was 15, clinically significant obsessive–compulsive symptoms were detected; he began repeatedly washing his hands and showering for hours due to constant contamination concerns. In addition, he repeatedly checked whether faucets were cleaned, to prevent contamination. He expressed a fair awareness of the senseless nature of these thoughts and behaviors but could not resist performing the rituals. Repetitive intrusive thoughts and ritualistic behaviors typical to OCD led to the diagnosis of DSM-IV OCD. From age 18, E exhibited preoccupations focused on his ears which according to him were "deformed and ugly," despite their obvious anatomic normality. E spent hours every day checking his reflection in the mirror and searching the internet for possible surgical interventions. These behaviors and his belief that other students made fun of his appearance eventually resulted in his dropping out of college. E described this preoccupation with his appearance as upsetting, but was too embarrassed to reveal the" real reason" for leaving school. He ultimately had cosmetic surgery for his "deformed" ears, but was not satisfied with the results and sought additional "ear corrections." He admitted that at this point he considered suicide the only solution for these "unbearable feelings." Notably, BDD content was not related to schizophrenic delusions and hallucinations. Neither BDD nor OCD symptoms were observed during the current psychotic episode, but both resurfaced after the resolution of psychosis.

Case 7.10. Body dysmorphic disorder in a schizophrenia patient.

Mr. S, a 25-year-old single man, had two younger siblings. Both of his siblings suffered from DSM-IV schizophrenic disorder. He grew up as a socially withdrawn boy, detached from his peers, and had exhibited marked schizoid personality traits since early adolescence. His school achievements were modest due to evident difficulties in concentration. From around age 17, he began to notice that his left wrist and fingers had a "feminine size and appearance." Every day he spent hours in front of the mirror checking and finding more reason for concern. He also began to camouflage his arm by wearing gloves, even during the summer. S was convinced that his concerns and associated behaviors were reasonable and rejected evidence to the contrary. Social avoidance was exacerbated because of his perceived left hand "inadequacy." He stopped going to a high school, and eventually became housebound because of his constant preoccupation with his "deformed appearance" and the belief that people made fun of his "defect." Finally, S tried to amputate the fingers on his left hand using a kitchen knife to deal with unbearable feelings of inadequacy. On examination, in addition to body dysmorphic beliefs of delusional intensity accompanied by corresponding delusions of reference, S exhibited marked thought disorganization, including cognitive slippage and idiosyncratic thinking. He admitted occasionally hearing voices of unfamiliar persons who used to comment on his "hand femininity," and exhibited Schneiderian symptoms of thought insertion and withdrawal. S met DSM-IV criteria for schizophrenic disorder, undifferentiated type, in addition to BDD.

Table 7.5 Screening questions for symptoms of body dysmorphic disorder in patients with schizophrenia

Were you ever worried about your appearance?

Were you ever concerned about the shape or size of any of your body parts such as face, nose, ears, or muscles?

How much time during the day are you preoccupied with the flaws you see in your appearance?

How frustrating are these concerns?

Do these concerns interfere with your daily routine?

Do you feel compelled to spend time camouflaging, mirror checking, excessive grooming, touching the disliked body areas, excessive exercising?

Source: Modified from Phillips (2009).

Recommendations for diagnosis and treatment of BDD in schizophrenia

Systematic investigation of the clinical features of OCD-related disorders in schizophrenia provide the basics for the following assumptions regarding BDD in schizophrenia:

- Despite its meaningful rate of occurrence and clinical significance BDD remains an under-recognized disorder. This seems to be particularly true for BDD comorbid to schizophrenia. BDD was not identified in any of our schizophrenia patients by their treating psychiatrists. Therefore, direct evaluation using screening questions, such as those suggested by Phillips (2009) for patients with BDD non-related to schizophrenia, may be useful (Table 7.5). Moreover, the revealed preferential aggregation of BDD in schizo-obsessive patients justifies a systematic search for this comorbidity particularly in the schizo-obsessive subgroup. Conversely, because the presence of BDD increases the odds of OCD in schizophrenia patients, targeting BDD may facilitate detection of obsessive–compulsive symptoms in schizophrenia. Repeated assessments during different stages of schizophrenic illness especially after resolution of acute psychosis are essential to optimize the detection of BDD.

- In general, BDD comorbid to schizophrenia has clinical characteristics that are similar to "ordinary" BDD. Thus, in schizophrenia patients BDD usually begins during adolescence, with mean age of onset around 18 (Table 7.6). In a majority (roughly 80%) of patients the onset of the first clinically significant BDD symptoms precedes the onset of the first psychotic symptoms. In schizo-obsessive patients BDD follows the occurrence of the first clinically significant obsessions and/or compulsions in approximately 70% of patients. Hence, a characteristic sequence of the appearance of disorders is OCD followed by BDD and finally schizophrenia. Furthermore, BDD in schizophrenia seems to usually have the same body areas of concern as "ordinary" BDD, that is skin, hair, and nose (Table 7.6). Almost half of the patients have two body areas of concern, and one-fifth have three areas. Additional similarities are reflected in patterns of behavior that are typical to BDD, such as preoccupation with appearance (e.g., mirror checking), safety behaviors (e.g., camouflaging disliked body parts), and avoidance behavior because of perceived ugliness.

Table 7.6 Clinical characteristics of schizo-obsessive patients who also have body dysmorphic disorder (BDD)

Patient	Age/gender	Schizophrenia subtype	Age of onset			OCD	BDD		Intervention	Consultation
			SCH	BDD	OCD	Insight[a]	Body areas of concern	Insight[b]		
1	24/M	Undifferentiated	16	13	16	Fair	Muscles	Delusional		Cosmetic surgeon
2	32/M	Residual	16	15	15	Fair	Ears	Delusional		
3	54/F	Paranoid	28	30	15	Lack	Hair, ears	Delusional		
4	25/M	Paranoid	16	16	21	Poor	Nose, hair, face	Delusional	Surgery	
5	30/M	Disorganized	17	25	25	Lack	Head shape	Delusional		Orthopedist
6	28/M	Disorganized	17	17	11	Poor	Hair, nose, face	Delusional		
7	18/M	Paranoid	18	15	15	Poor	Nose, ears, head shape	Delusional	Surgery	
8	46/M	Paranoid	25	25	19	Delusional	Nose	Delusional		Cosmetic surgeon
9	23/F	Paranoid	17	20	15	Delusional	Nose	Delusional		
10	53/F	Schizoaffective	20	32	25	Fair	Ears	Delusional		
11	33/M	Disorganized	14	14	22	Poor	Teeth	Poor		Dental surgeon
12	28/M	Schizoaffective	17	14	13	Fair	Ears	Poor		
13	21/F	Schizoaffective	18	15	13	Good	Mouth, ears	Fair		
14	22/F	Undifferentiated	16	16	12	Good	Skin, hair	Fair		
15	33/F	Schizoaffective	30	16	10	Good	Skin, chest	Poor		
16	23/F	Paranoid	17	16	12	Good	Face, nose, ear	Delusional	Surgery	
17	32/M	Paranoid	20	14	12	Fair	Arm/wrist	Delusional		Orthopedist
18	20/M	Undifferentiated	18	18	15	Fair	Nose, ears, leg	Delusional	Surgery	

[a] Insight for OCD was defined using the Yale–Brown Obsessive–Compulsive Scale.
[b] Insight for BDD was defined using the Yale–Brown Obsessive–Compulsive Scale modified for BDD.
Source: Poyurovsky et al, unpublished data.

- A majority of our schizophrenia patients with BDD sought and received cosmetic treatment for "flaws" in their appearance, and a remarkably high proportion (20%) underwent surgical procedures. Veale *et al.* (1996) found that 81% of 50 BDD patients without symptoms of schizophrenia were dissatisfied with past medical consultation or surgery. Surgical intervention appears to only rarely improve BDD symptoms in schizophrenia patients as well. Moreover, dissatisfaction with non-psychiatric treatment can have serious negative consequences for both patients and physicians. In a survey of cosmetic surgeons, 40% of responders indicated that dissatisfied BDD patients had threatened them physically or legally (Sarwer, 2002). This also appeared to be relevant to patients suffering from BDD associated with schizophrenia. It is therefore important for patients and their clinicians to be aware that non-psychiatric interventions appear unlikely to successfully treat BDD symptoms and may potentially trigger assaultive behavior.

- Suicidal behavior that is another expression of risk behaviors needs to be considered. There is compelling evidence indicating that rates of suicidal ideation, suicide attempts, and completed suicide are markedly elevated in BDD patients, and seem to be higher than that reported for nearly any other mental disorder (Phillips, 2009). Considering the suicide risk associated with schizophrenia, schizophrenia patients with comorbid BDD apparently have an increased risk for suicide. The high rate of co-occurring MDD is an additional contributing factor.

- Poor insight into the erroneousness of perceived appearance flaws as one of the key issues in "ordinary" BDD apparently poses extra diagnostic challenges in BDD associated with schizophrenia. A predominant majority of our patients exhibited lack of insight into BDD-related concerns and had unshakeable beliefs that their behaviors were reasonable. Only a few admitted ideas and behavior somewhat excessive ("fair insight," according to the Y-BOCS adopted for BDD), or alternatively maintained that they were not unreasonable and excessive, but acknowledged the validity of evidence to the contrary ("poor insight"). It seems that the presence of schizophrenia affects insight in BDD by causing even further deterioration. Noteworthy, insight into BDD was significantly worse than insight into OCD in schizophrenia patients, echoing a similar interrelation between insight in BDD and OCD in patients without schizophrenia (Table 7.6).

- In some patients (Case 7.9), the content of BDD concerns remains unrelated to a content of schizophrenic-related delusions and hallucinations and is usually not expressed during acute psychotic phases. In others (Case 7.10), BDD-related concerns predominate in a clinical picture forming a psychopathological "amalgam" with symptoms of schizophrenia. These cases are diagnostically the most challenging, specifically in distinguishing between BDD-related avoidant behavior from negative symptoms of schizophrenia, or referential thinking that accompanies both disorders. The presence of symptoms that meet DSM-IV Criterion A for schizophrenia is a prerequisite for establishing diagnosis of schizophrenia in addition to DSM-IV BDD.

- Treatment strategies for schizophrenia patients with BDD are yet to be developed. As noted, treatment with SRIs is recommended for "ordinary" BDD (Ipser *et al.*, 2009). The efficacy of antipsychotic medications remains controversial, with several case reports indicating successful SRI augmentation with an antipsychotic while one study found no advantage of pimozide augmentation vs. placebo when added to fluoxetine in BDD patients (Phillips, 2005). Clinical experience indicates that BDD in the context of schizophrenia may respond to an antipsychotic agent, especially when BDD psychopathologically intervenes with schizophrenic symptoms; The role of SRI augmentation to an antipsychotic agent for BDD in schizophrenia patients, particularly when BDD is unrelated to schizophrenic symptoms merits investigation. SRIs should be considered only in stabilized antipsychotic-treated patients during a remitted state, after careful evaluation of the potential risks and benefits, including pharmacokinetic interactions and potential side effects of antipsychotic–SRI combination. Cognitive–behavior therapy (CBT) may have therapeutic value in addressing BDD concerns and behaviors in remitted schizophrenia patients (Marks and Mishan, 1988). CBT comprising cognitive restructuring that focuses on changing appearance-related assumptions and beliefs, and exposure and response prevention to reduce avoidance and compulsive and safety behaviors were shown efficacious in non-schizophrenia BDD; its clinical utility in schizophrenia patients with BDD is yet unknown (Bjornsson et al., 2010).

Overall, systematic evaluation of psychiatric comorbidities in schizophrenia patients with and without OCD suggests that compared to patients with schizophrenia alone, those who have both schizophrenia and OCD exhibit higher rates of tic disorders and BDD which are believed to be related to the OCD-spectrum. From the clinical perspective, the findings of an aggregation of tic disorders and BDD in schizo-obsessive patients justify a systematic assessment of these comorbidities. Detection of additional OCD-spectrum disorders, should prompt a search for optimal therapeutic interventions, and their integration into the treatment of the primary schizophrenic disorder.

References

Albin R, Mink JW (2006) Recent advances in Tourette syndrome research. Trends in Neuroscience 29, 175–182.

American Psychiatric Association (1980) Diagnostic and Statistical Manual of Mental Disorders, 3rd edn. American Psychiatric Association, Washington, DC.

American Psychiatric Association (1987) Diagnostic and Statistical Manual of Mental Disorders, 3rd edn, revised. American Psychiatric Association, Washington, DC.

American Psychiatric Association (2000) Diagnostic and Statistical Manual of Mental Disorders, 4th edn, text revision. American Psychiatric Association, Washington, DC.

Begum M (2005) Clozapine-induced stuttering, facial tics and myoclonic seizures: a case report. Australian and New Zealand Journal of Psychiatry 39, 202.

Bejerot S, Humble M (2007) Low prevalence of smoking among patients with obsessive-compulsive disorder. Comprehensive Psychiatry 40, 268–272.

Bermanzohn PC, Porto L, Arlow PB, et al. (2000) Hierarchical diagnosis in chronic schizophrenia: a clinical study of co-occurring syndromes. Schizophrenia Bulletin 26, 517–525.

Berrios GE, Kan C-S (1996) A conceptual and quantitive analysis of 178 historical cases of dysmorphophobia. Acta Psychiatrica Scandinavica 94, 1–7.

Bienvenu OJ, Samuels JF, Riddle MA, et al. (2000) The relationship of obsessive-compulsive disorder to possible spectrum disorders: results from a family study. Biological Psychiatry 48, 287–293.

Bjornsson AS, Didie ER, Phillips KA (2010) Body dysmorphic disorder. Dialogues in Clinical Neuroscience 12, 221–232.

Bohlhalter S, Goldfine A, Matteson S, et al. (2006) Neural correlates of tic generation in tourette syndrome: an event related functioinal MRI study. Brain 129, 2029–2037.

Bohne A, Wilhelm S, Keuthen NJ, et al. (2002) Prevalence of body dysmorphic disorder in a German college student sample. Psychiatry Research 109, 101–104.

Buhlmann U, Etcoff NL, Wilhelm S (2006) Emotion recognition bias for contempt and danger in body dysmorphic disorder. Journal of Psychiatric Research 40, 105–111.

Bychowski G (1943) Disorders of the body image in clinical pictures of the psychosis. Journal of Nervous and Mental Disease 97, 310–334.

Cansever A, Uzun O, Dönmez E, Ozşahin A (2003) The prevalence and clinical features of body dysmorphic disorder in college students: a study in a Turkish sample. Comprehensive Psychiatry 44, 60–64.

Cath DC, Hedderly T, Ludolph AG, et al. (2011) European clinical guidelines for Tourette syndrome and other tic disorders: I. Assessment. European Child and Adolescent Psychiatry 20, 155–171.

Connoly FH, Gipson M (1978) Dysmorphophobia: a long-term study. British Journal of Psychiatry 132, 568–570.

Conroy M, Menard W, Fleming-Ives K, et al. (2008) Prevalence and clinical characteristics of body dysmorphic disorder in an adult inpatient setting. General Hospital Psychiatry 30, 67–72.

de Haan L, Sterk B, Wouters L, Linszen DH (2011) The 5-year course of obsessive-compulsive symptoms and obsessive-compulsive disorder in first-episode schizophrenia and related disorders. Schizophrenia Bulletin Jul 28. Epub ahead of print, schizophreniabulletin. oxfordjournals.org/content/early/2011/07/28/schbul.sbr077.full.

Deckersbach T, Savage CR, Phillips KA, et al. (2000) Characteristics of memory dysfunction in body dysmorphic disorder. Journal of the International Neuropsychological Society 6, 673–681.

Didie ER, Menard W, Stern AP, Phillips KA (2008) Occupational functioning and impairment in adults with body dysmorphic disorder. Comprehensive Psychiatry 49, 561–569.

Diniz JB, Rosario-Campos MC, Shavitt RG, et al. (2004) Impact of age at onset and duration of illness on the expression of comorbidities in obsessive-compulsive disorder. Journal of Clinical Psychiatry 65, 22–27.

Eapen V, Laker M, Anfield A, Dobbs J, Robertson MM (2001) Prevalence of tics and Tourette syndrome in an inpatient adult psychiatry setting. Journal of Psychiatry and Neuroscience 26, 417–420.

Eidelberg D, Moeller JR, Antonini A, et al. (1997) The metabolic anatomy of Tourette's syndrome. Neurology 48, 927–934.

Eisen JL, Phillips KA, Baer L, et al. (1998) The Brown Assessment of Beliefs Scale: reliability and validity. American Journal of Psychiatry 155, 102–108.

Eisen JL, Phillips KA, Coles ME, Rasmussen SA (2004) Insight in obsessive-compulsive disorder and body dysmorphic disorder. Comprehensive Psychiatry 45, 10–15.

Escobar R, Bernardo M (1993) Schizophrenia, obsessive-compulsive disorder, and Tourette's syndrome: a case of triple comorbidity. Journal of Neuropsychiatry 5, 108.

Fenichel O (1945). The Psycho-Analytic Theory of Neurosis. Norton, New York.

Fennig S, Neisberg-Fennig S, Pato M, Weizman A (1994) Emergence of symptoms of Tourette's syndrome during fluvoxamine treatment of obsessive-compulsive disorder. British Journal of Psychiatry 164, 839–841.

Feusner JD, Townsend J, Bystritsky A, Bookheimer S (2007) Visual information processing of faces in body dysmorphic disorder. Archives of General Psychiatry 64, 1417–1425.

Feusner JD, Moody T, Hemasher E (2010) Abnormalities of visual processing and fronto-striatal systems in body dysmorphic disorder. Archives of General Psychiatry 67, 197–205.

Freeman RD, Fast DK, Burd L, *et al.* (2000) An international perspective on Tourette syndrome: selected findings from 3500 individuals in 22 countries. *Developmental Medicine and Child Neurology* **42**, 436–447.

Glick ID, Poyurovsky M, Ivanova O, Koran LM (2008) Aripiprazole in schizophrenia patients with comorbid obsessive-compulsive symptoms: an open-label study of 15 patients. *Journal of Clinical Psychiatry* **69**, 1856–1859.

Grant JE, Kim SW, Crow SJ (2001) Prevalence and clinical feature of body dysmorphic disorder in adolescent and adult psychiatric inpatients. *Journal of Clinical Psychiatry* **62**, 517–522.

Hay GG (1970) Dysmorphophobia. *British Journal of Psychiatry* **116**, 399–406.

Hoch P, Polatin P (1949) Pseudoneurotic forms of schizophrenia. *Psychiatric Quarterly* **23**, 248–276.

Hollander E, Braun A, Simeon D (2008) Should OCD leave the anxiety disorders in DSM-V? The case for obsessive-compulsive related disorders. *Depression and Anxiety* **25**, 317–329.

Ipser JC, Sander C, Stein DJ (2009) Pharmacotherapy and psychotherapy for body dysmorphic disorder. *Cochrane Database of Systematic Reviews* (**1**): CD005332.

Janet P (1903) *Les Obsessions et Psychasthénie.* Alcan, Paris. (Reprinted: Arno, New York, 1976.)

Kapur S, Mamo D (2003) Half a century of antipsychotics and still a central role for dopamine D2 receptors. *Progress in Neuropsychopharmacology and Biological Psychiatry* **27**, 1081–1090.

Kerbeshian J, Peng CZ, Burd L (2009) Tourette syndrome and comorbid early-onset schizophrenia. *Journal of Psychosomatic Research* **67**, 515–523.

Klawans HL, Falk DK, Nausieda PA, Weiner WJ (1978) Gilles de la Tourette syndrome after long term chlorpromazine therapy. *Neurology* **28**, 1064–1068.

Koran LM, Abujaoude E, Large MD, Serpe RT (2008) The prevalence of body dysmorphic disorder in the United States adult population. *CNS Spectrums* **13**, 316–322.

Korkina MV (1959) The clinical significance of the syndrome of dysmorphophobia. *Zhurnal nevrologii i psikhiatrii imeni S.S. Korsakova* **59**, 994–1000.

Korkina MV (1984) Dysmorphomania in teenage and adolescent period. *Moscow: Medicina*, 224.

Kraepelin E (1915) *Psychiatrie*, 8th edn. J Barch, Leipzig, Germany.

Lindenmayer JP, Da Silva D, Buendia A, Zylberman I, Vital-Herne M (1995) Tic-like syndrome after treatment with clozapine. *American Journal of Psychiatry* **152**, 649.

Lyon GJ, Samar S, Jummani R, *et al.* (2009) Aripiprazole in children and adolescents with Tourette's disorder: an open-label safety and tolerability study. *Journal of Child and Adolescent Psychopharmacology* **19**, 623–633.

Lysaker PH, Marks KA, Picone JB, *et al.* (2000) Obsessive and compulsive symptoms in schizophrenia: clinical and neurocognitive correlates. *Journal of Nervous and Mental Disease* **188**, 78–83.

Lysaker PH, Whitney KA, Davis LW (2006) Obsessive-compulsive and negative symptoms in schizophrenia: associations with coping preference and hope. *Psychiatry Research* **141**, 253–259.

Marks I, Mishan J (1988) Dysmorphophobic avoidance with disturbed bodily perception: a pilot study of exposure therapy. *British Journal of Psychiatry* **152**, 674–678.

Mataix-Cols D, Pertusa A, Leckman JF (2007) Issues for DSM-V: how should obsessive-compulsive and related disorders be classified? *American Journal of Psychiatry* **164**, 1313–1314.

McElroy SL, Phillips KA, Keck PE (1994) Obsessive-compulsive spectrum disorders. *Journal of Clinical Psychiatry* **55** (Suppl. 10), 33–51.

Montgomery SA, Asberg M (1979) A new depression scale designed to be sensitive to change. *British Journal of Psychiatry* **134**, 382–389.

Morselli E (1891) Sulla dismorfofobia e sulla tafefobia. *Bulletinno della Reale Accademia di Genova* **6**, 110–119.

Muller N, Riedel M, Zawta P, Gunther W, Straube A (2002) Comorbidity of Tourette's syndrome and schizophrenia: biological and physiological parallels. *Progress in Neuropsychopharmacology and Biological Psychiatry* **26**, 1245–1252.

Munro A (1988) Delusional (paranoid) disorders. *Canadian Journal of Psychiatry* **33**, 399–404.

Murphy DL, Timpano KR, Wheaton MG, Greenberg BD, Miguel EC (2010) Obsessive-compulsive disorder and its related disorders: a reappraisal of obsessive-compulsive spectrum concepts. *Dialogues in Clinical Neuroscience* **12**, 131–148.

Nestadt G, Samuels J, Riddle MA, *et al.* (2001) The relationship between obsessive-compulsive disorder and anxiety and affective disorders: results from the Johns Hopkins OCD Family Study. *Psychological Medicine* **31**, 481–487.

Olson S (2004) Neurobiology: making sense of Tourette's. *Science* **305**, 1390–1392.

Pappert EJ, Goetz CG, Louis ED, Blasucci L, Leurgans S (2003) Objective assessments of longitudinal outcome in Gilles de la Tourette's syndrome. *Neurology* **61**, 936–940.

Phillips KA (2005) Placebo-controlled study of pimozide augmentation of fluoxetine in body dysmorphic disorder. *American Journal of Psychiatry* **162**, 377–379.

Phillips KA (2009) *Understanding Body Dysmorphic Disorder: An Essential Guide.* Oxford University Press, New York.

Phillips KA, McElroy SL, Keck PE Jr, Pope HG Jr, Hudson JI (1993) Body dysmorphic disorder: 30 cases of imagined ugliness. *American Journal of Psychiatry* **150**, 302–308.

Phillips KA, McElroy SL, Keck PE Jr, Hudson JI, Pope HG Jr (1994) A comparison of delusional and nondelusional body dysmorphic disorder in 100 cases. *Psychopharmacology Bulletin* **30**, 179–186.

Phillips KA, Gunderson CG, Mallya G, McElroy SL, Carter W (1998) A comparative study of body dysmorphic disorder and obsessive-compulsive disorder. *Journal of Clinical Psychiatry* **59**, 568–575.

Phillips KA, Pagano ME, Menard W, Stout RL (2006) A 12-month follow-up study of the course of body dysmorphic disorder. *American Journal of Psychiatry* **163**, 907–912.

Phillips KA, Stein DJ, Rauch SL, *et al.* (2010) Should an obsessive-compulsive spectrum grouping of disorders be included in DSM-V? *Depression and Anxiety* **27**, 528–555.

Pope CG, Pope HG, Menard W, *et al.* (2005) Clinical features of muscle dysmorphia among males with body dysmorphic disorder. *Body Image* **2**, 395–400.

Poyurovsky M, Bergman Y, Shoshani D, Schneidman M, Weizman A (1998) Emergence of obsessive-compulsive symptoms and tics during clozapine withdrawal. *Clinical Neuropharmacology* **21**, 97–100.

Poyurovsky M, Fuchs C, Faragian S, *et al.* (2006) Preferential aggregation of obsessive-compulsive spectrum disorders in schizophrenia patients with obsessive-compulsive disorder. *Canadian Journal of Psychiatry* **51**, 746–754.

Rajkumar RP, Reddy YC, Kandavel T (2008) Clinical profile of "schizo-obsessive" disorder: a comparative study. *Comprehensive Psychiatry* **49**, 262–268.

Reid SD (2004) Neuroleptic-induced tardive Tourette treated with clonazepam: a case report and literature review. *Clinical Neuropharmacology* **27**, 101–104.

Rief W, Buhlmann U, Wilhelm S, Borkenhagen A, Brahler E (2006) The prevalence of body dysmorphic disorder: a populatioin-based survey. *Psychological Medicine* **36**, 877–885.

Robertson MM (2000) Tourette syndrome, associated conditions and the complexities of treatment. *Brain* **123**, 425–462.

Roessner V, Plessen KJ, Rothenberger A, *et al.* (2011) European clinical guidelines for Tourette syndrome and other tic disorders: II. Pharmacological treatment. *European Child and Adolescent Psychiatry* **20**, 173–196.

Erratum *European Child and Adolescent Psychiatry* **20**, 377.

Ross MS, Moldofsky H (1978) A comparison of pimozide and haloperidol in the treatment of Gilles de la Tourette's syndrome. *American Journal of Psychiatry* **135**, 585–587.

Saccomani L, Fabiana V, Manuela B, Giambattista R (2005) Tourette syndrome and chronic tics in a sample of children and adolescents. *Brain and Development* **27**, 349–352.

Sandyk R, Bamford CR (1988) Gilles de la Tourette's syndrome associated with chronic schizophrenia. *International Journal of Neuroscience* **41**, 83–86.

Sarwer DB (2002) Awareness and identification of body dysmorphic disorder by aesthetic surgeons: results of a survey of American Society for Aesthetic Plastic Surgery members. *Aesthetic Surgery Journal* **22**, 531–535.

Saxena S, Feusner JD (2006) Toward a neurobiology of body dysmorphic disorder. *Primary Psychiatry* **13**, 41–48.

Saxena S, Brody AL, Schwartz JM, Baxter LR (1998) Neuroimaging and frontal-subcortical circuitry in obsessive-compulsive disorder. *British Journal of Psychiatry* **173** (Suppl. 35), 26–37.

Schneider K (1959) *Klinische Psychopathologie*, 12th edn. Georg Thieme, Stuttgart. (Transl. Hamilton MW (1976) *Clinical Psychopathology*. Grune and Stratton, New York.)

Sevincok L, Akoglu A, Kokcu F (2007) Suicidality in schizophrenic patients with and without obsessive-compulsive disorder. *Schizophrenia Research* **90**, 198–202.

Shapiro AK, Shapiro ES, Wayne H, Clarkin J (1972) The psychopathology of Gilles de la Tourette's syndrome. *American Journal of Psychiatry* **129**, 87–94.

Shapiro E, Shapiro E (1998) Treatment of tic disorders with haloperidol. In Cohen DJ, Bruun RD, Leckman JF (eds.) *Tourette Syndrome and Tic Disorders*. Wiley, New York, pp.267–280.

Siever LJ, Davis KL (2004) The pathophysiology of schizophrenia disorders: perspectives from the spectrum. *American Journal of Psychiatry* **161**, 398–413.

Singer HS (2005) Tourette's syndrome: from behavior to biology. *Lancet Neurology* **4**, 149–159.

Stekel W (1950) *Compulsion and Doubt*, vol. 2. Peter Nevill, London.

Stern E, Silbersweig DA, Chee KY, et al. (2000) A functional neuroanatomy of tics in Tourette syndrome. *Archives of General Psychiatry* **57**, 741–748.

Su JA, Tsang HY, Chou SY, Chung PC (2008) Aripiprazole treatment for risperidone-associated tic movement: a case report. *Progress in Neuropsychopharmacology and Biological Psychiatry* **32**, 899–900.

Swain JE, Scahill L, Lombroso PJ, King RA, Leckman JF (2007) Tourette syndrome and tic disorders: a decade of progress. *Journal of the American Academy of Child and Adolescent Psychiatry* **46**, 947–968.

Swerdlow NR, Weber M, Qu Y, Light GA, Braff D (2008) Realistic expectations of prepulse inhibition in translational models for schizophrenia research. *Psychopharmacology* **199**, 331–388.

Takeuchi K, Tamashita M, Morikyo M, et al. (1986) Gilles de la Tourette's syndrome and schizophrenia. *Journal of Nervous and Mental Disease* **174**, 247–248.

Vaghina GS (1966) Dysmorphophobia syndrome in the clinical treatment of schizophrenia. *Zhurnal nevrologii i psikhiatrii imeni S.S. Korsakova*, **66**, 1228–1234.

Veale D, Boocock A, Gournay K, Dryden W (1996) Body dysmorphic disorder: a survey of fifty cases. *British Journal of Psychiatry* **169**, 196–201.

Wagle AC, Staley CJ (1999) Gilles de la Tourette syndrome with schizophrenia and obsessive-compulsive disorder: a case report. *Journal of Neuropsychiatry and Clinical Neurosciences* **11**, 517.

Wang Z, Maia TV, Marsh R, et al. (2011) The neural circuits that generate tics in Tourette's syndrome. *American Journal of Psychiatry* **168**, 1326–1337.

Weiden P, Bruun R (1987) Worsening of Tourette's disorder due to neuroleptic-induced akathisia. *American Journal of Psychiatry* **144**, 504–505.

Wong DF, Brasic JR, Singer HS, *et al.* (2008) Mechanisms of dopaminergic and serotonergic neurotransmission in Tourette-syndrome: clues from an in vivo neurochemistry study with PET. *Neuropsychopharmacology* **33**, 1239–1251

World Health Organization (1992) *The ICD-10 Classification of Mental and Behavioral Disorders: Clinical Descriptions and Diagnostic Guidelines*. World Health Organization, Geneva.

Yamada M, Kobashi K, Shigemoto T, Ota T (1978) On dysmorphophobia. *Bulletin of the Yamaguchi Medical School* **25**, 47–54.

Ziemann U, Paulus W, Rothenberg A (1997) Decreased motor inhibition in Tourette's disorder: evidence from transcranial magnetic stimulation. *American Journal of Psychiatry* **154**, 1277–1284.

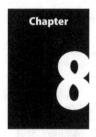

Schizotypal OCD

The interface of obsessive–compulsive and schizophrenic phenomena is not limited to the co-occurrence of DSM-IV schizophrenic disorder and obsessive–compulsive symptoms. Clinical experience and research findings have demonstrated that the two disorders may converge in an alternative complex clinical phenotype, DSM-IV OCD with schizotypal personality disorder ("schizotypal OCD").

The association between obsessive neurosis and obsessive–compulsive personality is arguably one of the best-known relationships between mental disorders and personality and can be traced back to the early days of psychoanalysis. However, systematic study of the association of OCD and personality disorders evolved with the establishment of a separate axis for personality disorders in DSM-III. Most individuals with OCD meet criteria for at least one comorbid personality disorder, but only a modest proportion of patients has obsessive–compulsive personality disorder. Other personality patterns appear to occur more frequently in OCD (Black and Noyes, 1997; Mataix-Cols et al., 2000; Matsunaga et al., 2000; Torres et al., 2006).

The assessment of personality disorders poses considerable challenges. Both personality disorder interviews and self-report inventories are susceptible to the over-reporting of personality pathology when mental illness is present. In addition, it is often difficult to distinguish between symptoms of psychiatric disorders and personality traits, especially in chronic disorders such as OCD, and many apparent dysfunctional personality traits may be secondary to OCD symptoms (Torres et al., 2006). Despite these obstacles, there is increasing evidence indicating that although OCD patients are ostensibly not at increased risk for developing schizophrenia (see Chapter 3), there is a substantial rate of co-occurrence of OCD and schizotypal personality disorder, an attenuated form of schizophrenia.

Schizotypal personality disorder

Schizotypal personality disorder was initially recognized as a specific personality disorder in DSM-III (Spitzer et al., 1979) to encompass the attenuated schizophrenia-like symptoms consistently observed in the relatives of patients with schizophrenia. The term "schizotypal" means "like schizophrenia" and was chosen to represent the concept of "borderline schizophrenia" introduced by Kety and colleagues (1971) to describe subtle psychopathological characteristics that are stable over time, and assumed to be genetically related to the schizophrenia spectrum.[1] Earlier, seminal observations by Kraepelin and Bleuler revealed that biological

---

[1] Alternatively, the term "borderline" referred to a constellation of relatively enduring personality features of unstable affect, interpersonal relationship, and sense of identity, and was reflected in definitions of the "borderline patient" (Gunderson and Singer, 1975), "borderline personality organization" (Kernberg, 1967), and currently retained in the DSM "borderline personality disorder."

relatives of schizophrenia patients often displayed subtle formal thought disorders and interpersonal oddities (Bleuler, 1911/1950; Kraepelin, 1919). Meehl (1990) proposed the term *schizotaxia* for the "genetically determined integrative defect, predisposing to schizophrenia," and the term *schizotypy* for a subtly deviant psycho-behavioral organization, reflective of interactions of schizotaxic vulnerability with environmental factors. Schizotaxic individuals manifest schizotypy on a dynamic continuum ranging from various degrees of subclinical deviance to schizophrenia-spectrum personality disorders to full-blown schizophrenia (Meehl, 1990).

Commonly used diagnostic instruments for the assessment of schizotypal personality disorder include the Structured Clinical Interview for DSM-IV Axis II personality disorders (SCID-II) (First *et al.*, 1995), and the Schizotypal Personality Questionnaire (Raine, 1991), based on DSM conceptualization of schizotypy. These instruments represent a categorical approach to schizotypy. In contrast, the "psychosis-proneness" scales of physical and social anhedonia (Chapman *et al.*, 1976) are used for evaluation of schizotypy based on the dimensional approach.

Individuals with schizotypal personality disorder share common phenomenological characteristics with those who suffer from schizophrenia (Siever and Davis, 2004; Raine, 2006; Skodol *et al.*, 2011). The DSM-IV diagnostic criteria for schizotypal personality disorder reflect both positive psychotic-like manifestations and negative deficit-like symptoms. Three major factors are common to schizotypal psychopathology and schizophrenia: *cognitive–perceptual* (magical thinking, unusual perceptual experiences, ideas of reference, paranoid ideation), *interpersonal* (no close friends, constricted affect, undue social society, paranoid ideation), and *disorganized* features (odd/eccentric behavior, odd speech) (Reynolds *et al.*, 2000; Raine, 2006). Notably, in the World Health Organization classification of diseases, ICD-10, schizotypal disorder is classified as a mental disorder associated with schizophrenia and not as a personality disorder as categorized in the DSM-IV. The phenotypic relationship to the obsessive–compulsive spectrum is highlighted by the inclusion of "obsessive ruminations without inner resistance, often with dysmorphophobic, sexual or aggressive contents" in the description of schizotypal disorder (Janca *et al.*, 1994).

In addition to phenomenological similarities, patients with schizotypal personality disorder share a number of neurophysiological, neurocognitive, and brain-imaging abnormalities found in schizophrenia patients. Shared information-processing abnormalities (e.g., a failure of pre-pulse inhibition) or the capacity to "gate" sensory input may result in sensory overload and cognitive disorganization (Siever and Davis, 2004). Cognitive impairments in executive function, working memory, and verbal learning are also comparable to those found in schizophrenia patients. Nevertheless, overall IQ is preserved, and neurocognitive deficits are less severe and persistent than in schizophrenia (Raine, 2006). These findings along with a lower striatal dopamine release mediated by amphetamine or by physiological stressors found in schizotypal personality disorder as compared to schizophrenia have been hypothesized to result in a significantly lower vulnerability for psychosis in patients with schizotypal personality disorder, and may account for the relatively low rate of progression to schizophrenia (Abi-Dargham *et al.*, 2002; Siever *et al.*, 2002; Mitropoulou *et al.*, 2004; Skodol *et al.*, 2011).

Schizotypal and obsessive–compulsive symptoms on a subclinical level

Does the increased prevalence of schizotypal personality disorder in OCD represent an epiphenomenon of a greater severity of OCD symptomatology? Examination of the relationship between schizotypal and obsessive–compulsive phenomena in *non-clinical* samples provides unique insight into the strength and nature of the relationship while avoiding the intervening factors of symptom severity, medication use, and chronic institutionalization typical to the clinical population.

Relationship between schizotypal and obsessive–compulsive symptoms has extensively been investigated in non-clinical samples of students and adolescents (Norman et al., 1996; Roth and Baribeau, 2000; Dinn et al., 2002; Rossi and Daneluzzo, 2002; Suhr et al., 2006; Chmielewski and Watson, 2008; Fonseca-Pedrero et al., 2011). Intercorrelation between the two dimensions was strongly supported when factor and cluster analyses were used. Notably, positive symptoms (oddity, mistrust, unusual beliefs) were linked to obsessive–compulsive symptoms, while negative symptoms were not, underscoring a distinct pattern of association between positive/negative dimensions of schizotypy and obsessive–compulsive symptoms in a non-clinical population. In an attempt to explain this pattern, Lee and colleagues (2005) hypothesized that the magical thinking facet of schizotypy may increase the likelihood that thought–action fusion would heighten the risk for obsessive–compulsive symptoms. *Thought–action fusion* refers to a set of cognitive biases that involve faulty causal relationships between one's own thoughts and external reality, thereby increasing the sense of personal responsibility. For instance, the belief that having an unacceptable or disturbing thought will increase the likelihood that the thought will occur in reality (e.g., "If I think of a friend losing his job, this increases the risk that he will indeed lose his job"). Furthermore, a cognitive model classified obsessions into two subtypes, "autogenous" and "reactive," based on the differences in their respective contents, emotional reactions, evaluative appraisals, control strategies, trigger stimuli, and relatedness to schizotypal traits (Lee and Telch, 2005). *Autogenous obsessions* are characterized by aggressive, sexual, and blasphemous themes. They are activated without clear triggers, perceived as highly ego-dystonic, and are not associated with overt compulsive rituals. In contrast, "*reactive obsessions*" are relatively more realistic thoughts (e.g., contamination) and the perceived threat is not the obsession itself but the associated potential negative consequences. The significant association of autogenous, but not reactive obsessions, with schizotypal traits was shown in a non-clinical sample of college students, lending empirical support for the hypothesis (Lee and Telch, 2005). The authors also found decreased latent inhibition, one of the neurophysiological correlates of impaired attentional inhibitory mechanisms, in individuals with autogenous but not reactive obsessions (Lee and Telch, 2010). Attenuated latent inhibition has consistently been demonstrated in patients with schizophrenia and schizotypal personality disorder (Lubow and De la Casa, 2002), further supporting a possible proximity in underlying mechanisms of autogenous obsessions and schizotypy.

Schizotypal personality disorder in OCD patients
Prevalence
The rate of occurrence of schizotypal personality disorder in OCD remains unclear. The observed rates vary substantially (0–50%) (Table 8.1). This may be accounted for by different definitions of schizotypal features (categorical vs. dimensional), methods of evaluation (structured interview vs. chart review), and the patient populations studied. The British National Survey of Psychiatric Morbidity 2000 (Torres et al., 2006),

Table 8.1 Rate of occurrence of schizotypal personality disorder in patients with OCD

Reference	Study sample	Study design and diagnostic criteria	Prevalence of schizotypal personality disorder in OCD	Comments
Jenike et al. (1986)	43 OCD patients	Chart review, DSM-III for SPD	33% (14/43)	OCD–SPD patients had poorer prognosis
Rasmussen and Tsuang (1986)	44 OCD patients	Semistructured interview	0%	
Baer et al. (1990)	96 OCD patients	SCID for DSM-III personality disorders	5% (5/96)	SPD – a predictor of poor outcome in OCD
Steketee (1990)	26 OCD patients	PDQ-R, self-report questionnaire based on the DSM-III-R criteria for personality disorders	34.6% (9/26)	SPD was among the most frequently occurring comorbidites, along with dependent and avoidant personality disorders
Black et al. (1993)	32 OCD patients; 33 controls	SCID for DSM-III personality disorders	18.8% (6/32) in OCD; 3% (1/33) in controls	OCD patients also had more Cluster C personality disorders
Eisen and Rasmussen (1993)	475 OCD patients	Semistructured interview, DSM-III-R criteria for OCD and SPD	3% (14/475)	79% of OCD–SPD patients were men and 69% had a deteriorative course
Bejerot et al. (1998)	36 OCD patients	SCID-II for personality disorders	3% (1/36)	One-third of the sample was diagnosed with Cluster A (schizoid, schizotypal, paranoid) personality disorders
Samuels et al. (2000)	72 OCD probands, 72 controls, and their first-degree relatives	Direct interview, SADS-LA, SIDP-R	0% (0/72) of OCD and 1.4% (1/72) of control probands had SPD	OCD probands had a higher prevalence of OCPD
Matsunaga et al. (2000)	94 OCD patients	SCID-II for personality disorders	23% (9/40) of men and 4% (2/54) of women had SPD	

Table 8.1 (*cont.*)

Reference	Study sample	Study design and diagnostic criteria	Prevalence of schizotypal personality disorder in OCD	Comments
Sobin *et al.* (2000)	119 OCD patients	SIS for schizotypy, self-rated	50% had mild to severe positive schizotypy signs	OCD patients with schizotypy had earlier age of onset, more comorbid diagnoses, and learning disability
Torres *et al.* (2006)	108 OCD patients in the community	SCID-II for personality disorders	24.9% (27/108)	SPD was among the most common personality disorders screened

SPD, Schizotypal Personality Disorder; SCID, Structured Clinical Interview for DSM-IV; PDQ-R, the revised Personality Diagnostic Questionnaire; SIS, the Structured Interview for Schizotypy; SADS-LA, the Schedule for Affective Disorders and Schizophrenia-Lifetime Anxiety; SIDP-R, the Revised Structured Instrument for the Diagnosis of Personality disorders; OCPD, obsessive–compulsive personality disorder.

a large-scale epidemiological study, provided particularly compelling evidence for the strength of the association between OCD and schizotypal personality disorder. The prevalence of personality disorders was compared among participants with OCD ($N = 108$), with other neuroses (generalized anxiety disorder, depressive disorder, phobias, panic disorder, and mixed anxiety and depressive disorder; $N = 1353$) and non-neurotic controls ($N = 6938$). The prevalence of screen-positive personality disorders in the OCD group was substantial (74%), and greater than in both comparison groups. Schizotypal personality disorder (24.9%) was one of the most common personality disorders in OCD patients.

Despite methodological differences, prevalence studies consistently demonstrated that OCD patients with associated schizotypal personality disorder exhibited a more deteriorative course and poorer prognosis than those with "pure" OCD. Notably, comorbidity of schizotypal personality disorder is not exclusively with OCD; it is as high as 66.3% for major depression, 40.7% for panic disorder, and 31.4% for social phobia (Raine, 2006).

Clinical characteristics

There is increasing evidence of differences in demographic and clinical characteristics of OCD patients with and without schizotypal features, supporting the clinical validity of schizotypal OCD (Eisen and Rasmussen, 1993; Matsunaga *et al.*, 2000; Sobin *et al.*, 2000; Torres *et al.*, 2006; Catapano *et al.*, 2010) (Table 8.2). Early age of onset, male gender, counting compulsions, and a history of specific phobia have been shown to increase the risk of schizotypy in patients with lifetime OCD. In addition, schizotypal OCD patients are more likely to be unmarried and unemployed. Similar to studies in non-clinical samples, most clinical research links positive symptoms of schizotypy with obsessive–compulsive symptoms (Enright and Beech, 1993; Einstein and Menzies, 2004; Lee and Telch, 2005). Strong links have been found between positive symptoms and indicators of severity in clinically diagnosed OCD, including earlier age of onset, comorbid diagnoses, and

Table 8.2 Clinical characteristics of schizotypal OCD compared to "pure" OCD

Poorer prognosis

Earlier age of onset

Male preponderance

Poorer insight

Hoarding is common

Predominance of positive schizotypal symptoms

Familial aggregation of schizophrenia-spectrum disorders

Antipsychotic augmentation to SRIs may be warranted

CBT seems to be less effective

SRI, serotonin reuptake inhibitor; CBT, cognitive–behavioral therapy.

treatment resistance (Sobin *et al.*, 2000; Moritz *et al.*, 2004). Explicit comparison of clinical characteristics of treatment-seeking OCD patients with and without schizotypal personality disorder revealed schizophrenia symptom scores coupled with lower general functioning scores in the schizotypal OCD group (Poyurovsky *et al.*, 2008). In addition, schizotypal OCD patients exhibited significantly poorer insight.

Among the various manifestations of OCD, hoarding seems to be associated with somewhat higher levels of schizotypal personality disorder. Hoarders are significantly more likely to have more severe psychopathology, poorer insight, higher prevalence of comorbid schizotypal or obsessive–compulsive personality disorder, closer association with symmetry dimension, and poorer treatment outcome (Frost *et al.*, 2000; Matsunaga *et al.*, 2010). Moreover, the association of schizotypal personality disorder and hoarding behavior seems to be moderated by gender in patients with OCD, as revealed in the OCD Collaborative Genetics Study (Samuels *et al.*, 2008).

Axis I comorbid psychiatric disorders are highly prevalent in patients with schizotypal OCD, and are associated with additional morbidity. Similar to "pure" OCD patients, two-thirds of patients with schizotypal OCD have at least one additional comorbid disorder (Poyurovsky *et al.*, 2008). Major depressive disorder appeared to be the most common (roughly 50%), followed by anxiety disorders (panic disorder, social and simple phobias), and OCD-spectrum disorders (tic disorders, body dysmorphic disorder).

The following case vignettes illustrate major clinical features of schizotypal OCD.

Case 8.1. A patient with OCD and predominant positive symptoms of schizotypal personality disorder.

Mr. G, 45 years old, single, came for psychiatric evaluation due to a recently intensified fear of contracting HIV, that had caused him distress for the past 10 years. He reported repetitive checking rituals to ensure the sterility of his environment. In addition, he repeatedly cleaned the phone receiver and would not sit down on a chair before thoroughly cleaning the seat, whether on public transportation, park benches, or in an office. He was unaware of the excessiveness of his behavior. These compulsions occupied more than 3 hours a day, substantially interfering with his daily functioning. He completed his studies with good grades, and then worked as a clerk in a hospital. He mentioned that he was always suspicious, could not trust others, and always assumed that others were criticizing him, even though there was no objective basis for these claims. He also recalled that he sometimes sensed the presence of another person in the room, a feeling that prompted him to repeatedly check the doors at home and at his workplace. His speech and thought processes were vague and idiosyncratic, but without formal thought disorders. His affect lacked the full range of emotional expressions and he appeared detached from the interviewer. His ideas of reference and perceptual disturbances never reached the severity of delusions or hallucinations. Thus he met criteria for DSM IV schizotypal personality disorder, in addition to OCD.

Case 8.2. A patient with OCD and predominant negative symptoms of schizotypal personality disorder.

Ms. A, a 59-year-old single woman, was referred for psychiatric evaluation following complaints of depressed mood, anhedonia, and sleep disturbances that occurred approximately 3 months prior to evaluation. This psychiatric assessment was the first in her life. Family history of mental disorders was positive for schizophrenia in her sister, and OCD in her father. A never had close friends and had only superficial acquaintances. She had not been in touch with her nuclear family for years. At age 25, after finishing secretarial school, she began to work in an office where she continued to work for the next 35 years. She communicated only with her boss, was reluctant to establish relationships with her co-workers, and was known to be odd and to have a somewhat eccentric personality. She expressed no desire for intimate relationships and had never had a boyfriend. She recalled that from as early as age 10, she had repetitive, intrusive, and distressful thoughts that her mother put needles in her bed. These thoughts caused a great deal of anxiety, and prompted her to conduct numerous ordering, arranging, and checking rituals before going to sleep in order to make sure that there were no needles in her bed. Later on, she developed counting and ordering rituals to prevent harm from her obsessive thoughts of the possibility of harming people around her. She was unaware of the senseless and excessive nature of her obsessional thoughts and rituals. They occupied a considerable amount of time and caused distress; however, she never sought professional treatment and had never been formally diagnosed with OCD. At intake, in addition to symptoms of moderate depression, she exhibited odd and magical thinking, of the ability to influence the behavior of others and predict their intentions. However, there was no evidence of delusions, formal thought disorders, or hallucinations. Her appearance was extravagant and somewhat juvenile. Her choice of language was pathetic, she acknowledged having multiple obsessions and compulsions, and said that she was now ready for help. She met DSM-IV criteria for major depressive disorder, in addition to OCD and schizotypal personality disorder.

Family inheritance

Schizotypal OCD seems to have a distinct pattern of familial aggregation of schizophrenia-spectrum disorders compared to "pure" OCD.

Our group obtained family information regarding OCD and schizophrenia-spectrum disorders for 131 first-degree relatives of OCD patients, with and without schizotypal personality disorder (Poyurovsky *et al.*, 2008). Information was collected in direct interviews of relatives (54.2%, 71 of 131), using the modules for schizophrenia and OCD of the SCID-I and schizotypal personality disorder of the SCID-II. For the remaining 45% (60 of 131) information was gathered indirectly using the Family History Research Diagnostic Criteria (FH-RDC) (Andreasen et al., 1977). Since the FH-RDC do not include OCD and schizotypal personality disorder modules, we used the SCID-I OCD and the SCID-II schizotypal personality disorder modules adapted to a third-person format.

As expected, there was a substantial aggregation of OCD cases in the relatives of both groups (13% in each), supporting a well-established familial transmission of the disorder (Pauls, 2008). In contrast, one-third of the schizotypal OCD patients had at least one first-degree relative with schizophrenia-spectrum disorders as compared to only 3% in the "pure" OCD group. The fact that the schizotypal OCD group had a family load of schizophrenia-spectrum disorders indicates that in this subset of patients, OCD and schizophrenia-spectrum disorders co-transmit in families. From the clinical perspective, detection of schizophrenia-spectrum disorders in first-degree relatives may contribute to better identification of schizotypal personality disorder in OCD patients.

Cognitive function and neuroimaging

Neurocognitive and neuroimaging findings lend some credence to the division of OCD into subgroups based on the presence of schizotypy. While patients with "pure" OCD display impaired performance on measures sensitive to the orbitofrontal cortex (alternation learning, response inhibition, delayed memory), OCD patients with schizotypal personality disorder perform poorly on tests sensitive to both the orbitofrontal and dorsolateral prefrontal cortex (Harris and Dinn, 2003; Shin et al., 2008). Similar to findings in schizophrenia patients, deficits in cognitive performance on tests sensitive to the dorsolateral prefrontal cortex are consistently found in patients with schizotypal personality disorder (Mitropoulou et al., 2002). OCD patients with schizotypal personality traits ($N = 20$), as assessed by the self-report Personality Disorder Questionnaire-4 (PDQ-4) (Hyler et al., 1988), also showed a significant gray matter volume reduction compared to their "pure" OCD counterparts ($N = 47$) (Jin Lee et al., 2006). Consistent with neurocognitive findings, the schizotypal OCD group is located mid range on the spectrum between OCD without schizotypy and the schizophrenia groups, based on gray matter volume reductions. Replication of these findings in a larger sample with clinically defined schizotypal personality disorder is needed.

Differential diagnosis
Psychotic disorders

Schizotypal personality disorder in OCD patients is distinguished from schizophrenia, delusional disorder, and affective disorder with psychotic features by a stable course and lack of pervasive positive symptoms. However, when brief psychotic episodes do emerge (lasting minutes to hours) the distinction becomes complicated. Noteworthy, clinical manifestations within schizotypal personality disorder are heterogeneous in terms of their prevalence and temporal stability (McGlashan et al., 2005). Paranoid ideation, ideas of reference, odd beliefs, and unusual experiences are the most common and stable expressions of the disorder. These features might represent milder variants of the cognitive distortion of reality that is central to the schizophrenia spectrum (Liddle and Barnes, 1990). In schizotypal personality disorder cognitive distortion is attenuated and emerges only intermittently as odd behavior or coldness, and is the least stable feature of the disorder (McGlashan et al., 2005).

In contrast to schizophrenia patients with clear-cut delusions of reference, individuals with schizotypal personality disorder often incorrectly interpret causal events, by assuming particular personal meanings, that is ideas of reference not associated with delusional conviction. They may be preoccupied with paranormal phenomena and may feel that they have special powers to predict events or to read others' thoughts. However, typical Schneiderian symptoms of mind-reading, thought insertion, or withdrawal and passivity phenomena are lacking. Perceptual distortions are not rare (e.g., sensing another person is present or hearing a voice murmuring his or her name), yet true auditory hallucinations are absent. Speech and thought processes are usually vague and idiosyncratic, but without actual incoherence, blocking, or derailment typical to formal thought disorders of schizophrenia. In patients with schizotypal personality disorder, affect usually lacks the full range of emotions. Schizotypal individuals often appear to interact with others in a stiff and constricted fashion, are uncomfortable in social situations particularly those involving unfamiliar people, and prefer to keep to themselves, feeling that they just do not "fit in." As a result they have few or no close friends. They also have decreased desire for intimate relationships. When the features of restricted affect, social isolation, and detachment are predominant, differential diagnosis between OCD-related schizotypal personality disorder and a subgroup of schizo-obsessive disorder with marked deficit symptoms becomes particularly challenging. Lack of prominent positive symptoms, chronic non-exacerbated course, social isolation, and low level of functioning are shared by the two conditions.

The following case exemplifies difficulties in the differential diagnosis of schizophrenia-spectrum disorders in an OCD patient and corresponding treatment challenges.

Case 8.3. Mr. A, a 46-year-old man, was characterized as a prudent and unsociable person. Since early adolescence he had felt uncomfortable in social situations particularly those involving unfamiliar people, and he had no close friends. He expressed no desire for intimate relationships and had never had a girlfriend. His peers considered him an odd and detached individual. His only strong attachment was to a computer; he spent hours programming new sites. He graduated from school with average grades, was recruited to the army and served as a computer technician. From the age of 18 he exhibited obsessive–compulsive symptoms along the themes of exactness and order. He developed what he described as "just right" compulsions: for example, turning the electricity on and off, getting his hair "just right," putting his belongings in the right place and in a special order. He also collected an exact number of the same writing pens; although he acknowledged that one was sufficient, it felt "right" to have more than one in case one got lost. He expressed fair insight into his obsessive–compulsive symptoms, but could not resist performing rituals. After discharge from the army he "abandoned" the idea of getting a job, and he remained single, unsociable, and aloof. His aging parents supported him financially. Prompted by his parents' concerns about his lifestyle and possible mental ailment, at age 32 he agreed to be seen by a psychiatrist. Their concerns were intensified by the fact that A's uncle had schizophrenia.

According to a psychiatric record, A appeared to be suspicious and expressed ideas of reference assuming that his parents wanted to put him in a psychiatric facility "to get rid of him." In addition, his affect was restricted, and his speech was vague and pathetic. He claimed that he was able to predict events based on his accentuated "sixth sense." No clear-cut delusions, hallucinations, or Schneiderian symptoms were revealed. Obsessive–compulsive symptoms were acknowledged, but not considered clinically significant. As recorded in his medical file, he was diagnosed with DSM-IV schizophrenic disorder, based on suspiciousness, ideas of reference, and prominent negative symptoms. Treatment with the antipsychotic haloperidol was initiated, but as no improvement was noted the dose was gradually increased. Since then A was prescribed regimens of various antipsychotics, including olanzapine, ziprasidone, and risperidone with gradually increasing doses due to "lack of response." When A was finally admitted to our research unit which specialized in treating patients with schizophrenia-spectrum disorders and OCD, he was taking haloperidol (10 mg/day) once again. Serious neuroleptic adverse effects, such as slow thinking, difficulty in concentration, decrease in emotional reaction, dysphoria, parkinsonism, and mild akathisia were recognized. A's psychiatric history was re-evaluated and his diagnosis of schizophrenia was changed to DSM-IV schizotypal personality disorder, based on the lack of pervasive positive symptoms and a stable course over decades without psychotic exacerbations. In addition, a diagnosis of OCD was established due to the presence of time-consuming and distressful ordering and collecting obsessions and compulsions that interfered with his daily functioning. We gradually decreased the dose of haloperidol and administered a low dose of risperidone (1 mg/day). During the follow-up no emergence of psychotic symptoms was noted. In contrast, there was marked improvement and eventual disappearance of neuroleptic-induced dysphoria and extrapyramidal side effects. Finally sertraline (up to 200 mg/day) was added to risperidone to address OCD symptoms. After 12 weeks of combined treatment a clinically significant improvement of obsessive–compulsive symptoms was noted and maintained during a 2-year follow-up (total Y-BOCS score dropped 50% from 24 to 12).

Pervasive developmental disorders

An additional diagnostic challenge is the distinction of children and adolescents with OCD and schizotypal personality disorder from the heterogeneous group of children and adolescents whose behavior is characterized by social isolation, eccentricity, and peculiarities in language similar to those seen in children with autistic disorders and Asperger's syndrome. The latter are distinguished primarily based on more severely impaired social interactions and stereotypical behaviors and interests (Svrakic and Cloninger, 2005).

Other personality disorders

When OCD patients present with schizotypal personality disorder, the latter should be distinguished from other personality disorders. Hence, schizoid and paranoid personality disorders are rarely associated with magical thinking, unusual perceptual experiences, or oddities in speech, appearance, and thought processes. Avoidant personality disorder is not characterized by disinterest and detachment, and is rarely associated with oddities in appearance and behavior. It is characterized by fear of embarrassment, which leads to social avoidance and isolation. Borderline personality disorder is characterized by affective instability and stormy relationships, as well as impulsive and manipulative behavior. It is of note that there is considerable co-occurrence of schizotypal personality disorder with schizoid, avoidant, and borderline personality disorders in patients with or without OCD, possibly because of overlapping diagnostic criteria (McGlashan *et al.*, 2005).

Treatment

Schizotypal personality disorder as a predictor of poor treatment response

Schizotypal personality disorder predicts poor response to standard pharmacological and behavioral intervention in OCD patients. Jenike *et al.* (1986) were among the first to retrospectively examine characteristics of 43 treatment-resistant obsessive–compulsive patients and to show that those with concomitant schizotypal personality disorder had an extremely high rate of treatment failure. Of the 29 treated OCD patients without schizotypal personality disorder, 26 (90%) improved at least moderately; and only one of 14 (7%) schizotypal patients improved. The same authors conducted a controlled 12-week trial of clomipramine hydrochloride in 55 patients with OCD and found that the presence of schizotypal personality disorder was a strong predictor of poor treatment outcome (Baer *et al.*, 1992). The results of an investigation of clinical factors related to drug treatment response in OCD patients treated with either clomipramine or fluoxetine for a period of 6 months (Ravizza *et al.*, 1995) support these findings. Response was defined as a decrease of at least 40% in the Y-BOCS total score and a rating of "improved" or "very much improved" on the Clinical Global Impression scale. By the sixth month of treatment, 22 (41.5%) of 53 patients did not respond to either clomipramine or fluoxetine. Non-responders had lower age at onset and longer duration of the disorder. They also showed higher frequency of compulsions, washing rituals, chronic course, concomitant schizotypal personality disorder, and previous hospitalizations. Poorer response to drug treatment was predicted in a stepwise multiple regression by (1) concomitant schizotypal personality disorder, (2) presence of compulsions, and (3) longer illness length. Similarly, in a 3-year prospective naturalistic study of patients that met DSM-IV criteria for OCD, significant predictors of poor outcome included longer duration of illness, a greater severity of obsessive–compulsive symptoms at intake, and the presence of comorbid DSM-IV schizotypal personality disorder (Catapano *et al.*, 2006).

Not all studies found an association between schizotypal personality disorder and non-response to treatment in patients with OCD. It was hypothesized that a binary approach (presence vs. absence of schizotypal personality) may obscure the relation between schizotypal personality disorder and treatment outcome (Moritz *et al.*, 2004). The authors investigated whether the predictive importance of schizotypal personality is confined to a subset of symptoms or whether it is shared by all of its features to the same extent. Fifty-three patients with OCD underwent multimodal cognitive–behavioral therapy with or without adjunctive SSRIs. Therapy response was defined as a 35% reduction in the Y-BOCS total score. Stepwise regression analysis revealed that indeed elevated scores in the positive but not negative schizotypal factor, especially perceptual aberrations, as assessed by the Schizotypal Personality Questionnaire and the Perceptual Aberration Scale (Chapman *et al.*, 1978), strongly predicted treatment failure.

Overall, the presence of schizotypal personality disorder, particularly its positive psychopathological dimension, seems to increase the risk of treatment failure in OCD patients prompting a search for adequate therapeutic strategies. Noteworthy, roughly 40–60% of non-schizotypal OCD patients do not respond adequately to SRI therapy and an even greater proportion of patients fail to experience complete symptom remission.

Even those patients who are judged to be clinical responders based on stringent response criteria (i.e., typically a greater than 25% or 35% decline in Y-BOCS scores) continue to experience significant impairment from residual OCD symptoms. Furthermore, as many as 25% of schizotypal patients with OCD fail to experience any improvement from initial SRI monotherapy (Ravizza et al., 1995; Erzegovesi et al., 2001).

Augmentation with low-dose antipsychotic agents

Two pharmacological augmentation strategies for non-responders to SRI monotherapy have been studied. The first strategy involved the use of serotonin-enhancing agents (e.g., lithium, clonazepam, or buspirone) to maximize treatment response, and yielded unanimously discouraging results. The second involved the addition of low-dose dopamine antagonists to SRIs. The rationale for adding dopamine antagonists is based on the assumption of the involvement of the dopaminergic system in addition to the serotonergic system in the mediation of obsessive–compulsive symptoms and putative treatment resistance. This seems to be particularly relevant in schizotypal personality disorder comorbid to OCD (Coccaro, 1998; Koenigsberg et al., 2003). Indeed, starting with small open-label studies, the presence of schizotypal personality disorder seemed to herald positive response to antipsychotic augmentation in SRI-resistant OCD.

McDougle et al. (1990) explicitly examined whether comorbid schizotypal personality disorder and tic spectrum disorders were associated with a positive response to the addition of a neuroleptic in 17 OCD patients who did not respond to the SSRI fluvoxamine (mean dose = 291 ± 26.4 mg/day for a mean of 7.7 ± 2.3 weeks). Fourteen patients received pimozide (mean dose 6.5 ± 5.4 mg/day), two patients received thioridazine (100 mg/day and 75 mg/day, respectively), and one patient received thiothixene (6 mg/day). Neuroleptic treatment lasted 2–8 weeks (mean 4.7 ± 1.9 weeks). On the basis of the Clinical Global Impression scale criterion of improvement, 9 (53%) of 17 participants responded: 7 (88%) of 8 patients with comorbid tic or schizotypal personality disorder responded; however, only 2 (22%) of 9 patients without these disorders responded ($p = 0.02$, Fisher's exact test). The addition of antipsychotic agents however was not without cost: more than half of the patients experienced mild-to-moderate extrapyramidal side effects after the addition of the neuroleptic agent. One patient developed dystonic symptoms requiring discontinuation of pimozide.

Promising results were also obtained when the efficacy of olanzapine addition to fluvoxamine-refractory OCD patients was investigated (Bogetto et al., 2000). Twenty-three OCD non-responders to a 6-month, open-label trial with fluvoxamine (300 mg/day) entered a 3-month open-label trial of augmentation with olanzapine (5 mg/day). Three OCD patients (13.04%) had comorbid chronic motor tic disorder, and four (17.39%) had a co-diagnosis of schizotypal personality disorder. Ten patients (43.5%) were rated as responders, and concomitant schizotypal personality disorder was the only factor significantly associated with response. The most common side effects were mild-to-moderate weight gain and sedation.

Saxena et al. (1996) substantiated therapeutic efficacy of low-dose risperidone (mean dose = 2.75 mg/day) in an open-label study of 21 OCD patients who had failed to respond to at least one adequate trial of an SRI. Of the 16 patients who tolerated combined treatment, 14 (87%) had substantial reductions in obsessive–compulsive symptoms within 3 weeks. Patients with comorbid psychotic disorders improved gradually over 2 to 3 weeks. The authors revealed that despite the low dose, risperidone addition was associated with a meaningful rate of extrapyramidal side effects; 5 (24%) of the 21 patients experienced akathisia, which forced discontinuation of risperidone.

McDougle *et al.* (2000) conducted a double-blind placebo-controlled study of risperidone addition in OCD patients refractory to SRIs. Seventy adult patients with a primary DSM-IV diagnosis of OCD received 12 weeks of treatment with an SRI. Thirty-six patients were refractory to the SRI and were randomized in a double-blind manner to 6 weeks of risperidone ($N = 20$) or placebo ($N = 16$) addition. There was no difference in response between OCD patients with and without comorbid diagnoses of schizotypal personality disorder or tic disorder: 50% of the risperidone-treated study completers (9 of 18) were responders (mean daily dose, 2.2 ± 0.7 mg/day) compared with none of 15 in the placebo addition group ($p < 0.005$).

Our comparative study of treatment-seeking OCD patients with and without schizotypal personality disorder revealed a significant difference between the two groups in the proportion of patients who required antipsychotic augmentation (Poyurovsky *et al.*, 2008). Thus, 73% (11 of 15 patients) in the schizotypal OCD group compared to 26% (8 of 31) patients were prescribed antipsychotic augmentation by their physicians (haloperidol, 2.5 mg/day, risperidone 0.5–1.5 mg/day, or olanzapine 5–10 mg/day). According to the treatment guidelines for OCD patients in our center, antipsychotic augmentation is undertaken only after two unsuccessful adequate trials with SRIs. This study supported clinical experience that indicated that treatment-seeking schizotypal OCD patients most probably require an SRI and antipsychotic agent combination to address both components of their complex psychiatric condition.

In a comprehensive systematic review, Bloch *et al.* (2006) strongly support the clinical utility of low-dose antipsychotic augmentation as an effective intervention for treatment-refractory OCD patients. However, the evaluation of the role of comorbid schizotypal personality disorder was notably absent because of the insufficient number of studies with randomized controlled trial methodology required to be included in this review. Some conclusions derived from this meta-analysis may be pertinent to treatment of schizotypal OCD patients as well. *First*, Bloch and colleagues found strong evidence for the efficacy of low-dose haloperidol and risperidone augmentation. Evidence regarding the efficacy of adjunctive quetiapine and olanzapine in treatment-refractory OCD is inconclusive, as is the efficacy of other antipsychotics (e.g., amisulpiride, aripiprazole, ziprasidone). The greater D_2-dopamine receptor affinity of haloperidol and risperidone compared to other antipsychotics may account for the revealed differences. Alternatively, differences between the trial designs that compare different antipsychotic augmentation agents to placebo could explain the discrepancy in efficacy. Head-to-head comparisons between antipsychotic augmentation agents in OCD patients with and without schizotypal personality disorder would show which antipsychotic agents are more effective, and whether comorbid schizotypal personality disorder plays a role in treatment response to a particular antipsychotic agent. *Second*, antipsychotic augmentation is effective relatively quickly in treating OCD, and patients are unlikely to improve if they have not responded after 1 month of intervention, since there was no difference in the number of treatment responders after 4 weeks of treatment. *Third*, the subgroup of OCD patients with comorbid tics appeared to have a particularly beneficial response to treatment with antipsychotic augmentation. As previously noted, tic disorders may be observed in a substantial proportion of schizotypal OCD patients highlighting the importance of an antipsychotic augmentation strategy in this subgroup of patients.

Antiglutamatergic agents as potential treatment of schizotypal OCD

Among novel treatment options glutamatergic agents are the promising new candidates for the treatment of OCD. This seems to be particularly pertinent to schizotypal OCD in view of the revealed glutamatergic dysfunction in both OCD and schizophrenia-spectrum disorders (see Chapter 1). Agents that attenuate glutamatergic neurotransmission, memantine and riluzole, produced promising results, but none has achieved sufficient empirical evidence to become recommended in treatment guidelines for OCD (Bandelow et al., 2008).

The following case vignette highlights the potential therapeutic efficacy of anti-glutamatergic drugs in patients with treatment-refractory OCD and comorbid schizotypal personality disorder (Poyurovsky and Koran, 2005). The therapy includes off-label use of memantine, and efficacy has not yet been confirmed in controlled trials.

Case 8.4. Ms. M, 34 years old, presented with incapacitating ego-dystonic obsessions, including fear that harm would come to her daughter, and fear of losing her mind. She developed compulsive checking behavior to decrease the associated anxiety. Obsessive–compulsive symptoms were initially detected at age 16, and remitted spontaneously 2 years later. Subsequent postpartum exacerbation of DSM-IV OCD symptoms associated with major depression occurred at age 30. She also met DSM-IV criteria for schizotypal personality disorder. Subsequent adequate trials with paroxetine and sertraline were ineffective. Add-on risperidone caused marked akathisia and was discontinued. At presentation, oral clomipramine was initiated and titrated to 300 mg/day. However, 10 weeks later there was no significant clinical improvement (Y-BOCS = 35). The addition of a selective dopamine D_2 antagonist, sulpiride (up to 400 mg/day for 4 weeks), was also ineffective (Y-BOCS = 34). At this point an off-label therapy of add-on memantine, an N-methyl-D-aspartate (NMDA) glutamatergic receptor antagonist, to her regimen of clomipramine (300 mg/day) and sulpiride (400 mg/day) was proposed. After receiving a detailed explanation for this novel treatment the patient signed informed consent to receive the treatment. Memantine was started at 5 mg/day, and titrated to 20 mg within 2 weeks. The patient reported initial relief on day 7 of combined treatment, and a significant decrease in symptom severity was noted 3 weeks later (Y-BOCS = 22). There was substantial reduction in distress and the time occupied by rituals, followed by increased control over obsessions. No clinically significant side effects were noted.

Clozapine

When there is no improvement with any of the available pharmacological strategies, and before considering invasive interventions (e.g., deep brain stimulation), clozapine therapy may be attempted in severe treatment-refractory OCD patients with schizotypal personality disorder. Clozapine monotherapy is beneficial in treatment-resistant schizophrenia, but not OCD (McDougle et al., 1995). An OCD-provoking effect of clozapine in schizophrenia patients is well established, but clozapine-related amelioration of schizophrenia-related obsessive–compulsive symptoms has also been revealed (Reznik et al., 2004). Indeed, relatively low doses of clozapine resulted in clinically significant improvement in some treatment-refractory OCD patients with comorbid schizotypal personality disorder, as shown in the following case vignettes (Poyurovsky et al., 2008). The therapy includes off-label use of clozapine, and efficacy has not yet been confirmed in controlled trials.

Case 8.5. Ms. R was first hospitalized at age 54 for contamination fears and incapacitating compulsive washing (Y-BOCS = 40, maximum score). She met DSM-IV criteria for OCD and schizotypal personality disorder at age 24. In ambulatory care she had adequate monotherapy trials (≥12 weeks) with SRIs (fluvoxamine 250 mg/day, paroxetine 60 mg/day, clomipramine 300 mg/day) and combined with typical (perphenazine 16 mg/day, haloperidol 2 mg/day) or atypical (risperidone 2 mg/day) antipsychotics, which were ineffective and resulted in tardive dyskinesia. Clozapine was initiated at 12.5 mg/day and titrated to 75 mg/day within 2 weeks. She reported substantial relief of OC symptoms (Y-BOCS = 29). Subsequent clozapine titration to 150 mg/day within 4 weeks led to a marked reduction in OCD severity (Y-BOCS = 15). Moderate sedation was the only side effect. Tardive dyskinesia completely disappeared.

Case 8.6. Mr. S, age 36, exhibited obsessive–compulsive symptoms from age 8. At age 22 he met DSM-IV criteria for OCD and schizotypal personality disorder. Adequate trials (≥12 weeks) with fluvoxamine (250 mg/day), sertraline (200 mg/day), and clomipramine (250 mg/ day) were ineffective, as were trials with ziprasidone (80 mg/day) or haloperidol (1 mg/day) augmentation. He eventually refused medications due to tardive dyskinesia. Mr. S was hospitalized for severe exacerbation of OCD. Clozapine was initiated at 12.5 mg/day and gradually titrated to 250 mg/day within 6 weeks. He regained control over rituals and the intensity of OCD substantially subsided. Y-BOCS dropped from 40 to 26 at week 8 and tardive dyskinesia disappeared. Clozapine side effects were hypersalivation and drowsiness. Weekly laboratory white blood cell count tests were normal for both patients.

Non-pharmacological interventions

Exposure and ritual prevention is an additional first-line treatment for OCD. Is it effective treatment for patients with OCD and schizotypal personality disorder? Minichiello et al. (1987) retrospectively reviewed the treatment outcome of OCD patients treated with behavior therapy either alone or in combination with pharmacotherapy, and determined which patients met DSM-III criteria for schizotypal personality disorder. Eighty-four percent (16 of 19) of the OCD patients without schizotypal personality disorder and only 10% (1 of 10) of those with schizotypy achieved at least moderate improvement in their OCD symptoms with combined behavioral and pharmacological treatment. The number of schizotypal features strongly negatively correlated with treatment outcomes ($r = -0.68$; $p = 0.001$). Schizotypal personality encompasses several factors that predict poor outcome. Most noticeably, a substantial proportion of these patients has poor insight and strongly believes that rituals are necessary to prevent the occurrence of terrible events. They frequently have difficulty complying with prescribed treatment and with record-keeping tasks assigned in CBT. Family involvement and support is essential in behavioral therapy, but schizotypal patients typically have poor social relations and chaotic family situations. Generally, it seems that schizotypal OCD patients do not benefit from CBT. Some schizotypal OCD patients have actually become more dysfunctional following CBT (Walker et al., 1994).

What alternative non-pharmacological interventions might address the substantial morbidity associated with the schizotypal component of the disorder? Social skills training is a behavioral procedure based on shaping appropriate responses, and extinguishing inappropriate or socially maladaptive behaviors and has proven to be an efficacious rehabilitative approach for schizophrenia-spectrum disorders. Conversation skills, appropriate facial expressions, eye contact, and reciprocity are some of the areas commonly targeted for social skills training.

The following case illustrates clinical utility of social skills training for a patient with schizotypal OCD (Mckay and Neziroglu, 1996).

Case 8.7. Mr. I is a 33-year-old man with a 17-year history of DSM-III-R OCD and schizotypal personality disorder. His schizotypal symptoms included poor interpersonal relations, ideas of reference (not delusional), social anxiety, unusual perceptual experiences (such as seeing things in the periphery that are not present when viewed directly), constricted affect, and some paranoid ideations. Mr. I performed rituals that included showering three times a day. He also showered after each time he voided his bowels or bladder for fear of contracting an illness. He also had extensive rituals for cooking meals to avoid contracting food-borne diseases, and he did not go to restaurants because he was wary of the sanitary conditions in the food preparation. He also engaged in checking rituals to determine whether doors were locked. The deficits in I's social skills were primarily in conversation, inappropriate affect, poor assertion, and lack of eye contact. He was also prone to aggressive outbursts in the home, and often broke objects out of frustration. Although none of his compulsions involved social situations, these deficits contributed to his ongoing obsessions and compulsions. Sessions were once a week for 45 minutes. The trial of social skills training lasted about 6 months. Skills training included sessions that addressed eye contact, assertion skills, introductions and beginning of conversations, maintaining conversations and identifying non-verbal cues to change topics, ending conversations, and setting social appointments . . . Following social skills treatment and at 6-month follow-up, the patient had considerable obsessive–compulsive symptom reduction.

Social skills training may result not only in the improvement of behaviors associated with the patient's schizotypy, but also with a meaningful decrease in the severity of obsessive–compulsive symptoms (Mckay and Neziroglu, 1996). This in turn may enable the initiation of exposure and ritual prevention to deal directly with obsessive–compulsive symptoms. It is reasonable to suggest social skills training contributes to an increased desire for socialization and the patient's ability to overcome anxiety associated with exposure. Social skills training promotes effective socialization and enables patients to initiate exposure to previously feared situations that involve interpersonal exchanges.

Diagnostic and treatment recommendations

Overall, schizotypal OCD seems to have clinical and predictive validity and putative etiological specificity. Lacking evidence-based guidelines, the following may be considered when formulating diagnosis, treatment plan, and prognosis in patients with schizotypal OCD:

- Schizotypal personality disorder is commonly observed in patients with OCD. Clinicians should be aware that as many as *one-quarter* of all individuals with OCD may have comorbid symptoms of schizotypy or DSM-IV schizotypal personality disorder. This high estimate, and the additional morbidity associated with the presence of schizotypal personality disorder in OCD patients, underscores the clinical relevance of schizotypal OCD.
- Diagnosis of schizotypal OCD is warranted for those patients who meet full DSM-IV criteria for both OCD and schizotypal personality disorder (Cases 8.1 and 8.2). Identification of schizophrenia-spectrum disorders in first-degree relatives of patients with OCD might contribute to the diagnosis. Patients with schizotypal OCD often come

for an initial psychiatric evaluation following a major depressive episode or other comorbid condition (Case 8.2), though thorough evaluation reveals the "primary" disorder.

- Differential diagnosis of schizotypal OCD from schizophrenia with obsessive–compulsive symptoms is challenging, but critical for better delineation and effective treatment of these patients. Stringent adherence to DSM criteria for schizophrenia, schizotypal personality disorder, and OCD and repeated evaluations to establish diagnostic stability is crucial for correct diagnosis (Case 8.3).
- Treatment of OCD patients with schizotypal personality disorder is a difficult endeavor.

Regardless of the presence of schizotypal personality disorder, owing to the meaningful rate of treatment response to continued SRI monotherapy, OCD patients should first be treated with at least 3 months of the highest-tolerated dose of an anti-obsessive agent before considering initiation of antipsychotic augmentation (American Psychiatric Association, 2007). Antipsychotic augmentation is necessary for schizotypal OCD patients who have not responded to an adequate trial with an SRI. Administration of the lowest effective dose of antipsychotic medication is essential to minimize the risk for extrapyramidal side effects and akathisia to which patients with schizotypal OCD seem to be especially sensitive (Case 8.3). Long-term gains and risks of adjunctive antipsychotic therapy for schizotypal OCD patients remain to be clarified. Social skills training might attenuate maladaptive behaviors associated with schizotypy, and might potentially enable the initiation of exposure and ritual prevention to deal directly with obsessive–compulsive symptoms.

References

Abi-Dargham A, Mawlawi O, Lombardo I, et al. (2002) Prefrontal dopamine D1 receptors and working memory in schizophrenia. Journal of Neuroscience 22, 3708–3719.

American Psychiatric Association (1994) Diagnostic and Statistical Manual of Mental Disorders, 4th edn. American Psychiatric Association, Washington, DC.

Andreasen NC, Endicott J, Spitzer RL, Winokur G (1977) The family history method using diagnostic criteria: reliability and validity. Archives of General Psychiatry 34, 1229–1235.

Baer L, Jenike MA, Ricciardi JN 2nd, et al. (1990) Standardized assessment of personality disorders in obsessive-compulsive disorder. Archives of General Psychiatry 47, 826–830.

Baer L, Jenike MA, Black DW, et al. (1992) Effect of Axis II diagnoses on treatment outcome with clomipramine in 55 patients with obsessive-compulsive disorder. Archives of General Psychiatry 49, 862–866.

Bandelow B, Zohar J, Hollander E, et al. (2008) World Federation of Societies of Biological Psychiatry (WFSBP) guidelines for the pharmacological treatment of anxiety, obsessive-compulsive and post-traumatic stress disorders: first revision. World Journal of Biological Psychiatry 9, 248–312.

Bejerot S, Eskelius L, Van Knorring L (1998) Comorbidity between obsessive–compulsive disorder (OCD) and personality disorders. Acta Psychiatrica Scandinavica 97, 398–402.

Black DW, Noyes R Jr (1997) Obsessive-compulsive disorder and axis II. International Review of Psychiatry 9, 111–118.

Black DW, Noyes R Jr, Pfohl B, Goldstein RB, Blum N (1993) Personality disorder in obsessive-compulsive volunteers, well comparison subjects, and their first-degree relatives. American Journal of Psychiatry 150, 1226–1232.

Bleuler E (1911/1950) Dementia Praecox or the Group of Schizophrenias, transl. Zinkin J. International Universities Press, New York.

Bloch MH, Landeros-Weisenberger A, Kelmendi B, et al. (2006) A systematic review: antipsychotic augmentation with treatment refractory obsessive-compulsive disorder. *Molecular Psychiatry* 11, 622 632.

Bloch MH, Landeros-Weisenberger A, Rosario MC, Pittenger C, Leckman JF (2008) Meta-analysis of the symptom structure of obsessive-compulsive disorder. *American Journal of Psychiatry* 165, 1532–1542.

Bogetto F, Bellini S, Vaschetto P, Ziero S (2000) Olanzapine augmentation of fluvoxamine-refractory obsessive-compulsive disorder (OCD): a 12-week open trial. *Psychiatry Research* 96, 91–98.

Catapano F, Perris F, Masella M, *et al.* (2006) Obsessive-compulsive disorder: a 3-year prospective follow-up study of patients treated with serotonine reuptake inhibitors – OCD follow-up study. *Journal of Psychiatric Research* 40, 502–510.

Catapano F, Perris F, Fabrazzo M, *et al.* (2010) obsessive-compulsive disorder with poor insight: a three-year prospective study. *Progress in Neuropsychopharmacology and Biologicalo Psychiatry* 34, 323–330.

Chapman LJ, Chapman JP, Raulin ML (1976) Scales for physical and social anhedonia. *Journal of Abnormal Psychology* 85, 374–382.

Chapman LJ, Chapman JP, Raulin ML (1978) Body-image aberration in schizophrenia. *Journal of Abnormal Psychology* 87, 399–407.

Chmielewski M, Watson D (2008) The heterogeneous structure of schizotypal personality disorder: item-level factors of the Schizotypal Personality Questionnaire and their associations with obsessive-compulsive disorder symptoms, dissociative tendencies, and normal personality. *Journal of Abnormal Psychology* 117, 364–376.

Claridge G, Broks P (1984) Schizotypy and hemisphere function: I. Theoretical considerations and the measurement of schizotypy. *Personality and Individual Differences* 5, 633–648.

Coccaro EF (1998) Clinical outcome of psychopharmacologic treatment of borderline and schizotypal personality disordered subjects. *Journal of Clinical Psychiatry* 59 (Suppl. 1), 30–35.

Einstein DA, Menzies RG (2004) Role of magical thinking in obsessive-compulsive symptoms in an undergraduate sample. *Depression and Anxiety* 19, 174–179.

Eisen JL, Rasmussen SA (1993) Obsessive-compulsive disorder with psychotic features. *Journal of Clinical Psychiatry* 54, 373–379.

Enright SJ, Beech AR (1993) Reduced cognitive inhibition in obsessive-compulsive disorder. *British Journal of Clinical Psychology* 32, 67–74.

Erzegovesi S, Cavallini MC, Cavedini P, *et al.* (2001) Clinical predictors of drug response in obsessive-compulsive disorder. *Journal of Clinical Psychopharmacology* 21, 488–492.

First MB, Spitzer R, Gibbon M, Williams JBW (1995) *Structured Clinical Interview for Axis I DSM-IV Disorders, Patient Edition (SCID-I/P, Version 2.0).* Biometrics Research Department, New York State Psychiatric Institute, New York.

Fonseca-Pedrero E, Paino M, Lemos-Giráldez S, Muñiz J (2011) Schizotypal traits and depressive symptoms in nonclinical adolescents. *Comprehensive Psychiatry* 52, 293–300.

Frost RO, Steketee G, Williams LF, Warren R (2000) Mood, personality disorder symptoms and disability in obsessive compulsive hoarders: a comparison with clinical and nonclinical controls. *Behaviour Research and Therapy* 38, 1071–1081.

Gunderson JG, Singer MT (1975) Defining borderline patients: an overview. *American Journal of Psychiatry* 132, 1–9.

Harris CL, Dinn WM (2003) Subtyping obsessive-compulsive disorder: neuropsychological correlate. *Behavioural Neurology* 14, 75–87.

Hyler SE, Rieder RO, Williams JBW, *et al.* (1988) The Personality Diagnostic Questionnaire: development and preliminary results. *Journal of Personality Disorders* 2, 229–237.

Janca A, Ustun TB, van Drimmelen J, Dittmann V, Isaac M (1994) *ICD-10 Symptom Checklist for Mental Disorders,*

Version 1.1. Division of Mental Health, World Health Organization, Geneva.

Jenike MA, Baer L, Minichiello WE, Schwartz CE, Carey RJ Jr (1986) Concomitant obsessive-compulsive disorder and schizotypal personality disorder. *American Journal of Psychiatry* 143, 530–532.

Jin Lee K, Wook Shin Y, Wee H, Youn Kim Y, Kwon JS (2006) Gray matter volume reduction in obsessive-compulsive disorder with schizotypal personality trait. *Progress in Neuropsychopharmacology and Biological Psychiatry* 30, 1146–1149.

Kernberg O (1967) Borderline personality organization. *Journal of the American Psychoanalytic Association* 15, 641–685.

Kety SS, Rosenthal D, Wender PH, Schulsinger F (1971) Mental illness in the biological and adoptive families of adopted schizophrenics. *American Journal of Psychiatry* 128, 302–306.

Koenigsberg HW, Reynolds D, Goodman M, et al. (2003) Risperidone in the treatment of schizotypal personality disorder. *Journal of Clinical Psychiatry* 64, 628–634.

Kraepelin E (1919) *Dementia Praecox.* Krieger, New York.

Lee HJ, Telch MJ (2005) Autogenous/reactive obsessions and their relationship with OCD symptoms and schizotypal personality features. *Anxiety Disorders* 19, 793–805.

Lee HJ, Telch MJ (2010) Differences in latent inhibition as a function of the autogenous-reactive OCD subtype. *Behaviour Research and Therapy* 48, 571–579.

Lee HJ, Cougle JR, Telch MJ (2005) Thought–action fusion and its relationship to schizotypy and OCD symptoms. *Behaviour Research and Therapy* 43, 29–41.

Liddle PF, Barnes TR (1990) Syndromes of chronic schizophrenia. *British Journal of Psychiatry* 157, 558–561.

Lubow RE, De la Casa G (2002) Latent inhibition as a function of schizotypality and gender: implications for schizophrenia. *Biological Psychology* 59, 69–86.

Mataix-Cols D, Baer L, Rauch SL, Jenike MA (2000) Relation of factor-analyzed symptom dimensions of obsessive-compulsive disorder to personality disorders. *Acta Psychiatrica Scandinavica* 102, 199–202.

Matsunaga H, Kiriike N, Matsui T, et al. (2000) Gender differences in social and interpersonal features and personality disorders among Japanese patients with obsessive-compulsive disorder. *Comprehensive Psychiatry* 41, 266–272.

Matsunaga H, Hayashida K, Kiriike N, Maebayashi K, Stein DJ (2010) The clinical utility of symptom dimensions in obsessive-compulsive disorder. *Psychiatry Research* 30, 25–29.

McDougle CJ, Goodman WK, Price LH, et al. (1990) Neuroleptic addition in fluvoxamine-refractory obsessive-compulsive disorder. *American Journal of Psychiatry* 147, 652–654.

McDougle CJ, Barr LC, Goodman WK, et al. (1995) Lack of efficacy of clozapine monotherapy in refractory obsessive-compulsive disorder. *American Journal of Psychiatry* 152, 1812–1814.

McDougle CJ, Epperson CN, Pelton GH, Wasylink S, Price LH (2000) A double-blind, placebo-controlled study of risperidone addition in serotonin reuptake inhibitor-refractory obsessive-compulsive disorder. *Archives of General Psychiatry* 57, 794–801.

McGlashan TH, Grilo CM, Sanislow CA, et al. (2005) Two-year prevalence and stability of individual DSM-IV criteria for schizotypal, borderline, avoidant, and obsessive-compulsive personality disorders: toward a hybrid model of Axis II disorders. *American Journal of Psychiatry* 162, 883–889.

Mckay D, Neziroglu F (1996) Social skills training in a case of obsessive-compulsive disorder with schizotypal personality disorder. *Journal of Behavior Therapy and Experimental Psychiatry* 27, 189–194.

Meehl PE (1990) Toward an integrated theory of schizotaxia, schizotypy and schizophrenia. *Journal of Personality Disorders* 4, 1–99.

Minichiello WE, Baer L, Jenike MA (1987) Schizotypal personality disorder: a poor prognostic indicator for behavior therapy in the treatment of obsessive-compulsive disorder. *Journal of Anxiety Disorders* 1, 273–276.

Mitropoulou V, Harvey PD, Maldari LA, *et al.* (2002) Neuropsychological performance in schizotypal personality disorder: evidence regarding diagnostic specificity. *Biological Psychiatry* 52, 1175–1182.

Mitropoulou V, Goodman M, Sevy S, *et al.* (2004) Effects of acute metabolic stress on the dopaminergic and pituitary–adrenal axis activity in patients with schizotypal personality disorder. *Schizophrenia Research* 70, 27–31.

Moritz S, Fricke S, Jacobsen D, *et al.* (2004) Positive schizotypal symptoms predict treatment outcome in obsessive-compulsive disorder. *Behaviour Research and Therapy* 42, 217–227.

Norman RM, Davies F, Malla AK, Cortese L, Nicholson IR (1996) Relationship of obsessive-compulsive symptomatology to anxiety, depression and schizotypy in a clinical population. *British Journal of Clinical Psychology* 35, 553–566.

Pauls DL (2008) The genetics of obsessive-compulsive disorder: a review of the evidence. *American Journal of Medical Genetics Part C Seminars in Medical Genetics* 148, 133–139.

Poyurovsky M, Koran LM (2005) Obsessive-compulsive disorder (OCD) with schizotypy vs. schizophrenia with OCD: diagnostic dilemmas and therapeutic implications. *Journal of Psychiatric Research* 39, 399–408.

Poyurovsky M, Faragian S, Pashinian A, *et al.* (2008) Clinical characteristics of schizotypal-related obsessive-compulsive disorder. *Psychiatry Research* 159, 254–258.

Raine A (1991) The SPQ: a scale for the assessment of schizotypal personality based on DSM-III-R criteria. *Schizophrenia Bulletin* 17, 555–564.

Raine A (2006) Schizotypal personality: neurodevelopmental and psychosocial trajectories. *Annual Review of Clinical Psychology* 2, 291–326.

Rasmussen SA, Tsuang MT (1986) Clinical characteristics and family history in DSM-III obsessive-compulsive disorder. *American Journal of Psychiatry* 143, 317–322.

Ravizza L, Barzega G, Bellino S, Bogetto F, Maina G (1995) Predictors of drug treatment response in obsessive-compulsive disorder. *Journal of Clinical Psychiatry* 56, 368–373.

Reynolds CA, Raine A, Mellingen K, Venables PH, Mednick SA (2000) Three-factor model of schizotypal personality: invariance across culture, gender, religious affiliation, family adversity, and psychopathology. *Schizophrenia Bulletin* 26, 603–618.

Reznik I, Yavin I, Stryjer R, *et al.* (2004) Clozapine in the treatment of obsessive-compulsive symptoms in schizophrenia patients: a case series study. *Pharmacopsychiatry* 37, 52–66.

Rossi A, Daneluzzo E (2002) Schizotypal dimension in normals and schizophrenic patients: a comparison with other clinical samples. *Schizophrenia Research* 1, 67–75.

Roth RM, Baribeau J (2000) The relationship between schizotypal and obsessive-compulsive features in university students. *Personality and Individual Differences* 29, 1083–1093.

Samuels J, Nestadt G, Bienvenu OJ (2000) Personality disorders and normal personality dimensions in obsessive-compulsive disorder. *British Journal of Psychiatry* 177, 457–462.

Samuels JF, Bienvenu OJ, Pinto A, *et al.* (2008) Sex-specific clinical correlates of hoarding in obsessive-compulsive disorder. *Behavioral Research and Therapy* 46, 1040–1046.

Saxena S, Wang D, Bystritsky A, Baxter LR Jr (1996) Risperidone augmentation of SRI treatment for refractory obsessive-compulsive disorder. *Journal of Clinical Psychiatry* 57, 303–306.

Shin NY, Lee AR, Park HY, *et al.* (2008) Impact of coexistent schizotypal personality traits on frontal lobe function in obsessive-compulsive disorder. *Progress in Neuropsychopharmacology and Biological Psychiatry* 32, 472–478.

Siever LJ, Davis KL (2004) The pathophysiology of schizophrenia disorders: perspectives from the spectrum. *American Journal of Psychiatry* 161, 398–413.

Siever LJ, Koenigsberg HW, Harvey P, *et al.* (2002) Cognitive and brain function in schizotypal personality disorder. *Schizophrenia Research* **54**, 157–167.

Skodol AE, Bender DS, Morey LC, *et al.* (2011) Personality disorder types proposed for DSM-5. *Journal of Personality Disorders* **25**, 136–169.

Sobin C, Blundell ML, Weiller F, *et al.* (2000) Evidence of a schizotypy subtype in OCD. *Journal of Psychiatric Research* **34**, 15–24.

Spitzer RL, Endicott J, Gibbon M (1979) Crossing the border into borderline personality and borderline schizophrenia: the development of criteria. *Archives of General Psychiatry* **36**, 17–24.

Steketee G (1990) Personality traits and disorders in obsessive-compulsive disorder. *Journal of Anxiety Disorders* **4**, 351–364.

Suhr JA, Spitznagel MB, Gunstad J (2006) An obsessive-compulsive subtype of schizotypy: evidence from a nonclinical sample. *Journal of Nervous and Mental Disease* **194**, 884–886.

Svrakic DM, Cloninger CR (2005) Personality disorders. In: Sadock BJ, Sadock, VA (eds.) *Kaplan and Sadock's Comprehensive Textbook of Psychiatry*, 8th edn. Lippincott Williams & Wilkins, Philadelphia, PA, vol. 2, pp.2063–2104.

Torres AR, Moran P, Bebbington P, *et al.* (2006) Obsessive-compulsive disorder and personality disorder: evidence from the British National Survey of Psychiatric Morbidity 2000. *Social Psychiatry and Psychiatric Epidemiology* **41**, 862–867.

Walker WR, Freeman RF, Christensen DK (1994) Restricting environmental stimulation (REST) to enhance cognitive behavioral treatment for obsessive-compulsive disorder with schizotypal personality disorder. *Behavior Therapy* **25**, 709–719.

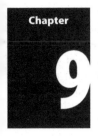

OCD with poor insight

The degree of insight into the senseless and excessive nature of obsessive–compulsive symptoms distinguishes obsessions from delusions and psychosis, and has traditionally been considered a defining feature of OCD. Patients with OCD exhibit a wide range of insight and a sizable proportion of OCD patients are characterized by partial or complete lack of insight. According to the DSM-IV patients reveal varying degrees of insight into the validity of their beliefs, and there is specification *"with poor insight"* for patients who "for most of the time" do not recognize that their symptoms are excessive or unreasonable. The following subcategories of insight are proposed in the forthcoming edition of DSM-V: *good or fair insight* (patients recognize that OCD beliefs are definitely or probably not true, or that they may or may not be true), *poor insight* (think OCD beliefs are probably true), *absent insight* (completely convinced that OCD beliefs are true) (Leckman *et al.*, 2010). Poor-insight patients firmly believe that if they do not ritualize, the feared consequence would actually occur. They are convinced that only ignorance prevents others from sharing their beliefs and they defend their beliefs despite contrary arguments and evidence, and some never try to resist their compulsive urges (Lelliott *et al.*, 1988). There is not always recognition of the absurdity of beliefs, and some OCD patients have particularly bizarre content of thoughts and ritualistic actions. How do OCD patients with poor insight differ from their fair-to-good insight counterparts? Do fixity and bizarreness of beliefs indicate the presence of schizophrenia or delusional disorder, as would be implied by the current diagnostic nomenclature? The answers to these questions have considerable diagnostic, treatment, and prognostic implications.

Assessment of insight in OCD

There is currently no gold standard for assessing insight in OCD (Carmin *et al.*, 2008). Item 11 of the Yale–Brown Obsessive–Compulsive Scale (Y-BOCS) ("Do you think your concerns or behaviors are reasonable?") is rated on a five-point scale ranging from 0 ("I think my obsessions or compulsions are unreasonable or excessive") to 4 ("I am sure my obsessions or compulsions are reasonable, no matter what anyone says"), and is the single reference to insight in OCD that has been extensively used in research studies. Multi-item instruments have been developed to examine the construct of insight in OCD. Foa and Kozak (1995) developed the Fixity of Beliefs Questionnaire (FBQ) for use in a DSM-IV OCD field trial. The FBQ contains seven items that measure the degree to which OCD patients recognize their obsessional fears as unreasonable. Each item is rated on a five-point scale ranging from 0 to 4. Foa *et al.* (1999) reported that two items (presence of feared consequences and certainty that feared consequences will occur) predicted OCD treatment outcome. Eisen *et al.* (1998) developed the Brown Assessment of Beliefs Scale (BABS) to assess the degree of poor insight and delusions in a variety of psychiatric conditions, including OCD (see Chapter 4). Neziroglu *et al.* (1999) developed the Overvalued Ideas Scale (OVIS) which contains items assessing bizarreness, belief accuracy, fixity of belief, reasonableness, perceived effectiveness of compulsions, pervasiveness of belief, reasons others do not share the belief, stability of belief, degree of resistance of the belief, and duration of belief stability. Item ratings are summed into a total score ranging from 0 to 10. The level of convergence among the available measures and the evidence that the scales predict treatment outcome in a consistent manner is yet to be examined (Carmin *et al.*, 2008).

Clinical correlates of OCD with poor insight

The majority of OCD patients with poor insight are otherwise indistinguishable from their counterparts with good insight. There is ample evidence that the demographic and clinical characteristics of OCD patients with poor insight do not differ substantially from those with full insight (Eisen and Rasmussen, 1993; Marazziti *et al.*, 2002; Eisen *et al.*, 2004). In addition, in a majority of studies the investigators found that OCD patients with poor insight are as likely to respond to SRIs as patients with better insight (Lelliott *et al.*, 1988; Neziroglu *et al.*, 1999; Eisen *et al.*, 2001). Insight in OCD may fluctuate with environmental influences (e.g., stress) or may parallel response to treatment. Thus, in an open-label 16-week study with sertraline, a decrease in OCD symptom severity with corresponding improvement in insight was observed (Eisen *et al.*, 2001). Similarly, at the end of a 6-month trial with combined clomipramine and cognitive–behavioral therapy, 56% (14 of 25) of patients no longer exhibited poor insight, and this improvement was associated with severity reduction of obsessive–compulsive and depressive symptoms (Matsunaga *et al.*, 2002).

The following vignette highlights the clinical features of an OCD patient with poor insight.

Case 9.1. Mr. F is a 23-year-old student. His family history was unremarkable. He achieved developmental milestones without delay, and was characterized by his family and peers as sociable but with a tendency to control and dominate during adolescence. At age 16, after the death of his grandfather, he began to fear that all family members would die unless he completed specific rituals. His belief was unshakeable, and attempts to convince him otherwise constantly failed. To appease his thoughts and fears, F developed complex checking and touching rituals that pervaded his daily activities. He also counted to seven, and avoided specific numbers, colors, and geometric forms throughout the day "to prevent death or harm" to his family. He felt compelled to perform rituals and was unwilling to resist them due to his belief in the inevitable negative consequences of abandonment of the rituals. Eventually, rituals occupied all of his time until he fell asleep. F was unable to concentrate enough to continue university studies or to pursue his usual home activities.

On evaluation, F reported that he was "exhausted" from the constant urge to ritualize, but expressed complete certainty of the "deadly consequences" of not performing rituals. He defended his belief despite arguments to the contrary, and expressed unwillingness to stop ritualizing. Aside from the fixity of that specific belief, he did not reveal any signs of formal thought disorders, typical delusional themes such as reference or persecution, or hallucinations, and had no symptoms of major affective disorders. The diagnoses of schizophrenia and other psychotic disorders were ruled out, and the DSM-IV diagnosis of OCD with poor insight was suggested. F did not have a clinically meaningful response to a trial with sertraline (up to 200 mg/day for 10 weeks), but responded positively to a trial with clomipramine (300 mg/day). The beneficial effect of clomipramine was associated with an attenuation of the fixity of F's beliefs and a reduction of time spent on compulsions (Y-BOCS score dropped from 32 to 19). Psychotherapy focused on assertiveness and control. Three years later, at follow-up, F revealed persistent obsessive–compulsive symptoms; however, his condition had improved enough to enable him to continue his education.

Quite contrary to study findings that underscored similarities between OCD with and without insight, some investigators reported that OCD with poor insight is associated with a graver clinical picture: earlier age of onset, longer duration of illness, more severe symptomatology, hoarding obsessions and compulsions, co-occurring depression, and poorer prognosis (Catapano *et al.*, 2001; Erzegovesi *et al.*, 2001; Matsunaga *et al.*, 2002; Turksoy *et al.*, 2002; Hollander *et al.*, 2003; Ravi Kishore *et al.*, 2004; De Berardis *et al.*, 2005). Thus, in a 3-year follow-up investigation of 106 OCD patients, Catapano and colleagues (2010) found that poor-insight patients were less likely to achieve even a partial remission throughout the study duration, required a significantly greater number of therapeutic trials, and were more likely to receive augmentation with low-dose antipsychotics. These inconsistent findings may be attributed to some extent to the methodological differences between studies, such as different methods for measuring insight, the use of a categorical vs. dimensional definition of insight, or cross-sectional vs. longitudinal study designs.

An additional possible explanation for discrepant findings is that some OCD patients with poor insight and poor prognosis are distinguished from good-insight patients by the relatedness of patients with poor insight to the schizophrenia spectrum (Eisen and Rasmussen, 1993; Poyurovsky and Koran, 2005). In support of this hypothesis, in a large sample of 475 OCD patients, those with poor insight and complete conviction about the true nature of their obsessions had remarkably similar demographic and clinical variables to their good-insight counterparts; however both subgroups differed substantially from the OCD subgroup with comorbid schizotypal personality disorder (Eisen and Rasmussen, 1993). Seventy percent of the schizotypal OCD patients had a deteriorative course, as apposed to only 17% in the poor-insight subgroup. A discriminant function analysis confirmed that compared to patients with poor insight, OCD patients with schizotypal personality disorder were significantly more likely to be single, to have earlier age of onset of illness, and to have poorer prognoses (Eisen and Rasmussen, 1993). It was later shown that patients with OCD and associated schizotypal personality disorder were more likely to have poor insight after treatment with SSRIs than patients with poor insight without schizotypy (Matsunaga *et al.*, 2002). In another study, OCD patients with poor insight (29.5%, 39 of 132) revealed more depressive symptoms ($p < 0.001$) and schizotypal personality disorder ($p < 0.001$) than patients with good insight; however, no significant between-group differences in treatment response were exhibited (Alonso *et al.*, 2008). In fact, three variables were significantly and independently associated with the degree of insight measured by the BABS in a large-scale study: presence of comorbid schizotypal personality disorder in OCD patients, severity of obsessions, and presence of schizophrenia-spectrum disorders in first-degree relatives (Catapano *et al.*, 2010). These findings imply that the co-occurrence of schizophrenia-spectrum disorders may account for some differences in clinical characteristics, treatment response, and prognosis between OCD patients with poor and good insight.

Bizarreness of content

Bizarreness of content poses an additional clinical challenge in the distinction between obsessive–compulsive and psychotic experiences. DSM-IV defines delusions as "bizarre" when they are clearly implausible, are not understandable, and do not derive from ordinary life experiences (an example is the belief that Martians have invaded one's mind in order to manipulate one's thoughts and behaviors). In fact, in the DSM-IV bizarreness of delusional content is a diagnostic criterion for schizophrenia, and diagnosis of schizophrenia can be based solely on the presence of a "bizarre" delusion. Clinicians may intuitively "empathize" with this concept and consider bizarre content synonymous with delusions. However, categorization of obsessions based upon their bizarreness has not been suggested. There is no empirical justification to subcategorize obsessions as "bizarre" and "non-bizarre" (O'Dwyer and Marks, 2000; Hudak and Dougherty, 2011). On contrary, Kendler *et al.* (1983) and Maj (1998) reported poor inter-rater reliability in the assessment of the bizarreness of delusions.

Following are extracts from case vignettes that highlight bizarre content of obsessions and compulsions in patients with OCD (O'Dwyer and Marks, 2000).

Case 9.2. Mr. Y developed beliefs about a "power" at age 13. He felt that everyone had a certain "quality" or "goodness" which was stored in the brain as a "power." He believed that other people drained the power from him and replaced it with their own rubbish. The exchange of power was triggered by an image in his mind of a face or object. When it happened he felt distressed, "dirty" and "horrible." He could only regain the power by doing complex rituals. He imagined the person's face and that he had detached their head from their body and sucked the power from the major vessels of their neck or from their eyes. He then transferred the power back into himself by banging his palm on a particular spot on his forehead, and exhaling repeatedly. This made him feel relieved and "good", but as the events recurred up to several times a minute the relief was short-lived. He felt compelled at times to take revenge on people who stole his power by drawing deformed and ugly representations of those people on a wall, with his finger. If he touched anything he left a "power" trace behind and then had to touch it repeatedly to get the "power" back. Y's belief in the experience was absolute. He knew it might seem strange to others but believed that if they experienced it, they would understand.

Case 9.3. At the age of 7, W began to fear that harm would come to his relatives. He engaged in hand-washing and touching rituals to prevent this harm. Gradually he began to believe that "spirits" or an outside force "reminded" him to carry out his rituals to avoid harm. He associated the numbers 13 and 66 with harm and, if he saw them, he believed they were inserted by an external force to remind him to carry out his rituals. He defended his belief absolutely but said he could not be 100% sure "because one can never be sure about anything." He was unable to resist his rituals, and his belief in the negative consequences of not performing them was absolute. His rituals centered around numbers, complex counting, and avoidance of specific numbers. At age 31 he developed a fear of contamination associated with many rituals of avoidance and hand-washing.

Case 9.4. For 20 years V had had a fear of being transported to another world. At age 17 he worried that reflections in mirrors represented another world, and had complex checking rituals involving mirrors. This gradually spread to all reflective surfaces. He believed that turning on electrical switches, using the television remote control, or hearing car engines turned on could cause him to be "transported" and constantly checked to make sure that this would not happen. He believed that if he ate while in another world, he would be forced to stay there, and so either avoided eating, or ate with complex rituals, or induced vomiting. Other rituals involved switching electrical switches on and off and wearing particular clothes. The "other" world was tangibly the same as the real one, but "felt" different – he felt that friends and family, although appearing the same, were "different" and might have been replaced by "doubles"...

Despite the bizarre content of obsessive–compulsive symptoms, a key feature in the presented cases is the "clear link" between the thoughts and the rituals (O'Dwyer and Marks, 2000). The rituals were all cued by intrusive thoughts and the patients felt compelled to carry them out to relieve associated distress. The patients were severely disabled by obsessive–compulsive symptoms but were otherwise intact, and had no paranoid delusions, hallucinations, or Schneiderian symptoms. Hence, it is the nature of the thought (i.e., the way the patient experiences the thought) rather than the content of the thought (i.e., what the thought is about) that discriminates between obsessional and psychotic phenomena (Hudak and Dougherty, 2011). If the presenting thought is determined to be intrusive, distressful, and inappropriate to the patient, the thought should be labeled obsessional, and in contrast to the delusion no further subtyping on whether the concern is "bizarre" or "non-bizarre" is warranted.

OCD with psychotic features

A more vexing diagnostic dilemma arises from a subset of severely ill OCD patients who develop psychotic symptoms during the course of illness. (Poor-insight OCD patients and those with associated schizotypal personality disorder are not included in this subgroup.) Although systematic evaluation of OCD associated with psychotic transformation is lacking, such cases were already documented in the initial stages of OCD research (Lewis, 1935; Straus, 1948: Gordon, 1950).

Robinson and colleagues (1976) reported the longitudinal course of 36 patients among whom obsessive–compulsive symptoms reached delusional intensity. Patients' attitudes to their obsessions varied, from doubtful and hesitant at times, i.e., ego-dystonic, to ego-syntonic at other times. Hallucinations were never observed. The course of illness was characterized by episodic psychotic deteriorations with symptom-free remissions. Despite the long duration of illness no emotional or intellectual impairment could be found, and during remissions most of the patients could carry on with their occupations. The disorder observed clearly differed from schizophrenia on both clinical and psycho-diagnostic levels and this appeared to justify the definition of "obsessive psychosis". The intriguing aspect of this investigation is that one-third of the patients had mixed obsessive and schizophrenic heredity, suggesting that the presence of schizophrenia in first-degree relatives might affect the clinical expression of OCD in probands, "driving" it to a severe extreme on the OCD spectrum.

The following is a case vignette portraying "obsessive psychosis," as reported by Robinson et al. (1976).

Case 9.5. A female, age 19. When admitted to the hospital, she was depressed due to obsessive ruminations over having caused severe physical harm to a child that she hit lightly. She was preoccupied with these thoughts for weeks although the child's parents had told her that the child was unharmed. After some time this obsession was spontaneously replaced by the obsession that she was pregnant. This went on for a few weeks despite the fact that her physician reassured her that there was no pregnancy. Then she suddenly recalled that 7 years earlier her neighbor's baby had fallen out of his carriage when she was taking him for a walk, and it now occurred to her that the child might have hurt his head when he fell. There were days when her own attitude towards her imaginations was one of doubt and she laughed at herself: however, at other times she believed in her obsessions ... She later began to think that she must have killed somebody in the department where she was working. She could give no explanation, she merely thought that it was a man, and although at times the idea appeared to her to be bizarre and unreal, she would look around again and again in an effort to remember who was missing from the department ... Finally, after an additional period of remission, she came to the hospital again with guilt feelings about her relations with a married man and about her wishes to be rid of his wife. These thoughts subsequently changed into an obsession that she had induced her lover to kill his wife.

In another investigation, Solyom and colleagues (1985) found that a subset of 45 OCD patients appeared to be atypical due to severely debilitating and near-delusional obsessive-compulsive symptoms. Aside from being more severely ill, this subgroup with *atypical obsessive–compulsive neurosis* was distinguished by an earlier age at onset and poorer social adjustment. Notably, although delusion-like experiences in the atypical OCD group suggested a psychotic form of illness, schizophrenia was not ascribed to any of the patients.

The following extract from the case vignette demonstrates a delusional-like phenomenon in a patient with "atypical obsessive–compulsive neurosis" (Solyom *et al.*, 1985).

Case 9.6. Mr. C, a 26-year old stationary engineer, suffered from obsessive fears of aggressive intent towards himself and others since age 12, which he attempted to mitigate with ritualistic behavior. C was convinced that he caused his employer's heart attack with unfriendly thoughts, despite all contrary evidence. C's thoughts about his employer's ailment were repetitive, intrusive, and were accompanied by repetitive questions for reassurance ...

In their seminal paper entitled "Obsessive–compulsive disorder with psychotic features: phenomenological analysis" Insel and Akiskal (1986) also highlighted the non-schizophrenic nature of psychotic transformations in OCD patients. When psychotic transformation does occur in OCD patients, it is typically precipitated by a stressful event, it is circumscribed and reversible, and there is no subsequent evidence of schizophrenic disorder. In such cases, the psychosis is generally a transient understandable complication arising from a background of typical obsessive–compulsive symptoms. The authors suggested that this shift may take either "an *affective form*, when the fear of contamination is replaced by the delusional guilt that one has contaminated others, or a *paranoid form*, when doubts about having committed some reprehensible act are replaced by the delusion that one is being subjected to persecution as if one had actually committed such acts."

The following vignettes demonstrate both the affective and the paranoid deterioration of obsessions. Note that psychotic episodes are preceded by stressful events, they are reversible, and thus appear to respond to an anti-obsessive medication (Case 9.7) or environmental changes (Case 9.8) (Insel and Akiskal, 1986).

Case 9.7. Mr. A, a married 57-year-old man, traced the onset of illness to a leave of absence from work because of an elbow injury 4 years before. Prior to that event, he had no psychiatric history. At that time he became concerned about bits of metal or glass on his skin. He began checking and washing compulsively, although he recognized that this behavior was bizarre and unreasonable. He also expressed fear that the particles on his skin might contaminate others and cause injury ... Upon admission to the hospital, he admitted to several symptoms of depression including poor appetite and sleep disturbances, all of which he explained as secondary to his rituals. He adjusted superficially to the ward milieu and was noted to be passive ... He later absconded from the ward, only to be returned by his wife. Upon his return, he was totally immobilized by his "phobia." He stood naked for hours in the middle of his room complaining that he was unable to move because he would contaminate others. He made a suicidal gesture and described wishing he were dead so that he would be freed from the burden of making others suffer. He had no Schneiderian symptoms. The "obsessional storm" remitted within 3 weeks with clomipramine treatment. A follow-up interview 2 years later revealed persistent non-psychotic obsessive–compulsive symptoms that were severe enough to preclude his returning to work. A had only a scant recollection of his delusional interval.

Case 9.8. Mr. B, a 25-year-old man, was referred for hospitalization because of compulsive checking that had continued for 8 years. He worked in a day-care center, where he became obsessed with thinking that he had inadvertently poisoned the children's juice. He repetitively tasted the juice from each can but could not resolve a nagging doubt that somehow he had spilled cleaning fluid into each container. At admission to the hospital, he described his obsessional thoughts about poisoning as "embarrassing" and "irrational." During the second week of hospitalization, he became increasingly agitated. He began washing compulsively for the first time and was unable to sleep ... B began insisting that he had not poisoned the children, but he was convinced that the hospital staff – in collusion with his referring therapist and the FBI – believed that he was guilty and that he was going to be jailed, beaten, and abused for crimes he had not committed. B was then treated with haloperidol but did not improve. He was transferred to another hospital and in the new environment, the delusional symptoms quickly resolved.

In another subset of OCD patients, as described in the next case vignette, obsessive thoughts are so intrusive that they were experienced as inner (accusatory) voices. At their worst, however, these voices remained repetitive and thought-like, lacking the conversational or imperative quality of true auditory hallucinations, and are best described as "pseudo-hallucinations" (Pies, 1984; Insel and Akiskal, 1986). Actually, perceptual disturbances in any modalities, such as auditory, visual, tactile, and olfactory, can sometimes be detected in severe cases of OCD; patients described their experiences as "hearing voices," "seeing dots of feces in hands," "sensing twinges of infected needles all over the body," or "smelling fetid odors" (Fontenelle *et al.*, 2008). These symptoms should be distinguished from "sensory phenomena," such as uncomfortable sensations in the skin, muscles, or body that may appear before or along with repetitive behaviors in patients with OCD and/or Tourette's syndrome (Miguel *et al.*, 2000).

Case 9.9. Mr. M, a 23-year-old man, was brought to our clinic because he was "hearing voices," was not able to concentrate, and suffered from severe anxiety. He had been diagnosed with DSM-IV schizophrenic disorder and was unsuccessfully treated with antipsychotic agents (perphenazine, olanzapine) for 2 years. On examination he suggested that the "voices" he complained about were intrusive thoughts, such as distressful and unpleasant cursing words and phrases. M recognized these "voices" as internal, although they often had the imperative and three-dimensional quality of auditory hallucinations. The "voices" were accompanied by compulsive urges to neutralize them; M thus began undoing rituals such as touching, counting, and checking to counteract the "hallucinations." During the evaluation, M recalled that at age 14 he had intrusive, distressful thoughts with aggressive and sexual content that he was reluctant to share with his parents or peers. Although he reported no complaints from age 16 to 20 years, the obsessive–compulsive symptoms re-emerged abruptly with the experience of hearing "voices." At this stage, though there was no evidence of formal thought disorders, paranoid delusions, or negative symptoms, he received the diagnosis of schizophrenic disorder. His physical and neurological examinations, blood tests, and toxicology analysis were normal. Based on the clinical presentation and anamnestic data, a diagnosis was re-evaluated and DSM-IV OCD was suggested. Treatment with the SRI sertraline (up to 200 mg/day) was initiated. After 12 weeks of treatment there was a clinically significant decrease in the intensity of M's intrusive experiences (Y-BOCS score dropped from 29 to 21).

Recommendations for the identification and management of poor-insight OCD patients

OCD with or without insight seems to represent the same disorder, and patients who exhibit poor insight and associated schizotypy or psychotic features have a more severe form of the illness (Box 9.1). Some of these patients are as disabled as their schizophrenia counterparts; and may be misdiagnosed as schizophrenic and receive long-term antipsychotic agents. Differential diagnosis between poor-insight OCD and psychotic disorders, primarily schizophrenia, is sometimes challenging. Obsessions held with delusional conviction can be distinguished from schizophrenic and manic delusions by the absence of other signs and symptoms of these disorders, as well as the characteristic course of illness. In addition, "delusional obsessions" have typical OCD content rather than content related to persecution, grandiosity, passivity experiences, or ideas of reference. A useful, although not definitive, distinction is that the OCD patient is more likely to fear hurting others, and the paranoid patient is preoccupied with harm to himself. More important, patients with OCD have a history of recognizing the senselessness of their obsessions even though they may fail

---

Box 9.1 OCD with poor insight

1. Patients with OCD exhibit a wide range of insight with a sizable proportion characterized by partial or complete lack of insight.
2. The majority of OCD patients with poor insight have similar demographic and clinical characteristics and treatment response to SRIs as their counterparts with good insight.
3. A subgroup of poor-insight OCD patients with comorbid schizotypal personality disorder tends to have graver clinical characteristics and poorer prognosis.
4. A small subset of OCD patients may develop psychotic symptoms during the course of illness. This psychotic transformation is typically a transient understandable complication arising from a background of typical obsessive–compulsive symptoms; it is generally precipitated by a stressful event; it is circumscribed and reversible; and there is no subsequent evidence of schizophrenic disorder.
5. A misdiagnosis of schizophrenia or delusional disorder may lead to unnecessary long-term exposure to an antipsychotic medication and reluctance to consider other, more effective, interventions. These OCD patients usually respond to anti-obsessive medications, SSRIs, or clomipramine. If an antipsychotic agent is used, it should be as a therapeutic trial, rather than long-term treatment. Response should be carefully monitored.

to resist them. It is the recognition of senselessness that defines the idea as an obsession rather than a true delusion. In addition, though thought processes are disturbed by the intrusive ideas, true thought derailment, thought insertion, and thought broadcasting are not present. Occasionally, an intrusive thought takes on the quality of an "inner voice." However, these "voices," in contrast to auditory hallucinations typical to schizophrenia, are repetitive, intrusive, and distressful, and may be associated with compulsive behaviors aimed to neutralize them. Doubt and reassurance-seeking are additional symptoms indicative of OCD. Magical thinking, namely the belief that one's thoughts, words, or actions might somehow cause or prevent a specific outcome in a way that defies the normal laws of cause and effect, should also be emphasized (Ayd, 1995). Magical thinking is a phenomenon that is contrary to paranoid delusions that are associated with the conviction that outside forces affect the individual. Distinguishing magical thinking from other thought disorders, such as thought broadcasting, however is less clear-cut. Finally, a misdiagnosis of schizophrenia or delusional disorder may lead to a lifetime of antipsychotic medication and reluctance to consider other, more effective, interventions (O'Dwyer and Marks, 2000). These OCD patients usually respond poorly to an antipsychotic medication but may improve with anti-obsessive medications, SSRIs, or clomipramine. If an antipsychotic agent is used, it should be as a therapeutic trial, rather than long-term treatment. Response should be carefully monitored.

References

Alonso P, Menchon JM, Segalas C, et al. (2008) Clinical implications of insight assessment in obsessive-compulsive disorder. Comprehensive Psychiatry 49, 305–312.

Carmin C, Wiegartz PS, Wu K (2008) Obsessive-compulsive disorder with poor insight. In: Abramowitz JS, McKay D, Taylor S (eds.) Clinical Handbook of Obsessive-Compulsive Disorder and Related Problems. Johns Hopkins University Press, Baltimore, MD, pp.109–125.

Catapano F, Sperandeo R, Perris F, Lanzaro M, Maj M (2001) Insight and resistance in patients with obsessive-compulsive disorder. Psychopathology 34, 62–68.

Catapano F, Perris F, Fabrazzo M, et al. (2010) Obsessive-compulsive disorder with poor insight: a three-year prospective study. Progress in Neuropsychopharmacology and Biological Psychiatry 34, 323–330.

De Berardis D, Campanella D, Gambi F, et al. (2005) Insight and alexithymia in adult outpatients with obsessive-compulsive disorder. European Archives of Psychiatry and Clinical Neuroscience 255, 350–358.

Eisen JI, Rasmussen SA (1993) Obsessive-compulsive disorder with psychotic features. Journal of Clinical Psychiatry 54, 373–379.

Eisen JL, Phillips KA, Baer L, et al. (1998) The Brown Assessment of Beliefs Scale: reliability and validity. American Journal of Psychiatry 155, 102–108.

Eisen JL, Rasmussen SA, Phillips KA, et al. (2001) Insight and treatment outcome in obsessive-compulsive disorder. Comprehensive Psychiatry 42, 494–497.

Eisen JL, Phillips KA, Coles ME, Rasmussen SA (2004) Insight in obsessive-compulsive disorder and body dysmorphic disorder. Comprehensive Psychiatry 45, 10–15.

Erzegovesi S, Cavallini MC, Cavedini P, et al. (2001) Clinical predictors of drug response in obsessive-compulsive disorder. Journal of Clinical Psychopharmacology 21, 488–492.

Foa EB, Kozak MJ (1995) DSM-IV field trial: obsessive-compulsive disorder. American Journal of Psychiatry 152, 90–96.

Foa EB, Abramowitz JS, Franklin ME, Kozak MJ (1999) Feared consequences, fixity of belief, and treatment outcome in patients with obsessive-compulsive disorder. Behavior Therapy 30, 717–724.

180 | Chapter 9: OCD with poor insight

Fontenelle LF, Lopes AP, Borges MC, et al. (2008) Auditory, visual, tactile, olfactory, and bodily hallucinations in patients with obsessive-compulsive disorder. CNS Spectrums 13, 125–130.

Goodman WK, Price LH, Rasmussen SA, et al. (1989) The Yale–Brown Obsessive Compulsive Scale: I. Development, use, and reliability. Archives of General Psychiatry 46, 1006–1011.

Gordon A (1950) Transition of obsessions into delusions: evaluation of obsessional phenomena from the prognostic standpoint. American Journal of Psychiatry 107, 455–458.

Hollander E, Rossi NB, Sood E, Pallanti S (2003) Risperidone augmentation in treatment-resistant obsessive-compulsive disorder: a double-blind, placebo-controlled study. International Journal of Neuropsychopharmacology 6, 397–401.

Hudak R, Dougherty DD (eds.) (2011) Clinical Obsessive-Compulsive Disorders in Adults and Children. Cambridge University Press, Cambridge, UK.

Insel TR, Akiskal HS (1986) Obsessive-compulsive disorder with psychotic features: a phenomenological analysis. American Journal of Psychiatry 143, 1527–1533.

Kendler KS, Glazer WM, Morgenstern H (1983) Dimensions of delusional experience. American Journal of Psychiatry 140, 466–469.

Leckman JF, Denys D, Simpson HB, et al. (2010) Obsessive-compulsive disorder: a review of the diagnostic criteria and possible subtypes and dimensional specifiers for DSM-V. Depression and Anxiety 27, 507–527.

Lelliott PT, Noshirvani HF, Basoglulu M, Marks IM, Monteiro WO (1988) Obsessive-compulsive beliefs and treatment outcome. Psychological Medicine 18, 697–702.

Lewis A (1935) Problems of obsessional illness. Proceedings of the Royal Society of Medicine 29, 325–336.

Maj M (1998) Critique of the DSM-IV operational diagnostic criteria for schizophrenia. British Journal of Psychiatry 172, 458–460.

Marazziti D, Dell'Osso L, Di Nasso E, et al. (2002) Insight in obsessive-compulsive disorder: a study of an Italian sample. European Psychiatry 17, 407–410.

Matsunaga H, Kiriike N, Matsui T, et al. (2002) Obsessive-compulsive disorder with poor insight. Comprehensive Psychiatry 43, 150–157.

Miguel EC, de Rosario-Campos MC, Prado HS, et al. (2000) Sensory phenomena in obsessive-compulsive disorder and Tourette's disorder. Journal of Clinical Psychiatry 61, 150–156.

Neziroglu F, McKay D, Yaryura-Tobias J, Stevens K, Todaro J (1999) The Overvalued Ideas Scale: development, reliability and validity in obsessive-compulsive disorder. Behavior Research and Therapy 37, 881–902.

O'Dwyer AM, Marks I (2000) Obsessive-compulsive disorder and delusions revisited. British Journal of Psychiatry 176, 281–284.

Pies R (1984) Distinguishing obsessional from psychotic phenomena. Journal of Clinical Psychopharmacology 4, 345–347.

Poyurovsky M, Koran LM (2005) Obsessive-compulsive disorder (OCD) with schizotypy vs. schizophrenia with OCD: diagnostic dilemmas and therapeutic implications. Journal of Psychiatry Research 39, 399–408.

Ravi Kishore V, Samar R, Janardhan Reddy YC, Chandrasekhar CR, Thennarasu K (2004) Clinical characteristics and treatment response in poor and good insight obsessive-compulsive disorder. European Psychiatry 19, 202–208.

Robinson S, Winnik HZ, Weiss AA (1976) Obsessive psychosis: justification for a separate clinical entity. Israel Annals of Psychiatry 14, 39–48.

Solyom L, Di Nicola VF, Phil M, Sookman D, Luchins D (1985) Is there an obsessive psychosis? Aetiological and prognostic factors of an atypical form of obsessive-compulsive neurosis. Canadian Journal of Psychiatry 30, 372–380.

Straus EW (1948) On Obsession: A Clinical and Methodological Study. Nervous and Mental Disease Monograph 73, New York.

Turksoy N, Tukel R, Ozdemir O, Karali A (2002) Comparison of clinical characteristics in good and poor insight obsessive-compulsive disorder. Journal of Anxiety Disorders 17, 233–242.

Chapter 10

Neurobiology of schizo-obsessive disorder

In contrast to the considerable amount of research that has been undertaken to uncover the neurobiological foundation of both schizophrenia and OCD, investigation of the neurobiology of a schizo-obsessive subgroup is still in its infancy. To date, all reports are of an exploratory nature rendering conclusions preliminary. Nevertheless, several initial clues concerning putative neurobiological mechanisms underlying a schizo-obsessive disorder have recently emerged.

Structural and functional brain alterations

Initial brain imaging studies implied that the presence of obsessive–compulsive symptoms in schizophrenia may contribute to a specific pattern of structural and functional brain abnormalities in a schizo-obsessive subgroup. Hence, a smaller volume of the left hippocampus was detected in patients with juvenile-onset schizophrenia and obsessive–compulsive symptoms as compared to schizophrenia patients without OCD (Aoyama et al., 2000). In another MRI study researchers revealed significant enlargement of the anterior horn of the lateral ventricle and the third ventricle in schizophrenia patients with obsessive–compulsive symptoms relative to those without these symptoms (Iida et al., 1998). Significant differences were also detected between two small groups of patients with obsessive–compulsive disorder: one group with OCD symptoms in the prodromal phase of schizophrenia, and a second group with "pure" OCD (Kurokawa et al., 2000). The ventricle–brain ratio (VBR) of the schizo-obsessive group was significantly larger than that of the OCD group: the minimum VBR in the schizophrenia group was larger than the maximum VBR in the OCD group. If these findings are replicated, they may assist in the differential diagnosis of patients who manifest OCD symptoms early in the course of schizophrenia and typical OCD patients who are not at risk of developing schizophrenia.

In the only exploratory study of functional MRI (fMRI) published to date, Levine and colleagues (1998) analyzed brain activation parameters from the left dorsolateral prefrontal cortex (DLPFC) in schizophrenia patients with varying degrees of obsessive–compulsive symptoms while they performed a cognitive challenge paradigm that included a verbal fluency task. Though no relationship was found between obsessive–compulsive symptom severity and fMRI signal change for the entire group, a significant relationship was detected in a small subgroup of the participants. In these patients, there was a significant negative correlation between a severity of OCD symptomatology and activation of the left DLPFC; that is, as OCD severity increased, the activation of the DLPFC decreased. This pattern of brain activation parallels the pattern seen in schizophrenia patients.

Although preliminary findings show certain differences in structural and functional brain abnormalities between schizophrenia patients with and without obsessive–compulsive symptoms, they have not yet been replicated. Moreover, the next generation of studies will most likely concentrate on an abnormal distribution of activity and functional connectivity using both resting-state and task-based fMRI, rather than focus on "region of interest" analyses. These studies are currently under way.

Neuropsychological dysfunction

Does the presence of obsessive–compulsive symptoms in schizophrenia account for a unique pattern of cognitive dysfunction, or alternatively does it contribute to a more severe neurocognitive impairment stemming from the two disorders? These hypotheses were tested in a series of comparative investigations including schizophrenia, schizo-obsessive, and OCD patient groups. Similar to brain imaging studies the findings are equivocal. Overall, most but not all studies have revealed that rather than having a unique "schizo-obsessive" neurocognitive profile, a combined group exhibits more severe cognitive dysfunction, supporting a "pathophysiological double jeopardy" in this overlap group (Bottas et al., 2005). Hence, schizo-obsessive patients demonstrated delayed non-verbal memory and cognitive set-shifting abilities and performed worse in the areas of visuospatial skills than their counterparts with schizophrenia only (Berman et al., 1998; Patel et al., 2010). Similarly, Whitney and colleagues (2004) administered a range of cognitive tests sensitive to DLPFC and orbitofrontal dysfunction among 54 schizophrenia patients with and without obsessive–compulsive symptoms, and found that though no statistically significant between-group differences were noted, the profile of the schizo-obsessive patients reflected poorer performance across nearly all neuropsychological domains (Figure 10.1).

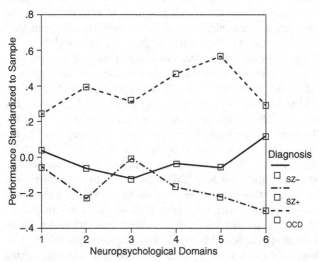

Figure 10.1 Profile analysis of neuropsychological performance by group. (1) Dorsolateral prefrontal function (WCST % perseverative errors *T*-Score). (2) Orbitofrontal function (BGT advantageous–disadvantageous selections). (3) Visual spatial skills (Visual spatial skills index). (4) Visual memory (RCFT percent recalled). (5) Verbal memory/learning (CVLT trials 1–5 total *T*-Score). (6) Attention (CPT attentiveness score). Diagnoses: SZ–, schizophrenia/schizoaffective disorder without OC symptoms; SZ+, schizophrenia/schizoaffective disorder with OC symptoms. Tests: WCST, Wisconsin Card Sorting Test; BGT, Bender Gestalt Test; RCFT, Rey Complex Figure Test and Recognition Trial; CVLT, California Verbal Learning Test; CPT, Continuous Performance Test. (From Whitney KA, Fastenau PS, Evans JD, Lysaker PH (2004) Comparative neuropsychological function in obsessive–compulsive disorder and schizophrenia with and without obsessive–compulsive symptoms. *Schizophrenia Research* **69**, 75–83. Reprinted with permission.)

The same authors followed up on this study and, using factor analysis, determined a single score that estimated overall executive function (Lysaker *et al.*, 2008). Poorer executive function predicted higher levels of obsessive–compulsive symptoms both concurrently and prospectively even when general levels of anxiety were controlled.

In contrast to reports pointing towards somewhat more severe cognitive impairment in a combined group, lack of a difference between schizophrenia patients with and without obsessive–compulsive symptoms has also been shown (Ongür and Goff, 2005; Tumkaya *et al.*, 2009). Noteworthy, schizo-obsessive patients showed better performance on selected frontal lobe tests than schizophrenia patients without OCD (Borkowska *et al.*, 2003). In an attempt to reconcile these discrepancies, it was suggested that the effect of obsessive–compulsive symptoms in schizophrenia may depend upon the stage of schizophrenic illness, with OCD conferring greater impairment in chronic schizophrenia but possibly a "protective" effect in the early stages of schizophrenia (Borkowska *et al.*, 2003). This hypothesis is in accord with a mitigating effect of obsessive–compulsive symptoms on the severity of schizophrenic symptoms across several psychopathological domains revealed in first-episode psychosis but not in patients with chronic schizophrenia (Poyurovsky *et al.*, 1999).

Neurological soft signs

Neurological deficits were observed in a majority of patients with schizophrenia: these include both "hard" signs that reflect impairments in motor, sensory, and reflex functions which may be localized to a particular brain area, and "soft" non-localizing deficits that do not implicate a specific brain region or demarcate a specific neurological syndrome (Heinrichs and Buchanan, 1988). Hard neurological signs include among others impaired olfactory function, oculomotor abnormalities, and hypoalgesia. Neurological soft signs (NSS) include impairments in motor dexterity, presence of primitive reflexes or cortical release signs, difficulties in proper sequencing of complex motor tasks, and deficits in sensory integration (Tandon *et al.*, 2009).

Neurological soft signs are prevalent in schizophrenia patients, representing valid and reliable indicators of brain dysfunction in schizophrenia, and were found to be associated with cognitive deficits and with negative and disorganized symptoms of the disorder (Bombin *et al.*, 2005). NSS are considered an intrinsic feature of schizophrenia rather than a side effect of antipsychotic agents, since they have been observed in drug-naïve first-episode schizophrenia patients (Browne *et al.*, 2000; Dazzan and Murray, 2002; Bachmann *et al.*, 2005). NSS were found in high-risk individuals, monozygotic twins discordant for schizophrenia, and first-degree relatives, findings that support their role as trait markers for schizophrenia (Bombin *et al.*, 2005).

Although studies on NSS in OCD are scarce, patients with OCD seem to have an increased rate of NSS compared to healthy controls (Hollander *et al.*, 1990; Khanna, 1991; Anderson and Savage, 2004; Jaafari *et al.*, 2011). Moreover, the severity of some of the soft signs in OCD patients (e.g., deficits in motor speed and sequencing) are comparable to those seen in schizophrenia, suggesting frontal–striatal dysfunction common to both disorders (Bolton *et al.*, 1998).

Explicit evaluation of the rate and the pattern of distribution of NSS in schizophrenia patients with OCD has also been performed (Poyurovsky *et al.*, 2007). The study group included 59 patients who met DSM-IV criteria for both schizophrenic disorder and OCD; 20 (33.4%) patients in this group represented a subset of first-episode schizophrenia patients. The comparison groups included 51 schizophrenia patients without OCD (first-episode: 16 of 51 [31.4%]), matched for age (± 3 years) and number of hospitalizations to the schizo-obsessive group. Twenty OCD patients were also recruited to test the hypothesis regarding the "additive" effect of schizophrenia- and OCD-related neurological deficits in the schizo-obsessive group, as were 51 healthy individuals.

Neurological soft signs were assessed using the Neurological Evaluation Scale (NES) (Buchanan and Heinrichs, 1989). NES is a structured scale presenting scores in subscales of motor coordination, sensory integration, sequencing of complex motor acts, and "others" signs. There are 26 items rated on the scale of 0–2 (0 = normal, 1 = some disruption, 2 = major disruption) according to standardized instructions. The motor coordination subscale includes tandem walk, rapid alternation movements, finger/thumb opposition and the finger-to-nose test. The sensory integration subscale includes audio-visual integration, stereognosis, graphesthesia, extinction, and right/left confusion. Sequencing of complex motor acts includes the first-ring test, the first-edge-palm test, the Ozeretski test, and rhythm-taping test. The "others" signs include short-term memory, eye movement abnormalities, frontal release signs, and primitive reflexes.

The major finding of this study is that NSS did not differentiate between schizophrenia patients with and without OCD (Table 10.1). Regardless of the presence of OCD, roughly half of the patients in the two schizophrenia groups had a substantial and remarkably similar "soft neurological deficit" in motor and sensory areas, in comparison to healthy individuals. Remarkably the rate and the pattern of NSS did not differ between a subgroup of first-episode schizophrenia patients and patients with repeated hospitalizations, supporting growing evidence that NSS are biological trait markers, detectable early in the illness (Keshavan et al., 2003; Whitty et al., 2003; Bachmann et al., 2005). It is unlikely that the relatively small sample size of the two schizophrenia groups accounted for lack of detection of a between-group difference (type II error), since not even a minor signal indicating a possible group difference was noted. In addition, a number of studies using identical

Table 10.1 Neurological soft signs in schizophrenia patients with and without OCD, patients with OCD, and healthy subjects

Variable	Schizo-obsessive (N = 59)	Schizophrenia (N = 51)	OCD (N = 20)	Healthy controls (N = 51)	F (df = 3,177)	p
Motor coordination	1.25 (1.34)[a]	1.18 (1.65)[a]	0.45 (0.69)	0.10 (0.30)	10.90	0.00
Sensory integration	1.93 (1.59)[a]	1.88 (1.54)[a]	1.60 (0.82)	0.73 (0.83)	9.26	0.00
Motor sequencing	2.68 (1.97)[a]	2.73 (2.02)[a]	2.85 (2.00)[a]	1.80 (1.64)	16.82	0.00
"Others"	2.64 (1.86)[a]	2.63 (1.93)[a]	1.80 (1.64)	1.20 (1.28)	8.48	0.00

[a] $p < 0.001$ vs. healthy controls, significant after the Bonferroni correction.
Source: Poyurovsky M, Faragian M, Pashinian A, Levi A, Viosburd A, Stryjer R, Weizman R, Fuchs C, Weizman A (2007) Neurological soft signs in schizophrenia patients with obsessive–compulsive disorder. Journal of Neuropsychiatry and Clinical Neurosciences 19, 145–150. Reprinted with permission from the Journal of Neuropsychiatry and Clinical Neurosciences (copyright 2007, American Psychiatric Association).

research methodology also failed to find any significant group differences (Sevincok et al., 2006; Thomas and Tharyan, 2011; Tumkaya et al., 2012). Hence, it is conceivable that a pervasive schizophrenia-related "soft neurological deficit" superimposes any additional deficits related to a comorbid disorder, such as OCD.

Neurophysiological alterations

Neurophysiological evaluation involves assessment of brain electrical activity using scalp electrodes at rest or during participation in experimental paradigms. The major advantage of these techniques is the high temporal resolution that enables tracking the various stages of information processing from primary sensory to association brain regions (Javitt et al., 2008). Neurophysiological approaches include among others (Braff and Light, 2005; Keshavan et al., 2008):

• P300 event-related potentials (ERP), which involve averaging EEG epochs time-locked to repeated presentations of specific stimuli (typically auditory or visual) with the positive wave occurring about 300 ms after the delivery of a task-relevant stimulus considered to reflect higher cognitive functions; schizophrenia is associated with blunted amplitude of the auditory P300 response to salient stimuli.

• P50 auditory-evoked response, the ability of the brain to attenuate the P50 response (a positive ERP component about 50 ms after each click) to the second stimulus when presented with two clicks separated by 500 ms; this inhibitory effect is reduced in schizophrenia.

• Pre-pulse inhibition (PPI), startle response, such as blinking, typically elicited by a sudden auditory stimulus is normally inhibited when the stimulus is preceded by a pre-pulse 60–120 ms earlier; this pre-pulse inhibition, thought to reflect the process of sensorimotor gating, that is reduced in schizophrenia.

• Mismatch negativity (MMN) is a negative voltage component of ERPs, elicited when a train of uniform auditory stimuli are presented, interspersed with unique or deviant stimuli; it represents a pre-attentive stage of auditory information processing and is reduced in schizophrenia.

Markedly, neurophysiological abnormalities observed in OCD patients have also been associated with deficits in focusing and directing attention, though, differently. Deficits in shifting attentional focus on objective neuropsychological tasks has been observed in OCD patients (Chamberlain et al., 2005). Reduced P300 amplitudes for target stimuli but enlarged amplitudes for non-target stimuli in OCD patients as well as shorter latencies have been shown (Pallanti et al., 2009). Collectively, specific ERP abnormalities in OCD have been interpreted in terms of over-focused attention to random details putatively associated with cerebral hyperactivation of the frontal lobe.

In the only study to date, ERPs were used to probe neurophysiological correlates of cognitive and emotional disturbances in a group of schizo-obsessive patients (Pallanti et al., 2009).

The study groups included 11 schizo-obsessive patients, 14 schizophrenia patients, 16 OCD patients, and 12 healthy individuals. All diagnoses were established according to DSM-IV criteria. During the Discriminate Response Task (DRT) participants made simple motor responses to the visual Go (target) stimuli, but avoided responses to the No-Go (non-target) stimuli. ERPs were recorded using wideband EEG sampled continuously at

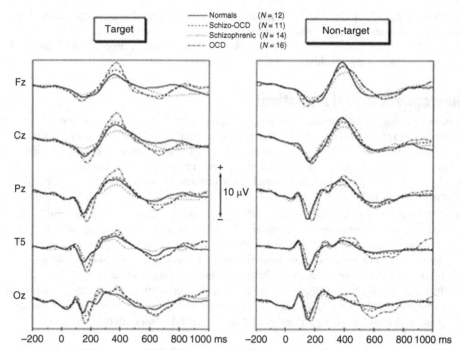

Figure 10.2 Grand average ERP in schizo-obsessive, schizophrenia, and OCD patients and healthy subjects for target (left panel) and non-target (right panel) conditions recorded in five selected electrodes. (From Pallanti S, Castellini G, Chamberlain SR, Querciolo L, Zaccara G, Fineberg NA (2009) Cognitive event-related potentials differentiate schizophrenia with obsessive–compulsive disorder (schizo-OCD) from OCD and schizophrenia without OC symptoms. *Psychiatry Research* **170**, 52–60. Reprinted with permission.)

2 ms/channel using NeuroScan Inc. software (SCAN v. 3.1). Peak amplitudes (relative to the pre-stimulus baseline) and peak latencies of major ERP components were calculated for the early components (P100, N100, P200) and for the late components (P300).

In this investigation, the schizo-obsessive patients exhibited a distinct ERP pattern, with abnormally increased target activation (akin to OCD patients, but unlike the pattern observed in schizophrenia patients) and reduced P300 amplitudes (akin to schizophrenia patients, but unlike OCD patients) (Figure 10.2).

Similar to the healthy subjects, the schizo-obsessive patients showed larger amplitudes in the non-target condition than in the target condition. It is plausible that distinct clinical characteristics of a schizo-obsessive disorder may have a distinguishable neurophysiological pattern and might contribute to identification of a valuable endophenotype for a schizo-obsessive subgroup.

Overall, preliminary studies that aimed to elucidate some of the neurobiological under-pinnings of a schizo-obsessive subgroup of schizophrenia yielded contradictory results: no difference between schizophrenia with and without OCD, poorer performance or a distinct pattern of abnormalities in a schizo-obsessive group. An integrative approach including neurocognitive evaluation, NSS, and brain imaging in schizophrenia patients with and without OCD could lead to better validation of a schizo-obsessive subgroup of schizophrenia.

The genetic basis for a schizo-obsessive disorder
Family studies

Family studies are important for establishing diagnostic validity of a psychiatric entity (Robins and Guze 1970; Kendler 2002). Both schizophrenia and OCD strongly aggregate in families. First-degree relatives of patients with schizophrenia not only have higher rates of schizophrenia than the general population, but also have higher rates of schizophrenia-spectrum disorders, including schizoaffective disorder, other non-affective psychoses, and schizotypal and paranoid personality disorders (Kendler and Diehl, 1993; Asarnow et al., 2001; Nicolson et al., 2003).

Similarly, contemporary family studies using rigorous controlled designs, structured clinical interviews, and DSM-IV diagnostic criteria revealed higher morbid risk for OCD in first-degree relatives of OCD probands compared to relatives of healthy controls (Pauls et al., 1995; Nestadt et al., 2000). In addition, both OCD probands and their first-degree relatives revealed a higher prevalence of obsessive–compulsive personality disorder (OCPD), indicating that OCPD might share a common familial etiology with OCD (Samuels et al., 2000).

Validity of a schizo-obsessive disorder may be further supported by a comparison of differential familial aggregation of schizophrenia-spectrum disorders versus OCD-associated disorders in first-degree relatives of schizophrenia probands with and without OCD. If the obsessive–compulsive component constitutes an independent dimension in schizophrenia, it can be predicted that the rate of occurrence of OCD-associated disorders in first-degree relatives of schizo-obsessive probands will be higher than among the relatives of schizophrenia probands. Indeed, our family study substantiated this hypothesis (Poyurovsky et al., 2005b).

In this study, 57 probands, consecutively admitted to Tirat Carmel Mental Health Center (Tirat Carmel, Israel) who met DSM-IV criteria for both schizophrenia and OCD were recruited, as were 60 comparative schizophrenia patients without OCD who were admitted to the same treatment facility, matched for gender, age, and number of hospitalizations, and 50 healthy individuals.

One hundred and eighty-two first-degree relatives of schizo-obsessive probands, 210 relatives of non-OCD schizophrenia probands, and 165 relatives of community controls were identified. Roughly 75% of the relatives were interviewed in person using the Structural Clinical Interview for DSM-IV (First et al., 1995). The Structured Clinical Interview for DSM-III-R Axis II Personality Disorders (Spitzer et al., 1990) was used for direct assessment of personality disorders. Family history information regarding the remaining participants was obtained from the best informant(s), primarily first-degree relatives, using the Family History Research Diagnostic Criteria (FH-RDC) (Andreasen et al., 1977). For the statistical analysis, the Kaplan–Meier method (Kaplan and Meier, 1958) was used to estimate age-corrected rate (morbid risk) for schizophrenia and OCD in relatives. "Survival time" was determined as the age of onset of illness for affected relatives, and the age of interview was used as "censored time" for unaffected relatives.

No between-group differences for morbid risks for schizophrenia-spectrum disorders were revealed (Table 10.2). As expected relatives of both schizophrenia groups (with and without OCD) had significantly higher morbid risks for schizophrenia-spectrum disorders (9.4% and 7.5%, respectively) than relatives of community-based control subjects (0.75%). These estimates are remarkably similar to the established average risk for schizophrenia in first-degree relatives found in contemporary family studies of schizophrenia (6–9%) (Gottesman, 1991;

Table 10.2 Morbid risk for schizophrenia-spectrum disorders and obsessive–compulsive associated disorders in first-degree relatives of schizophrenia probands with and without OCD and community control subjects

Diagnosis	Relatives of schizo-obsessive probands (N = 182)		Relatives of schizophrenia probands (N = 210)		Relatives of community subjects (N = 165)		Statistics for pairwise comparisons[a]		
	Morbid risk (%)	SE	Morbid risk (%)	SE	Morbid risk (%)	SE	Schizo-obsessive vs. schizophrenia	Schizo-obsessive vs. community controls	Schizophrenia vs. community controls
(A) Schizophrenia-spectrum disorders									
Schizophrenia	9.4	2.33	7.5	2.12	0.75	0.75	0.88	14.26**	8.79**
Schizoaffective disorder	0	0	0	0	0	0			
Other non-affective psychosis	0	0	0	0	0	0			
Schizotypal personality disorder	1.65	0.94	0.48	0.48	0	0	1.11	1.88	1.00
Paranoid personality disorder	3.30	1.32	1.43	0.82	1.82	1.04	1.20	0.94	0.29
Pooled schizophrenia-spectrum disorders	13.19	2.51	7.62	1.83	2.42	1.20	1.79	4.14**	2.38*
Schizo-obsessive disorder	2.20	1.10	0	0	0	0	4.57*	4.76*	
(B) OCD-associated disorders									
OCD	4.41	1.53	1.43	0.82	0.68	0.68	3.02	6.74**	0.99
OCPD	7.14	1.91	1.90	0.94	3.03	1.33	2.46*	1.88	0.69
OCD/OCPD/schizo-obsessive disorder	13.74	2.25	3.33	1.24	3.64	1.46	3.67**	3.61**	0.16
(C) Other Axis I disorders									
Major depressive disorder	8.31	2.21	3.99	1.48	2.24	1.28	1.63	2.08	0.87
Bipolar disorder	0.65	0.64	0	0	0	0	1.00	1.00	
Substance-use disorder	1.29	0.90	2.87	1.26	1.50	1.05	1.02	0.15	0.82

[a] Between-group comparisons for schizophrenia, schizo-obsessive disorder, and personality disorders performed by the log-rank test; for major depressive disorder, bipolar disorder and substance-use disorders by the abridged Weinberg method.
* $p < 0.05$; ** $p < 0.01$.
OCD, obsessive–compulsive disorder; OCPD, obsessive–compulsive personality disorder.
Source: From Poyurovsky M, Kriss V, Weisman G, Faragian S, Schneidman M, Fuchs C, Weizman A, Weizman R (2005b). Reprinted with permission.

Kendler, 2000). In contrast, we found a robust differentiation ($p = 0.0002$) between relatives of the two schizophrenia groups with respect to OCD-associated disorders evaluated in the study. Namely, relatives of schizo-obsessive probands had higher morbid risks for schizo-obsessive disorder, OCD, and OCPD than relatives of schizophrenia probands (Table 10.2). Finally, as in a majority of family studies of schizophrenia, the morbid risks for affective disorders and substance-use disorders did not differ between the two schizophrenia groups, and between the schizophrenia groups and community subjects.

The results of this large-scale family study strongly suggest that a schizo-obsessive disorder is associated with a *specific* elevation in familial rates of OCD-associated disorders rather than an elevation of psychopathology in general.

Some prevalence estimations concerning familial transmission of the disorders of interest are noteworthy. *First*, as mentioned above, the expected rate of schizophrenia in first-degree relatives of schizophrenia probands is approximately 6–9%. The expected rate of OCD in first-degree relatives of OCD probands is approximately 10% (Pauls *et al.*, 1995; Nestadt *et al.*, 2000). Thus, under the assumption of independence, the expected rate of schizo-obsessive disorder in first-degree relatives would have been approximately 0.6–0.9% (10% × 6–9%). In our study the morbid risk for schizo-obsessive disorder in relatives of schizo-obsessive probands is 2.2%, as compared to 0% in relatives of schizophrenia probands. This observed morbid risk is about threefold higher (2.2% vs. 0.6–0.9%) than expected based on the assumption of no linkage between the two disorders. Moreover, the rate of schizo-obsessive disorder in relatives of schizo-obsessive probands was 26.6%, that is remarkably similar to the prevalence of OCD in schizophrenia patients in studies on schizophrenia–OCD comorbidity. Overall, it seems that schizo-obsessive disorder is to some degree familial, i.e., if a patient suffers from schizo-obsessive disorder his/her first-degree relatives have increased risk for this disorder as well (or vice versa). *Second*, relatives of schizo-obsessive probands had a four-fold increase of morbid risk for OCD compared to relatives of schizophrenia patients. This morbid risk for OCD (6.63%) is considerably higher than in our community-based control group and that reported in the general population (1.2–2.4%) (Karno *et al.*, 1988), However it is lower than the rate reported in first-degree relatives of OCD patients (roughly 10%) (Pauls *et al.*, 1995; Nestadt *et al.*, 2000). In contrast, the morbid risk for OCD in relatives of schizophrenia probands (1.43%) was similar to the estimated rate of OCD in the general population. *Third*, there is an increased rate of OCPD in "pure" OCD patients (Malaix-Cols *et al.*, 2000; Samuels *et al.*, 2000). There are no data on the rate of OCPD in schizophrenia patients. Our finding of 7.14% morbid risk for OCPD in schizo-obsessive relatives (2.3 times more than the community relatives and 3.7 times more than the schizophrenia relatives) is in between that found in relatives of OCD probands (11.5%) (Samuels *et al.*, 2000) and in the general population (1–2%) (Torgensen *et al.*, 2001).

From a clinical perspective, the revealed preferential familial aggregation and transmission of OCD-related disorders in schizo-obsessive patients justifies a systematic search for these morbidities particularly in this subgroup of schizophrenia patients. The detection of OCD, OCPD, or schizo-obsessive disorder in a patient's relatives increases the likelihood of their presence in that patient.

Molecular genetics

Molecular genetics of a schizo-obsessive disorder is making important strides, and the first candidate gene studies have recently emerged. Thus the role of the catechol-O-methyltransferase

(COMT) gene for susceptibility to schizo-obsessive disorder has been evaluated. COMT, one of the major enzymes involved in the metabolic inactivation of catecholamines dopamine and norepinephrine, is located at the q11 band of human chromosome 22. The essential role of COMT in catabolism of dopamine, a neurotransmitter, which has been consistently implicated in the pathogenesis of both schizophrenia and OCD, made the COMT gene an attractive candidate gene for susceptibility to either disorder of interest. A common polymorphism (valine to methionine substitution at codon 158) in the membrane-bound form of the enzyme (MB-COMT), which causes a three- to fourfold variation in the COMT enzyme activity, was used to address the involvement of this gene in psychiatric disorders, including schizophrenia and OCD. The high-activity Val allele has been associated with poor cognitive performance in schizophrenia patients and normal controls (Goldberg et al., 2003). A meta-analysis of case-control studies, however, failed to show a major effect of either allele in schizophrenia, although meta-analysis of family-based studies found some evidence implicating high-activity Val allele (Glatt et al., 2003). Several studies suggested that the low-activity Met allele of the COMT gene is associated with susceptibility to OCD in a recessive and sexually dimorphic manner (Karayiorgou et al., 1997).

Our group conducted a case-controlled association study of the COMT Val[158]Met polymorphism in 113 schizo-obsessive patients compared to 79 OCD patients and 171 control subjects (Poyurovsky et al., 2005a). There was no significant difference in allele and genotype distribution of the COMT gene between schizo-obsessive patients and healthy controls. This report was followed by a study conducted by Zinkstok and colleagues (2008) who found a significant association between the COMT Val[158]Met polymorphism and the severity of OCD, as assessed by the Yale–Brown Obsessive–Compulsive Scale (Y-BOCS) in 77 male patients with recent-onset schizophrenia: the Val/Val genotype was associated with the highest Y-BOCS scores, whereas patients with the Met/Met genotype had the lowest Y-BOCS scores. The authors suggest that the COMT Val[158]Met polymorphism may be a modifier gene for the obsessive–compulsive symptomatology in schizophrenia. These are the first steps, and they are apparently inconsistent. More studies on candidate risk genes, as well as DNA structural variations, will likely follow to address different forms of genomic risk for complex schizo-obsessive disorder.

References

Anderson KE, Savage CR (2004) Cognitive and neurobiological findings in obsessive-compulsive disorder. Psychiatric Clinics of North America 27, 37–47, viii.

Andreasen NC, Endicott J, Spitzer RL, Winokur G (1977) The family history method using diagnostic criteria. Archives of General Psychiatry 34, 1229–1235.

Aoyama F, Iida J, Inoue M, et al. (2000) Brain imaging in childhood- and adolescence-onset schizophrenia associated with obsessive-compulsive symptoms. Acta Psychiatrica Scandinavica 102, 32–37.

Asarnow RF, Nuechterlein KH, Fogelson D, et al. (2001) Schizophrenia and schizophrenia-spectrum personality disorders in the first-degree relatives of children with schizophrenia: the UCLA family study. Archives of General Psychiatry 58, 581–588.

Bachmann S, Bottmer C, Schroder J (2005) Neurological soft signs in first-episode schizophrenia: a follow-up study. American Journal of Psychiatry 162, 2337–2343.

Berman I, Merson A, Viegner B, et al. (1998) Obsessions and compulsions as a distinct cluster of symptoms in schizophrenia: a neuropsychological study. Journal of Nervous and Mental Disease 186, 150–156.

Bolton D, Gibb W, Lees A, et al. (1998) Neurological soft signs in obsessive compulsive disorder: standardised assessment and comparison with schizophrenia. *Behavioral Neurology* **11**, 197 201.

Bombin I, Arango C, Buchanan RW (2005) Significance and meaning of neurological signs in schizophrenia: two decades later. *Schizophrenia Bulletin* **31**, 962–977.

Borkowska A, Pilaczyñska E, Rybakowski JK (2003) The frontal lobe neuropsychological tests in patients with schizophrenia and/or obsessive-compulsive disorder. *Journal of Neuropsychiatry and Clinical Neurosciences* **15**, 359–362.

Bottas A, Cooke RG, Richter MA (2005) Comorbidity and pathophysiology of obsessive-compulsive disorder in schizophrenia: is there evidence for a schizo-obsessive subtype of schizophrenia? *Journal of Psychiatry and Neuroscience* **30**, 186–193.

Braff D, Light GA (2005) The use of neuropsychological endophenotypes to understand the genetic basis of schizophrenia. *Dialogues in Clinical Neuroscience* **7**, 125–135.

Browne S, Clarke M, Gervin M, *et al.* (2000) Determinants of neurological dysfunction in first episode schizophrenia. *Psychological Medicine* **30**, 1433–1441.

Buchanan RW, Heinrichs DW (1989) The Neurological Evaluation Scale (NES): a structured instrument for the assessment of neurological signs in schizophrenia. *Psychiatry Research* **27**, 335–350.

Chamberlain SR, Blackwell AD, Fineberg NA, Robbins TW, Sahakian BJ (2005) The neuropsychology of obsessive-compulsive disorder: the importance of failures in cognitive and behavioural inhibition as candidate endophenotypic markers. *Neuroscience and Biobehavioral Reviews* **29**, 399–419.

Dazzan P, Murray RM (2002) Neurological soft signs in first-episode psychosis: a systematic review. *British Journal of Psychiatry* (Suppl.) **43**, S50–S57.

First MB, Spitzer RL, Gibbon M, Williams JBW (1995) *Structured Clinical Interview for Axis I DSM-IV Disorders, Patient Edition (SCID-I/P, Version 2.0)*. Biometrics Research Department, New York State Psychiatric Institute, New York.

Glatt SJ, Faraone SV, Tsuang MT (2003) Association between a functional catechol-*O* methyltransferase gene polymorphism and schizophrenia: meta-analysis of case-control and family-based studies. *American Journal of Psychiatry* **160**, 469–476.

Goldberg TE, Egan MF, Gscheidle T, *et al.* (2003) Executive subprocesses in working memory: relationship to catechol-*O*-methyltransferase Val[158]Met genotype and schizophrenia. *Archives of General Psychiatry* **60**, 889–896.

Gottesman II (1991) *Schizophrenia Genesis: The Origins of Madness*. W.H. Freeman, New York.

Heinrichs DW, Buchanan RW (1988) Significance and meaning of neurological signs in schizophrenia. *American Journal of Psychiatry* **145**, 11–18.

Hollander E, Schiffman E, Cohen B, *et al.* (1990) Signs of central nervous system dysfunction in obsessive-compulsive disorder. *Archives of General Psychiatry* **47**, 27–32.

Iida J, Matumura K, Aoyama F (1998) Cerebral MRI findings in childhood-onset schizophrenia, comparison of patients with prodromal obsessive-compulsive symptoms and those without symptoms. *Recent Progress in Child and Adolescent Psychiatry* **2**, 75–83.

Jaafari N, Baup N, Bourdel MC, *et al.* (2011) Neurological soft signs in OCD patients with early age at onset, versus patients with schizophrenia and healthy subjects. *Journal of Neuropsychiatry and Clinical Neurosciences* **23**, 409–416.

Javitt DC, Spencer KM, Thaker GK, Winterer G, Hajós M (2008) Neurophysiological biomarkers for drug development in schizophrenia. *Nature Reviews Drug Discovery* **7**, 68–83.

Kaplan EL, Meier P (1958) Nonparametric estimation from incomplete observations. *Journal of the American Statistical Association* **53**, 457–481.

Karayiorgou M, Altemus M, Galke BL, *et al.* (1997) Genotype determining low catechol-*O*-methyltransferase activity as a risk factor for obsessive-compulsive disorder. *Proceedings of the National Academy of*

Sciences of the United States of America **94**, 4572–4575.

Karno M, Golding JM, Sorenson SB, Burnam MA (1988) The epidemiology of obsessive-compulsive disorder in five US communities. *Archives of General Psychiatry* **45**, 1094–1099.

Kendler KS (2000) Schizophrenia: genetics. In: Sadock BJ, Sadock VA (eds.) *Kaplan and Sadock's Comprehensive Textbook of Psychiatry*, 7th edn. Lippincott, Williams & Wilkins, Philadelphia, PA, pp.1147–1158.

Kendler KS (2002) Hierarchy and heritability: the role of diagnosis and modelling in psychiatric genetics. *American Journal of Psychiatry* **159**, 515–518.

Kendler KS, Diehl SR (1993) The genetics of schizophrenia: a current, genetic-epidemiologic perspective. *Schizophrenia Bulletin* **19**, 261–285.

Keshavan MS, Sanders RD, Sweeney JA, *et al.* (2003) Diagnostic specificity and neuroanatomical validity of neurological abnormalities in first-episode psychoses. *American Journal of Psychiatry* **160**, 1298–1304.

Keshavan MS, Tandon R, Boutros NN, Nasrallah HA (2008) Schizophrenia, "just the facts": what we know in 2008 III. Neurobiology. *Schizophrenia Research* **106**, 89–107.

Khanna S (1991) Soft neurological signs in obsessive-compulsive disorder. *Biological Psychiatry* **29** (Suppl.), 442.

Kurokawa K, Nakamura K, Sumiyoshi T, *et al.* (2000) Ventricular enlargement in schizophrenia spectrum patients with prodromal symptoms of obsessive-compulsive disorder. *Psychiatry Research* **99**, 83–91.

Levine JB, Gruber SA, Baird AA, Yurgelun-Todd D (1998) Obsessive-compulsive disorder among schizophrenic patients: an exploratory study using functional magnetic resonance imaging data. *Comprehensive Psychiatry* **39**, 308–311.

Lysaker PH, Warman DM, Dimaggio G, *et al.* (2008) Metacognition in schizophrenia: associations with multiple assessments of executive function. *Journal of Nervous and Mental Disease* **196**, 384–389.

Malaix-Cols D, Baer L, Rauch SL, Jenike MA (2000) Relation of factor-analyzed symptom dimensions of obsessive-compulsive disorder to personality disorder. *Acta Psychiatrica Scandinavica* **102**, 199–202.

Nestadt G, Samuels J, Riddle M, *et al.* (2000) A family study of obsessive-compulsive disorder. *Archives of General Psychiatry* **57**, 358–363.

Nicolson R, Brookner FB, Lenane M, *et al.* (2003) Parental schizophrenia spectrum disorders in childhood-onset and adult-onset schizophrenia. *American Journal of Psychiatry* **160**, 490–495.

Ongór D, Goff DC (2005) Obsessive-compulsive symptoms in schizophrenia: associated clinical features, cognitive function and medication status. *Schizophrenia Research* **75**, 349–362.

Pallanti S, Castellini G, Chamberlain SR, *et al.* (2009) Cognitive event-related potentials differentiate schizophrenia with obsessive-compulsive disorder (schizo-OCD) from OCD and schizophrenia without OC symptoms. *Psychiatry Research* **170**, 52–60.

Patel DD, Laws KR, Padhi A, *et al.* (2010) The neuropsychology of the schizo-obsessive subtype of schizophrenia: a new analysis. *Psychological Medicine* **40**, 921–933.

Pauls DL, Alsobrook JP 2nd, Goodman W, Rasmussen S, Leckman JF (1995) A family study of obsessive-compulsive disorder. *American Journal of Psychiatry* **152**, 76–84.

Poyurovsky M, Fuchs K, Weizman A (1999) Obsessive-compulsive symptoms in patients with first-episode schizophrenia. *American Journal of Psychiatry* **156**, 1998–2000.

Poyurovsky M, Michaelovsky E, Frisch A, *et al.* (2005a) COMT Val[158]Met polymorphism in schizophrenia with obsessive-compulsive disorder: a case-control study. *Neuroscience Letters* **389**, 21–24.

Poyurovsky M, Kriss V, Weisman G, *et al.* (2005b) Familial aggregation of schizophrenia-spectrum disorders and obsessive-compulsive associated disorders in schizophrenia probands with and without OCD. *American Journal of Medical Genetics Part B Neuropsychiatric Genetics* **133**, 31–36.

Poyurovsky M, Faragian S, Pashinian A, *et al.* (2007) Neurological soft signs in schizophrenia patients with obsessive compulsive disorder. *Journal of Neuropsychiatry and Clinical Neurosciences* 19, 145–150.

Robins E, Guze SB (1970) Establishment of diagnostic validity in psychiatric illness: its application to schizophrenia. *American Journal of Psychiatry* 126, 983–987.

Samuels J, Nestadt G, Bienvenu J, *et al.* (2000) Personality disorders and normal personality dimension in obsessive-compulsive disorder. *British Journal of Psychiatry* 177, 457–462.

Sevincok L, Akoglu A, Arslantas H (2006) Schizo-obsessive and obsessive-compulsive disorder: comparison of clinical characteristics and neurological soft signs. *Psychiatry Research* 145, 241–248.

Spitzer RL, Janet W, Gibbon M, First MB (1990) *Structured Clinical Interview for DSM-III-R Personality Disorders (SCID-II, Version 1.0).* American Psychiatric Press, Washington, DC.

Tandon R, Nasrallah HA, Keshavan MS (2009) Schizophrenia, "just the facts": IV. Clinical features and conceptualization. *Schizophrenia Research* 110, 1–23.

Thomas N, Tharyan P (2011) Soft neurological signs in drug-free people with schizophrenia with and without obsessive-compulsive symptoms. *Journal of Neuropsychiatry and Clinical Neuroscience* 23, 68–73.

Torgensen S, Kringlen E, Cramer V (2001) The prevalence of personality disorders in a community sample. *Archives of General Psychiatry* 58, 590–596.

Tumkaya S, Karadag F, Oguzhanoglu NK, *et al.* (2009) Schizophrenia with obsessive-compulsive disorder and obsessive-compulsive disorder with poor insight: a neuropsychological comparison. *Psychiatry Research* 165, 38–46.

Tumkaya S, Karadag F, Oguzhanoglu NK (2012) Neurological soft signs in schizophrenia and obsessive compulsive disorder spectrum. *European Psychiatry* 27, 92–99.

Whitney KA, Fastenau PS, Evans JD, Lysaker PH (2004) Comparative neuropsychological function in obsessive-compulsive disorder and schizophrenia with and without obsessive-compulsive symptoms. *Schizophrenia Research* 69, 75–83.

Whitty P, Clarke M, Browne S, *et al.* (2003) Prospective evaluation of neurological soft signs in first-episode schizophrenia in relation to psychopathology: state versus trait phenomena. *Psychological Medicine* 33, 1479–1484.

Zinkstok J, van Nimwegen L, van Amelsvoort T, *et al.* (2008) Catechol-*O*-methyltransferase gene and obsessive-compulsive symptoms in patients with recent-onset schizophrenia: preliminary results. *Psychiatry Research* 157, 1–8.

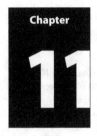

Chapter 11

Treatment of schizophrenia with obsessive–compulsive symptoms

Although there is general consensus that schizo-obsessive patients comprise a difficult-to-treat subgroup that requires a distinct therapeutic approach, research addressing treatment interventions for patients with schizo-obsessive disorder is still in the initial stages, and well-designed large-scale controlled treatment trials are notably lacking. While treating schizo-obsessive patients, physicians face the following questions that have yet to be adequately answered:

● For whom is monotherapy with an antipsychotic agent appropriate and who would benefit from the addition of anti-obsessive agents?
● At what stage of schizophrenia should anti-obsessive agents be initiated for patients with schizo-obsessive disorder?
● How should various phenomenological expressions of obsessive–compulsive phenomena in schizophrenia (e.g., typical vs. psychotic-related obsessions and/or compulsions) be addressed?
● What are the short- and long-term risks and benefits of antipsychotic–SRI combinations in schizo-obsessive patients?
● Which patients are susceptible to antipsychotic-induced obsessive–compulsive symptoms? How are antipsychotic-induced obsessive–compulsive symptoms detected in schizophrenia patients and how should they be dealt with?
● What is the role of non-pharmacological intervention (e.g., cognitive–behavioral therapy) in the management of schizo-obsessive patients?

Monotherapy with antipsychotic agents

Typical antipsychotic agents seem to be of limited therapeutic value for schizo-obsessive patients, presumably owing to their limited serotonergic properties (Green *et al.*, 2003). The bulk of reports to date indicate that atypical antipsychotics with their serotonin/dopamine antagonism might induce *de novo* or aggravate pre-existing obsessive–compulsive symptoms in schizophrenia patients (described in Chapter 12). Yet there is preliminary evidence indicating that monotherapy with atypical antipsychotics may in turn, alleviate obsessive–compulsive symptoms, pointing toward a potential *bidirectional (alleviating vs. provoking) effect* on obsessive–compulsive symptoms in schizophrenia.

Olanzapine versus risperidone

Van Nimwegen *et al.* (2008) conducted a large-scale randomized comparative study of olanzapine (59 patients) and risperidone (63 patients) in young patients with recent-onset schizophrenia-spectrum disorders. The primary outcome measure was the mean baseline-to-

194

endpoint change in total score on the Yale–Brown Obsessive–Compulsive Scale (Y-BOCS). By the end of a 6-week trial, olanzapine (mean dose 11.3 mg) but not risperidone (mean dose 3.0 mg) was associated with a meaningful decrease in the severity of obsessive–compulsive symptoms (-2.2 vs. -0.3, $z = -2.651$, $p < 0.01$). In contrast, though not statistically significant, more patients without pre-existing obsessive–compulsive symptoms (score 0 on the Y-BOCS) in the risperidone group than in the olanzapine group developed obsessive–compulsive symptoms (8 vs. 2). These results corroborate earlier reports suggesting that for some schizo-obsessive patients, monotherapy with olanzapine may improve both schizophrenic and obsessive–compulsive dimensions of psychopathology without running the risk of exacerbation of obsessive–compulsive symptoms (Baker et al., 1996).

In support of these findings, a positive therapeutic effect of olanzapine monotherapy (10–20 mg/day) was found in three schizo-obsessive patients who were unsuccessfully treated with various conventional neuroleptics in combination with anti-obsessive agents and subsequently showed intolerance to clozapine prior to the switch to olanzapine (Poyurovsky et al., 2000). The patients demonstrated significant improvement in both schizophrenia and obsessive–compulsive symptoms as measured by the Brief Psychiatric Rating Scale (decreased by 53%, 51%, and 48%, respectively) and Y-BOCS (decreased by 68%, 73%, and 85%). It is worthwhile to note, however, that the improvement of obsessive–compulsive symptoms during olanzapine monotherapy may have been attributed in part to the discontinuation of clozapine.

Sasson et al. (1997) also reported a beneficial effect of olanzapine (6.5 ± 2.3 mg/day for 8 weeks) in nine patients with comorbid schizophrenia and OCD. All nine patients completed an adequate trial of at least one SSRI or clomipramine combined with either typical or atypical antipsychotics prior to the addition of olanzapine. Four of the nine patients were responders (>40% decrease in Y-BOCS score), two patients were "partial responders," and only one patient reported worsening of obsessive–compulsive symptoms.

The following is an illustrative case vignette, showing a beneficial effect of olanzapine monotherapy on schizophrenic and obsessive–compulsive symptoms in a schizophrenia patient.

Case 11.1. Mr. D is a 25-year-old man. His psychiatric history was unremarkable except for stuttering until age 13. His first psychiatric hospitalization at age 20 was for a psychotic breakdown which warranted a DSM-IV diagnosis of schizophrenic disorder, paranoid type. Treatment with perphenazine (12 mg/day for 3 months) diminished the bizarre behavior, delusional ideas of reference and persecution, and third-person auditory hallucinations, leading to a clinical remission. However, 2 years later, he was rehospitalized, with both acute psychotic symptoms (psychomotor agitation, delusions of reference, Schneiderian symptoms) and emergent obsessive–compulsive symptoms. On interview, D reported recurring intrusive profane thoughts about God that were extremely distressful especially since he was a religious person. He was fully convinced of the "true nature" of his thoughts and even related them to God's voice that he heard from time to time. He also attempted to get these thoughts "out of his mind" with cleaning rituals that lasted as long as 3–5 hours a day. This complex psychopathological phenomenon appeared to be psychotic in content and obsessive–compulsive in form. Subsequent neuroleptic trials (perphenazine, risperidone) were partially effective but were associated with clinically significant extrapyramidal side effects and akathisia. Olanzapine was started and titrated up to 20 mg/day within 3 weeks. A relatively rapid improvement in all components of the patient's complex psychopathology was noted within 3 weeks. This included a substantial decrease in the severity of the delusions and hallucinations (total Positive and Negative Syndrome score dropped 40% from 80 to 48), accompanied by the alleviation of the obsessive–compulsive component. D's obsessive thoughts decreased in intensity and the related cleaning rituals also abated. Olanzapine's side effects included increased appetite and moderate weight gain.

The ameliorating effect of olanzapine on obsessive–compulsive symptoms in some schizophrenia patients should be weighed against a tendency to induce or aggravate obsessions and/or compulsions in others (Lykouras *et al.*, 2000). The potential side effects, primarily weight gain, metabolic syndrome, sedation, and orthostatic hypotension, should also be taken into account when considering treatment with olanzapine.

Aripiprazole

Atypical antipsychotics differ in their receptor pharmacology and corresponding effects on schizophrenia-related obsessive–compulsive symptoms. Glick *et al.* (2008) reported results of a preliminary investigation in schizo-obsessive patients of the administration of aripiprazole, an atypical antipsychotic with unique pharmacological properties. Aripiprazole is distinguished by its partial dopamine agonism coupled with a low 5-HT_2 to D_2 affinity ratio and a low 5-HT_{1A} receptor occupancy (Mamo *et al.*, 2007). In a 6-week, open-label, flexible-dose trial, monotherapy with aripiprazole (10–30 mg/day) resulted in a meaningful clinical improvement of obsessive–compulsive symptoms in schizophrenia patients who were partially responsive to a prior exposure to either typical or atypical antipsychotic agents. Six of the seven study completers showed a decrease of roughly 35% from baseline on the Y-BOCS, combined with an improvement of schizophrenia symptoms (Glick *et al.*, 2008). It is obvious that even modest improvement of functioning due to improvement in an obsessive–compulsive component, as revealed in this study, might be clinically meaningful for this challenging subset of schizophrenia patients.

The following is a case vignette showing a beneficial effect of aripiprazole monotherapy on schizophrenic and obsessive–compulsive symptoms in a schizophrenia patient.

Case 11.2. Mr. F, a 27-year-old single unemployed man living with his parents, had been under psychiatric supervision for 5 years since his first acute psychotic breakdown at age 22, when he was a freshman student of engineering. F was heterosexual, but developed fears of being homosexual, claiming that his male peers glared at him and made remarks and gestures with sexual context. He also heard a male voice whispering "homosexual" when he was alone in his room. This worry was intrusive and distressful, and led him to ask for recurring reassurance that he was not gay. He was compelled to make repeated attempts at checking whether his appearance indeed indicated homosexuality. In addition to this complex psychopathological presentation, delusional in content and obsessive–compulsive in form, F exhibited formal thought disorders, such as blocking, circumstantial and tangential thinking, and mind-reading and mind broadcasting phenomena, prompting a DSM-IV diagnosis of schizophrenic disorder. He also revealed ritualistic behavior unrelated to delusional themes, such as counting until 33 before leaving the house, touching door frames repeatedly to prevent dreadful events, and associating certain numbers with certain events. In contrast to "obsessive delusions" of homosexuality associated with full conviction of their validity, these time-consuming and distressful counting and touching rituals appeared to be typical to OCD and were associated with fair insight into their excessive and senseless nature. They first emerged roughly 3 years prior to the first episode of psychosis. An additional DSM-IV diagnosis of OCD was established.

Risperidone (up to 4 mg/day) was initiated. Within a few days the patient became increasingly agitated and his touching and counting compulsions worsened to the point that it took him several hours to be brought into the office for evaluation because of his rituals. Risperidone was discontinued and switched to quetiapine (up to 800 mg/day), which was intolerable to the patient because of excessive sedation and severe orthostatic hypotension. Subsequent gradual cross-tapering with aripiprazole (up to 20 mg/day) was associated with substantial improvement of schizophrenic symptoms, including auditory hallucinations and thought disorders (the total PANSS score dropped 40% from 90 to 54). There was a gradual de-actualization of "obsessive delusions" which finally disappeared after 4 weeks of aripiprazole treatment. Notably, no worsening of typical touching and counting compulsions was observed. In contrast, there was a modest improvement in their severity, in the time spent on rituals, and distress. After 8 weeks of treatment, the total Y-BOCS score dropped 18% from 26 to 21. Eventually, sertraline (up to 150 mg/day) was added to aripiprazole (20 mg/day) to deal with the remaining typical obsessions and compulsions, and a meaningful therapeutic effect of the combination was achieved within 10 additional weeks of treatment (total Y-BOCS score 13).

Despite the revealed beneficial effect of aripiprazole on both schizophrenic and obsessive–compulsive symptoms, its potential to aggravate obsessions or compulsions in susceptible individuals should not be disregarded (Desarkar et al., 2007; Mouaffak et al., 2007). Clinicians should also be aware that administration of aripiprazole may be associated, especially early in treatment, with agitation and akathisia with prevalence as high as 18% (Kane et al., 2010). Clinical experience revealed that the occurrence of these aripiprazole-induced adverse effects might be accompanied by the exacerbation of both psychotic and obsessive–compulsive symptoms. Starting with lower aripiprazole doses, slow up-titration and slow cross-tapering with the previous antipsychotic, as well as early recognition of these side effects, are essential to minimize their occurrence and to prevent early drug discontinuation. Aripiprazole's clinically meaningful advantages include low propensity to induce weight gain, metabolic syndrome, and prolactinemia.

Amisulpiride

Amisulpiride is distinguished from the majority of atypical antipsychotics by its highly selective dopamine D_2/D_3 receptor antagonism and a minimal affinity for the 5-HT_{2A} receptor (Lecrubier et al., 2001). It was hypothesized that owing to these pharmacological properties, amisulpiride would not induce or exacerbate obsessive–compulsive symptoms in patients with schizophrenia. Indeed, this was the case when 16 DSM-IV schizophrenia patients with additional obsessive–compulsive symptoms (Y-BOCS > 10) were switched to amisulpiride (dose range 200–1200 mg/day) from risperidone (13 patients, mean dose 4.5 mg/day) or aripiprazole (three patients, mean dose 30 mg/day) (Kim et al., 2008). The previous antipsychotic was tapered within the first 4 weeks of this 12-week open-label prospective trial, and amisulpiride was simultaneously up-titrated. At the end of the trial, the obsession, compulsion, and total subscale scores of the Y-BOCS significantly improved after switching to amisulpiride ($p < 0.01$, for all subscales). Twelve patients (75%) showed 50% or more improvement in the Y-BOCS score. The improvement in obsessive-compulsive symptoms was independent from a reduction in the severity of psychotic symptoms. No clinically significant adverse effects were reported in association with the medication switch. The fact that patients with pre-existing obsessive–compulsive symptoms tended to be less responsive to the switch to amisulpiride than those with obsessive-compulsive symptoms induced by prior administration of risperidone and aripiprazole suggests that discontinuation of a previous antipsychotic might be responsible for the amelioration of obsessive–compulsive symptoms. Nevertheless, potent and selective blockade of the D_2 receptor by amisulpiride, along with its negligible affinity for the serotonin 5-HT_{2A} receptor, might play a role in controlling obsessive–compulsive symptoms in schizophrenia patients. Amisulpiride's side effect profile, potential to induce hyperprolactemia, and a low propensity for weight gain and metabolic syndrome should also be considered.

The following case vignette demonstrates a positive effect of amisulpiride on a patient with schizo-obsessive disorder.

Case 11.3. Ms. P, a 30-year-old unmarried woman living with her parents. She was able to keep a full-time position as a medical secretary until 6 months prior to her hospitalization for an acute psychotic episode. Initial typical obsessive–compulsive symptoms were detected at age 15, when P began washing her hands repeatedly because of her fears of contamination. Since then the course of this disturbance waxed and waned. Partial remissions alternated with periods of deterioration when she performed washing rituals up to 2 hours a day. She had fair insight into the excessive and senseless nature of her obsessions and compulsions; however, she could not stop performing rituals. The functional impairment associated with her symptoms was substantial and P was prompted to take days off during exacerbations of her malady. She was seen by a psychiatrist at age 25, and received a DSM-IV diagnosis of OCD. P refused a trial with an SSRI; behavior therapy (exposure plus response prevention sessions) was of minimal therapeutic effect. Over the 6 months prior to her current hospitalization she became increasingly suspicious, expressing vague and persistent ideas of reference and persecution associated with hostility towards her family members. She began to claim that she was receiving special messages from a TV broadcaster who "deliberately affected her mind by inserting unwanted thoughts." She gradually became disorganized, and affect was grossly inappropriate as was her behavior. At this point a DSM-IV diagnosis of schizophrenic disorder, disorganized type, was established. In addition to positive and disorganized symptoms of schizophrenia, P was involved in repeated hand-washing which lasted for hours, to the point that she had to be forcibly pulled out of the bathroom. She also repeatedly checked her hair standing in front of a mirror for hours, again to the point that she had to be forcibly stopped. P had performed analogous rituals before hospitalization, but they were substantially less severe and time-consuming. In addition, insight into obsessive–compulsive symptoms expressed prior to hospitalization was lost during acute psychosis. Subsequent trials with perphenazine (up to 32 mg/day) and risperidone (up to 4 mg/day) were associated with a decrease of positive and disorganized schizophrenic symptoms, but were however associated with clinically significant extrapyramidal side effects and akathisia. Moreover, alleviation of psychotic symptoms was not accompanied by any improvement of compulsive-like behavior. Escitalopram (10 mg/day) was tried in addition to risperidone, but after 7 days of combined treatment there was a worsening of psychosis. Escitalopram was discontinued. Amisulpiride was initiated, while risperidone was discontinued. Monotherapy with amisulpiride (800 mg/ day) led to gradual improvement of both schizophrenic (the total PANSS score dropped 42.5% from 84 to 50) and obsessive-compulsive symptoms (pre-amisulpiride total Y-BOCS score dropped 50% from 22 to 11). Her compulsive hand-washing and checking improved with amisulpiride and she now spent roughly 30 minutes daily on the rituals. P reported that with this improvement she was able to control rituals which became substantially less intrusive and distressful.

Clozapine

Clozapine is currently the most effective available antipsychotic. However, due to a burden of adverse effects (e.g., potentially life-threatening agranulocytosis), clozapine is reserved for treatment-resistant schizophrenia patients. In contrast to apparent efficacy in schizophrenia patients, clozapine was found ineffective in patients with OCD (McDougle *et al.*, 1995). There is compelling evidence that links clozapine with precipitating or worsening obsessions and compulsions in individuals with schizophrenia (described below). However, there are also preliminary data indicating that clozapine in a relatively low dose range may exert a beneficial effect at least in some schizo-obsessive individuals.

A chart review of 200 patients (mean age at admission 21.5 years, SD = 5.03) with recent-onset schizophrenia-spectrum disorders treated by clozapine or other antipsychotic medications supports this observation (de Haan *et al.*, 2004). Though four out of 41 patients (9.8%) developed *de novo* OCD during clozapine therapy, disappearance of pre-existing OCD during treatment with clozapine was observed in another four (9.8%) patients. Though these findings are limited by retrospective chart review methodology, it seems that one subgroup of clozapine-treated schizophrenia patients is susceptible to induction or exacerbation of OCD, yet others may benefit from clozapine administration and show a reduction of OCD severity.

The following case vignettes demonstrate a considerable improvement of obsessions and compulsions in patients with chronic treatment-resistant schizophrenia treated with a relatively low dose of clozapine (Bermanzohn *et al.*, 1997; Tibbo and Gendemann, 1999).

Case 11.4. A 44-year-old married woman was diagnosed with schizophrenia and first hospitalized with paranoid ideation, ideas of reference, and auditory hallucinations. Psychotic symptoms were controlled, though not eliminated, with low-dose haloperidol. The patient also had contamination obsessions with compulsive hand-washing, cleaning, ordering, and checking; however, the patient was not sure whether or not these obsessions and compulsions predated the psychotic symptoms. She initially did not disclose these symptoms to her attending physician, since she felt they were "silly," yet acknowledged she could spend up to 4 hours daily performing the compulsive behaviors. Review of her history revealed that her previous obsessions and compulsions were not related to any delusional theme, and no specific anti-obsessional agents had been prescribed in the past. She had no other significant medical history, including alcohol or drug abuse, and she attended an outpatient schizophrenia program on a regular basis. Because of the side effects of haloperidol, she was switched to clozapine; at 75 mg daily her psychotic symptoms were under control, and in addition, she noticed a marked improvement in her obsessions and compulsions. It was only with this improvement and her subsequent participation in a research study that she disclosed her obsessions and compulsions. Her compulsive behavior had improved with clozapine and she was now spending less than 1 hour daily on the rituals. Although no previous rating scales were available, her present scores include Y-BOCS = 11, Positive and Negative Syndrome Scale total = 98, and Global Assessment of Functioning = 60.

Case 11.5. Mr. A is a 43-year-old man. At age 16 he began to be tormented by intrusive thoughts that people thought he was gay, and therefore noticed, talked about, and made fun of him. He also believed that people wanted to hurt him and make his life miserable. He left school because of these intrusive and distressing thoughts, and became virtually housebound for about 7 years, during which time he spent hours each day monitoring his walking in front of a mirror to be sure he did not walk in an "effeminate" manner. He heard a voice that kept a running commentary on his thoughts and actions and two or more voices that conversed with each other. He also heard laughter, his name being called, and "noises that didn't make sense." From age 17 to 20 A repeatedly combed his hair "until I got the part exactly right," usually taking between 15 and 20 minutes daily, but sometimes hours. He became occupied with violent, sexually aggressive, and homosexual thoughts, which led him to see his neighborhood priest daily to confess. He also had to blink in ritualistic ways, feeling that he had to synchronize his blinking with that of TV personalities. He said of his thoughts and actions: "I just couldn't stop," and recognized that they were taken to excess. Despite recurrent depressive episodes, he was about 37 years old before he clearly fulfilled criteria for a major depressive syndrome. At that time he was diagnosed and hospitalized with schizoaffective disorder. A variety of typical neuroleptics during his long course of illness had no effect on A's preoccupation that others thought he was gay and were ridiculing him. After he had been on haloperidol for several years, clomipramine up to 250 mg/day was added to his regimen. After this trial failed, clozapine was initiated and slowly increased to 200 mg/day. After 4 weeks of this regimen, he experienced a definite reduction in the intrusiveness of his thoughts and in the distress they caused him.

Describing the diversity of treatment response in schizo-obsessive patients, Bermanzohn et al. (1997) suggested that obsessive–compulsive symptoms in schizophrenia patients might originate from two sources. Schizophrenia patients for whom obsessive delusions grew out of pre-existing simple obsessions, for which they lost insight, tend to respond to adjunctive anti-obsessional agents (see below), and patients whose obsessive delusions grew out of "obsessive preoccupation with schizophrenic delusions" tend to respond to atypical antipsychotics (Cases 11.1, 11.3, and 11.5). It is also possible that the complex nature of the treatment response could be interpreted by viewing obsessive–compulsive symptoms in schizophrenia patients as either comorbid OCD or as an inherited obsessive–compulsive dimension of schizophrenic symptomatology. Conceivably, symptomatic anti-obsessive treatment with SRIs needs to be added to ongoing antipsychotics in schizophrenia patients for whom typical OCD represents a comorbid disorder and usually appears prior to the emergence of schizophrenic symptoms. However, schizophrenia patients whose obsessive–compulsive symptoms are "intimately linked" to psychotic symptoms, that is they emerge or are heightened during psychotic exacerbation, may benefit from monotherapy with antipsychotic agents associated with a low risk for worsening obsessive–compulsive symptoms, and with potential to improve them, such as amisulpiride (Case 11.3) or aripiprazole (Case 11.2). Despite the potential to provoke obsessive–compulsive symptoms other atypical antipsychotics, such as olanzapine and clozapine, may exert a beneficial effect in susceptible individuals as well. This seems to be particularly true when obsessive-compulsive symptoms form a "psychopathological hybrid" with psychotic symptoms (Cases 11.1 and 11.5). This hypothesis, however, has not been empirically tested, and predictors of such diverse responses have yet to be elucidated.

Addition of serotonin reuptake inhibitors

The independent nature of obsessive–compulsive symptoms in a vast majority of schizo-obsessive individuals and their clinical similarity with "pure" OCD prompted evaluation of adjunctive anti-obsessive agents for antipsychotic-treated schizo-obsessive patients. Fourteen schizo-obsessive patients who received fluvoxamine (100–200 mg/day for 8 weeks) added to a stable regimen of typical antipsychotics revealed a greater reduction in Y-BOCS total ($p = 0.02$) and compulsion subscale ($p < 0.05$) as compared to schizo-obsessive patients randomized to continue previous antipsychotic therapy (16 patients) (Reznik and Sirota, 2000). Adjunctive fluvoxamine also accounted for an improvement in OCD-related pathological slowness and doubt, an additional and clinically meaningful advantage. Clinical utility of the drug was supported by the results of an open-label study of fluvoxamine addition (up to 150 mg/day for 12 weeks) to typical antipsychotic agents for ten inpatients with clinically stable DSM-IV schizophrenic disorder and comorbid OCD (Poyurovsky et al., 1999). The investigators revealed a significant improvement in the obsessive component of OCD ($p < 0.02$) in addition to a modest improvement of both positive and negative schizophrenia symptoms. This study draws attention to fluvoxamine's potential to exacerbate psychosis and increase aggressiveness in schizo-obsessive patients with prior indications of impulsivity and aggressive behavior. It is plausible that patients with clinically significant aggressiveness may be at higher risk of psychotic exacerbation if treated with adjunctive fluvoxamine or possibly other SSRIs.

Escitalopram, the most selective serotonin reuptake inhibitor, also showed a beneficial effect on the obsessive–compulsive symptoms in a small open-label prospective trial of 12 weeks' duration in 15 DSM-IV schizophrenia patients (10 men, 5 women, mean age 39 ± 14, range 21–61) who were stabilized on antipsychotic medication for at least 3 months (R. Stryjer et al., unpublished data). Escitalopram (up to 20 mg/day) accounted for a significant improvement in Y-BOCS total scores (from baseline 28.9 ± 7.2 to study completion 23.3 ± 8.8, $p < 0.001$). In addition, a slight but statistically significant improvement was observed in general schizophrenia symptoms, as assessed by the Positive and Negative Syndrome Scale. The drug's well-tolerated side effect profile and paucity of drug–drug interactions was substantiated. No clinically significant side effects or worsening of psychosis were observed.

Adjunctive clomipramine, a tricyclic antidepressant and a non-selective SRI, was also evaluated as a putative therapeutic option. A small placebo-controlled cross-over study and a number of case reports revealed that clomipramine (dose range from 50 to 300 mg/day) was associated with a beneficial effect on obsessive–compulsive symptoms, reduction of anxiety accompanied by compulsive rituals, and improvement of positive and negative schizophrenia symptoms in some schizo-obsessive patients (Zohar et al., 1993; Berman et al., 1995; Poyurovsky and Weizman, 1998). However, lack of therapeutic effect of clomipramine and exacerbation of psychosis were also reported (Bark and Lindenmayer, 1992; Margetis, 2008). In addition, the anticholinergic properties of clomipramine, its cardiovascular side effects, and associated weight gain limit its utility in schizophrenia patients, particularly those who are treated with low-potency typical antipsychotic agents, anticholinergic agents, or clozapine.

The following are illustrative case vignettes that show a preferential effect of a specific SRI added to an antipsychotic agent in two schizophrenia patients (father and son) with obsessive–compulsive symptoms (Poyurovsky et al., 2003).

Case 11.6. Mr. A Jr., 23 years old, was hospitalized for a first psychotic episode, lasting 8 months, characterized by delusions of persecution, auditory hallucinations, and first-rank Schneiderian symptoms. He met DSM-IV criteria for schizophrenia disorder, paranoid type. Three years prior to the occurrence of his initial schizophrenia symptoms he exhibited repetitive ego-dystonic preoccupation with symmetry, accompanied by checking and touching rituals. He met DSM-IV criteria for OCD. Paroxetine (60 mg/day for 12 weeks) led to partial resolution of symptoms (Y-BOCS score decreased from 20 to 16). During hospitalization, psychotic symptoms remitted with olanzapine (up to 20 mg/day, within 5 weeks). No signs of OCD were noted during an acute psychotic episode with pervasive delusions. Four weeks after resolution of psychosis, OCD symptoms re-emerged. Addition of fluvoxamine (300 mg/day for 12 weeks) had no effect (Y-BOCS scores range 21–19) and was associated with troublesome sedation. Sertraline was given instead, in daily doses up to 150 mg, and within 4 weeks there was substantial improvement of OCD (Y-BOCS score = 6). The combination of olanzapine and sertraline was well tolerated. At 6-month follow-up the patient remained in remission of both psychosis and OCD.

Case 11.7. Mr. A Sr., 55 years old, had been diagnosed with DSM-IV schizophrenia, paranoid type, at age 30. During his current hospitalization, he was successfully treated with olanzapine (7.5 mg/day). While in remission, he revealed obsessive preoccupation with his bodily wastes accompanied by checking compulsions (Y-BOCS score = 16). Similar OCD symptoms had emerged in his early adulthood and resolved spontaneously. Notably, 10 months before hospitalization he also developed panic attacks. Paroxetine (40 mg/day) and alprazolam (up to 3 mg/day) were added to ongoing olanzapine therapy but discontinued after 4 months due to lack of improvement (Y-BOCS score = 18). Considering his son's robust response to sertraline, it was given at 150 mg/day with olanzapine (7.5 mg/day), and both OCD and panic attacks remitted within 10 weeks (Y-BOCS score = 7) and remained in remission at 6-month follow-up. The similar specific beneficial responses to sertraline–olanzapine treatment in father and son may indicate a possible pharmacogenetic component in OCD–schizophrenia comorbidity (see below).

Overall, the SRI class of drugs exerts a favorable effect on obsessive–compulsive symptoms in some schizophrenia patients. Nevertheless, the safety and tolerability profiles of individual compounds differ, as well as patients' preferential response to specific SRIs, similar to OCD patients without schizophrenia (Pigott et al., 1990). Moreover, the important question of therapeutic dose ranges for adjunctive SRIs while treating schizophrenia patients is yet to be addressed. The fact that a sizeable proportion of schizo-obsessive patients does not respond or is intolerant to an SRI addition indicates that obsessive–compulsive symptoms in schizophrenia are not readily amenable to anti-obsessional agents. No predictors of response and long-term treatment outcomes have yet been established. An additional pitfall of SRI–antipsychotic drug combination is the potential for clinically significant pharmacokinetic drug interactions. Elevated plasma concentrations of haloperidol and clozapine five- to tenfold with adjunctive fluvoxamine and roughly twofold with adjunctive fluoxetine and paroxetine have been reported (Hiemke, 1994). This in turn may increase the likelihood of antipsychotic-drug-induced side effects (e.g., extrapyramidal side effects, decreased seizure threshold).

Drug-induced motor side effects

Schizo-obsessive patients seem to be particularly vulnerable to developing motor side effects when treated with antipsychotic agents, SSRIs, and their combinations. SSRIs may induce extrapyramidal side effects and akathisia via indirect attenuation of dopamine neurotransmission, with an estimated rate of occurrence of roughly 10% in non-schizophrenia patients (Leo, 1998). When antipsychotic agents, especially those with potent dopamine D_2 receptor antagonism such as typical neuroleptics, are combined with SSRIs the risk of development of motor side effects is increased even more. Differential diagnosis of motor side effects in schizo-obsessive patients is challenging, since they may be masked or confounded by the symptoms of the primary disorders. Thus, restlessness and repetitive pacing associated with akathisia can be interpreted as stereotypic schizophrenic movements or ritualistic behavior related to OCD. Parkinsonian slowness may be confounded by schizophrenic ambivalence or pathological doubt typical to OCD, or by their co-occurrence in the most complicated cases. Thorough clinical examination and follow-up are necessary to establish temporal proximity between the administration of the offending agent and the emergence of extrapyramidal adverse events, as well as change over time. In cases of iatrogenic drug-induced motor side effects a dose reduction of the antipsychotic and/or the SSRI, initiation of anticholinergic agents for parkinsonian symptoms or dystonia, and beta-blockers for akathisia, or both strategies, may be required.

These clinical observations are supported by the findings of an explicit comparative examination of the significance of motor symptoms in schizophrenia patients with and without OCD (Krüger et al., 2000). Seventy-six schizophrenia patients, 12 with OCD and 64 without OCD, were comprehensively evaluated for the presence of motor symptoms using the Simpson–Angus Rating Scale (SAS) (Simpson and Angus, 1970) for extrapyramidal side effects, the Hillside Akathisia Scale (HAS) (Fleischhacker et al., 1989) for akathisia, the Abnormal Involuntary Movement Scale (AIMS) (Guy, 1976) for tardive dyskinesia, and the Catatonia Rating Scale (CRS) (Bräunig et al., 2000) for catatonic symptoms. Schizophrenia patients with OCD had more severe subjective and objective akathisia ($p < 0.05$) and were categorized on the clinical global impression item of the HAS as "markedly akathisic," in contrast to the non-OCD schizophrenia patients, who were rated as "borderline akathisic." Fifty-eight percent of the subjects with OCD developed abnormal involuntary movements, as opposed to 28% of subjects without OCD ($p < 0.05$). Similarly, 83% of patients with OCD fulfilled CRS criteria for catatonic symptoms as compared to only 8% of the non-OCD patients ($p < 0.001$). On the SAS, more schizo-obsessive patients revealed mild pseudoparkinsonism, but group differences in total SAS scores fell short of significance. When all of the scores were controlled for neuroleptic effect, significant main effects for OCD remained robust. Notably, the schizo-obsessive patients had more severe motor symptoms despite being treated with lower dosages of typical neuroleptics and more frequently with atypical antispsychotics than their non-OCD counterparts. These findings lend support to clinical observations that schizophrenia patients with OCD are particularly vulnerable to developing both antipsychotic-drug-induced neurological motor side effects as well as motor symptoms not related to a medication. The high prevalence of motor symptoms in schizo-obsessive individuals supports the hypothesis of a basal ganglia–frontal lobe connection linking OCD with schizophrenia (Krüger et al., 2000). The high frequency of catatonic symptoms (e.g., stereotypy, mannerisms, negativism, echophenomena, catalepsy, grimacing) in schizo-obsessive patients substantiates clinical observations made by authors prior to the neuroleptic era who introduced the concept of manneristic catatonia to describe a subtype of schizophrenia with catatonic and obsessive–compulsive symptoms (Huber and Gross, 1982).

Glutamatergic agents

An additional avenue in psychopharmacology research for schizo-obsessive disorder focuses on alternative underlying mechanisms shared by the two disorders. Recent findings implicate abnormalities in glutamatergic, in addition to dopaminergic and serotonergic, neurotransmission. Specifically, in schizophrenia, characteristic symptoms and cognitive deficits have been produced in remitted schizophrenia patients by the NMDA antagonist ketamine, and agents that stimulate glutamatergic neurotransmission appeared to have antipsychotic properties (Krystal et al., 2005). In OCD, elevated levels of a combined measure of glutamate and glutamine in brain regions relevant to OCD were found using magnetic resonance spectroscopy (Whiteside et al., 2006), and glutamate levels were increased in the cerebrospinal fluid (Chakrabarty et al., 2005). Preliminary data indicate a beneficial effect of agents with marked antiglutamatergic properties (memantine, riluzole) in patients with treatment-resistant OCD (Pittenger et al., 2006). These findings premised a pilot study of lamotrigine, an anticonvulsant with marked downstream effects on neuronal function including inhibition of glutamate release. In an 8-week, open-label trial, lamotrigine (25 mg/day for 1 week, 50 mg for 2 weeks, 100 mg for 2 weeks, 200 mg for 3 weeks) was added to ongoing psychotropic drug regimens in 11 schizophrenia patients with clinically significant obsessive–compulsive symptoms (Poyurovsky et al., 2010). The Y-BOCS score of the nine patients who completed the trial decreased significantly from baseline to week 8 (22.9 ± 6.1 vs.17.4 ± 3.6; $t = 2.33$, $p = 0.033$), and five (55.5%) patients were deemed responders ($\geq 35\%$ decrease in a total Y-BOCS score). In addition, depressive symptoms, assessed with the Calgary Depression Rating Scale, improved significantly (6.4 ± 1.5 vs. 4.0 ± 2.5; $t = 3.19$, $p = 0.013$), and this change positively correlated with improvement in obsessive–compulsive symptoms ($r = 0.69$, $p = 0.04$). Intriguingly, all responders in this small study were patients with schizoaffective disorder, bipolar or depressive type, who had depressive symptoms at trial entry. Lamotrigine was found efficacious in relieving depressive symptoms and maintaining euthymia in patients with bipolar disorder (Ketter et al., 2008). Hence, it is plausible that lamotrigine's beneficial effect on depressive symptoms accounted for a secondary improvement of obsessive–compulsive symptoms. Explicit evaluation of lamotrigine's effect on obsessive–compulsive symptoms in schizophrenia patients without depressive psychopathology would clarify whether lamotrigine exerts specific anti-obsessive properties in schizo-obsessive patients who have marked affective symptoms. The OCD-attenuating effect of lamotrigine was not accompanied by improvement of schizophrenia symptoms, corroborating findings regarding the lack of lamotrigine's effectiveness on schizophrenia symptoms revealed in two large-scale studies of lamotrigine addition to atypical antipsychotic agents (Goff et al., 2007). In contrast, some clozapine-resistant schizophrenia patients may further benefit from lamotrigine addition which appears safe and well tolerated (Tiihonen *et al.*, 2009; Porcelli *et al.*, 2012). The efficacy of lamotrigine in clozapine-treated schizophrenia patients with obsessive-compulsive symptoms needs to be elucidated.

Non-pharmacological interventions

Cognitive–behavioral therapy (CBT) along with pharmacotherapy is a first-line treatment for OCD. In contrast, the role of CBT in treating obsessive–compulsive symptoms related to schizophrenia remains unclear. This may reflect concerns that accentuated stress of exposure-based interventions may increase vulnerability to psychotic relapse. To address this issue, Tundo and colleagues (2012) conducted a small naturalistic study and enrolled 21 DSM-IV schizophrenia patients (13 males, 8 females; mean age 29.3 years), who were stabilized on antipsychotic agents (Positive and Negative Symptoms Scale total score ≤75). The presence of clinically significant obsessive–compulsive symptoms (Y-BOCS total score ≥16) in all participants justified therapeutic intervention. CBT consisted of imagined and in vivo exposure and ritual prevention, as well as cognitive therapy to supplement exposure and ritual prevention strategies. CBT was adjusted to each patient after considering the levels of insight and treatment adherence. Patients received an average of four sessions per month during the first 4 months and then continued therapy with one to four monthly sessions. Roughly 30 hours of CBT were provided to each patient during the 12-month period. Three patients dropped out from the study due to lack of effectiveness of CBT, and one patient was rehospitalized due to exacerbation of psychosis deemed unrelated to CBT. The remaining 17 patients showed clinically meaningful improvement in the severity of obsessive–compulsive symptoms, insight into illness, and general functioning (52% were rated "much/very much" improved with the Clinical Global Impression scale). These preliminary results are noteworthy because they indicate that schizophrenia patients with obsessive–compulsive symptoms do adhere to CBT, and that adjunctive CBT indeed may be an effective alternative to an SRI for at least some patients.

Following is a case vignette that illustrates successful adjunctive treatment with exposure and response prevention in a pharmacologically stabilized schizophrenia patient with clinically significant obsessive–compulsive symptoms (Ekers *et al.*, 2004).

Case 11.8. A patient was stabilized on a regimen of quetiapine (500 mg/day) over a 2-year remission period. Prior to remission, clear-cut psychotic symptoms including auditory hallucinations, delusions of reference, thought disorders, and social withdrawal had been present for almost 1 year justifying the diagnosis of DSM schizophrenic disorder. Prior to development of psychosis at age 16, the patient experienced symptoms of OCD that were not evident during the acute psychotic phase but resurfaced during remission. The main obsession was fear of making mistakes while performing daily activities, resulting in the possibility of a range of consequences from people being upset with him, disasters such as the house burning down, or death to himself or others. The patient performed numerous checking rituals, particularly of items such as cookers, kettles, and gas fires. At assessment his rituals took over 8 hours daily and caused extreme discomfort when interrupted.

Treatment consisted of graded exposure and response prevention (ERP). The patient received 20 hours of therapist time focused upon exposure to distressing obsessions and ritual prevention. Exposure targets were carried out at home independently and monitored by the patient using diaries. These consisted of holding the distressing thought and resisting the use of both cognitive and physical compulsions while engaging in anxiety-provoking activities. During initial treatment sessions the patient's community mental health nurse was involved in treatment to assist in the collaborative monitoring of psychotic symptoms. Modeling of targets took place in sessions with the therapist. The pace of therapy was carefully considered to prevent undue arousal, and initially this was slower than routinely delivered to patients with OCD. The patient, however, readily accepted the treatment rationale and was able to set his own targets and progressed substantially between sessions.

There was a significant reduction in the severity of OCD symptoms and associated distress, as measured by the Y-BOCS, by the end of the treatment period and was maintained at the 6-month follow-up. No evidence of psychotic exacerbation was noted; general mood and anxiety ratings reflected a low level of symptoms maintained throughout the ERP intervention.

CBT avoids drug-induced side effects and drug–drug interactions associated with adjunctive SRIs in schizophrenia patients, and may be beneficial for patients for whom SRIs are contraindicated or intolerable. Limitations are the need for an experienced therapist, cost, and the time-consuming nature of CBT. Ekers *et al.* (2004) suggested a more graded approach for schizo-obsessive patients than might be used for patients with OCD alone. The stability of effect over time and long-term compliance with treatment need to be determined. Close monitoring of mental state and regular assessments of symptoms are essential to address risks (especially the potential risk of worsening of psychosis) and benefits of combined pharmacotherapy and CBT in schizo-obsessive patients.

Electroconvulsive therapy

Electroconvulsive therapy (ECT) is not an approved therapy for OCD. ECT is indicated for schizophrenia patients in cases of catatonia or treatment-resistance and when pharmacotherapy is contraindicated. Case reports indicate the utility of ECT for schizo-obsessive patients who did not respond to or could not tolerate side effects associated with psychotropic agents (Lavin and Halligan, 1996; Hanisch *et al.*, 2009), and in cases in which the severity of the symptoms poses a serious threat to the patient's mental health and physical safety (Case 11.9) (Chaves *et al.*, 2005). Side effects (e.g., memory disturbances), stigma associated with ECT, and patients' preferences need to be taken into account prior to administration of ECT.

Case 11.9. Mr. A, a 17-year-old male, had a history of excessive concerns about cleanness and contamination, accompanied by checking and reassurance-seeking rituals, for a period of 3 years. He was admitted to the psychiatry emergency room of a university hospital, brought by firemen who convinced him to leave his bedroom, where he had been for the past 9 months. During that time, he urinated in bottles and defecated on the floor and rarely bathed. Other complaints included diffuse paranoid ideation, poor insight, and affective instability, in addition to significant OCD symptoms. After admission to an inpatient psychiatry ward, A continued to show isolation, paranoid ideas, obsessions, and compulsions. The patient met DSM-IV criteria for both schizophrenia and OCD. Treatment consisted of pharmacotherapy (fluoxetine, haloperidol, risperidone, clomipramine, and carbamazepine), occupational therapy, and family and group psychotherapy. Despite all of these attempts, he showed no improvement during the first

3 months of hospitalization. Instead, he began to have new obsessive thoughts of hitting family members and staff, destroying furniture, and finally biting his tongue.

After the patient had been physically restrained or pharmacologically sedated most of the time for 2 weeks due to his hyperactivity and impulsivity, ECT was tried. Bitemporal stimuli were delivered bilaterally by a Thymatron™ (Somatics, Lake Bluff, Ill.), DG-100% = 504 microcoulomb (brief-pulse) device. A total of six effective (generalized motor or electrographic seizures lasting more than 25 s and 30 s, respectively) ECT sessions were administered (twice a week) over a period of 3 weeks. During the period of treatment with ECT, A was independently evaluated by two psychiatrists using the Brief Psychiatric Rating Scale (BPRS), the Y-BOCS, and Clinical Global Impression (CGI). Aggressive, psychotic, and OCD symptoms markedly decreased on all rating scales. BPRS score decreased from 27 to 8; Y-BOCS score, from 50 to 16; and CGI score, from 6 to 2. Clomipramine and risperidone were administered after the treatment with ECT, which resulted in improvement in A's quality of life. A 6-month follow-up showed no relapse of the patient's positive psychotic symptoms, compulsions, or impulsivity although some isolation and obsessive thoughts remained.

Treatment recommendations

Overall, progress has been made during the last decade in the search for effective pharmacotherapy for the distinct subgroup of schizo-obsessive patients. Preliminary signs of efficacy were detected; however, the putatively efficacious treatments might well represent an observer- and/or patient-expectancy effect that is not uncommon in uncontrolled pilot studies. Small sample sizes, absence of a control group, and lack of a measure to ensure participants' adherence to the prescribed medication in the majority of studies pose even greater limitations to the generalizability of the findings. Large-scale randomized controlled trials are needed to substantiate the initial encouraging results. Presently in the absence of evidence-based data, the following recommendations may be considered when treating schizo-obsessive patients (Figure 11.1).

1. Monotherapy with atypical antipsychotic agents is a first-line treatment for schizo-obsessive patients. Preliminary reports indicate that olanzapine, aripiprazole, and amisulpiride may exert beneficial effect on both schizophrenia and obsessive–compulsive symptoms in some patients. Schizophrenia patients whose obsessive–compulsive symptoms emerge or are accentuated during psychotic exacerbation seem to be good candidates for treatment with atypical antipsychotic monotherapy, whereas those with a full-blown OCD that usually precedes the development of schizophrenia would most probably require the addition of an SSRI. Data regarding therapeutic utility of other atypical antipsychotics (quetiapine, ziprasidone, risperidone) as well as newly available antipsychotic agents (asenapine, lurasidone, illoperidone) in schizo-obsessive patients are still lacking. Therapeutic benefit should be weighed against the side effect profile for each atypical antipsychotic.
2. Addition of an SSRI to an atypical antipsychotic agent is the next step following insufficient response to monotherapy with an atypical antipsychotic. Obsessive–compulsive symptoms in schizophrenia may be considered a target for an anti-obsessive drug intervention only when the severity of obsessive–compulsive symptoms reaches a threshold for clinical significance, and their clinical features are similar to typical OCD. Anti-obsessive agents should be administered only in stabilized antipsychotic-treated

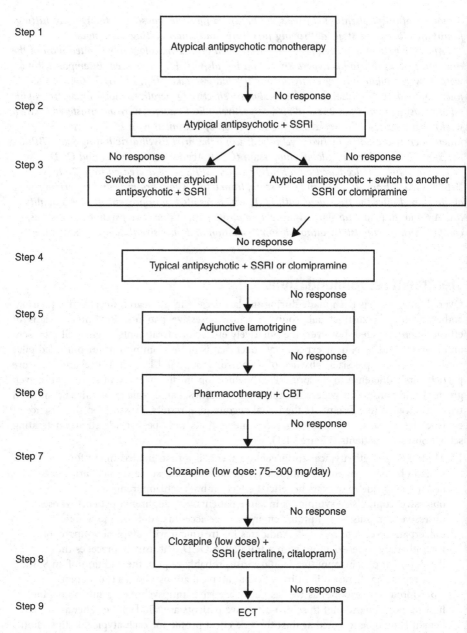

Figure 11.1 Proposed treatment algorithm for patients with schizo-obsessive disorder. SSRI, selective serotonin reuptake inhibitor; CBT, cognitive–behavioral therapy; ECT, electroconvulsive therapy.

patients. Lower doses of anti-obsessive agents than typically used in treatment of OCD seem to be required when dealing with obsessive–compulsive symptoms in the context of psychotic disorder; however, the evidence base is still lacking. In addition, schizo-obsessive patients with a history of impulsivity and aggressiveness may be at higher risk of psychotic exacerbation during adjunctive SSRI treatments. Noteworthy, schizo-obsessive patients seem to be particularly vulnerable to developing extrapyramidal side effects and akathisia when treated with antipsychotic agents, SSRIs, and especially combination of the two drug types. Careful evaluation of the potential risks and benefits of adjunctive pharmacotherapy in schizo-obsessive patients, and the administration of the minimal effective dose of an SRI, is a prerequisite for successful pharmacotherapy.

3. Lack of response to the first atypical antipsychotic/SSRI combination may justify switching to an alternative atypical antipsychotic/SSRI or clomipramine combination.

4. Since monotherapy with typical antipsychotic agents appears to be of limited value in schizo-obsessive patients, the typical antipsychotic/SSRI combination may be a reasonable next step prior to initiation of treatment with clozapine.

For steps 2–4, pharmacokinetic interactions and potential side effects of combinations should be closely monitored. SSRIs with minimal drug–drug interactions, such as citalopram/escitalopram and sertraline, may be preferable as adjunctive agents.

5. Adjunctive lamotrigine, and potentially other glutamatergic agents, may be of therapeutic value, particularly in a subgroup of schizo-obsessive patients with marked affective, primarily depressive, symptoms and comorbid OCD.

6. Clozapine monotherapy should be reserved for treatment-resistant schizo-obsessive patients. Although the majority of case reports dealt with *de novo* emergence or exacerbation of obsessive–compulsive symptoms in schizophrenia, clozapine in a relatively low dose range (75–300 mg) may exert a beneficial effect at least in some schizo-obsessive individuals. Until findings from controlled studies regarding clozapine's beneficial effect in schizo-obsessive individuals are available, slow up-titration of clozapine and close monitoring of its potential improving vs. provoking effect on obsessive–compulsive symptoms in schizophrenia patients is recommended.

7. Lack of therapeutic effect of clozapine monotherapy justifies a trial of clozapine/SSRI combination. SSRIs should be added to clozapine with caution, and those that are devoid of clinically significant drug–drug interactions (escitalopram, citalopram, or sertraline) seem to be safer.

8. Cognitive–behavioral therapy (CBT) may contribute to an integrative treatment approach for schizo-obsessive patients. CBT should be considered only in pharmacologically stabilized patients who experience typical to OCD obsessive–compulsive symptoms. CBT would seem particularly appropriate for patients who are compliant with treatment and who are capable of understanding cognitive therapy and its rationale. Regular assessments are necessary to address potential risks (e.g. worsening of psychosis) and benefits of combined pharmacotherapy and CBT.

9. Electroconvulsive therapy is the last resort when pharmacotherapy fails.

A beneficial effect of deep brain stimulation for a schizophrenia patient with highly treatment-resistant obsessive–compulsive symptoms has also been reported (Plewnia *et al.*, 2008).

References

Baker RW, Ames D, Umbricht DS, Chengappa KN, Schooler NR (1996) Obsessive-compulsive symptoms in schizophrenia: a comparison of olanzapine and placebo. *Psychopharmacology Bulletin* 32, 89–93.

Bark N, Lindenmayer JP (1992) Ineffectiveness of clomipramine for obsessive-compulsive symptoms in a patient with schizophrenia. *American Journal of Psychiatry* 149, 136–137.

Berman I, Kalinowski A, Berman S, Lengua J, Green AI (1995) Obsessive-compulsive symptoms in chronic schizophrenia. *Comprehensive Psychiatry* 36, 6–10.

Bermanzohn PC, Porto L, Arlow PB, et al. (1997) Are some neuroleptic refractory symptoms of schizophrenia really obsessions? *CNS Spectrums* 2, 51–57.

Bräunig P, Krüger S, Shugar G, Höffler J, Börner I (2000) The catatonia rating scale: I. Development, reliability, and use. *Comprehensive Psychiatry* 41, 147–158.

Chakrabarty K, Bhattacharyya S, Christopher R, Khanna S (2005) Glutamatergic dysfunction in OCD. *Neuropsychopharmacology* 30, 1735–1740.

Chaves MPR, Crippa JAS, Morais SL, Zuardi AW (2005) Electroconvulsive therapy for coexistent schizophrenia and obsessive-compulsive disorder. *Journal of Clinical Psychiatry* 66, 542–543.

de Haan L, Oekeneva A, Van Amelsvoort T, Linszen D (2004) Obsessive-compulsive disorder and treatment with clozapine in 200 patients with recent-onset schizophrenia or related disorders. *European Psychiatry* 19, 524.

Desarkar P, Das A, Nizamie SH (2007) Aripiprazole-induced obsessive-compulsive disorder: a report of 2 cases. *Journal of Clinical Psychopharmacology* 27, 305–306.

Ekers D, Schlich T, Carmen S (2004) Successful outcome of exposure and response prevention in the treatment of obsessive compulsive disorder in a patient with schizophrenia. *Behavioral and Cognitive Psychotherapy* 32, 375–378.

Fleischhacker WW, Bergmann KJ, Perovich R, et al. (1989) The Hillside Akathisia Scale: a new rating instrument for neuroleptic-induced okathisia. *Psychopharmacology Bulletin* 25, 222–226.

Glick ID, Poyurovsky M, Ivanova O, Koran LM (2008) Aripiprazole in schizophrenia patients with comorbid obsessive-compulsive symptoms: an open-label study of 15 patients. *Journal of Clinical Psychiatry* 69, 1856–1859.

Goff DC, Keefe R, Citrome L, et al. (2007) Lamotrigine as add-on therapy in schizophrenia: results of 2 placebo-controlled trials. *Journal of Clinical Psychopharmacology* 27, 582–589.

Green AI, Canuso CM, Brenner MJ, Wojcik JD (2003) Detection and management of comorbidity in patients with schizophrenia. *Psychiatric Clinics of North America* 26, 115–139.

Guy W (1976) *ECDEU Assessment Manual for Psychopharmacology*, revised edn. US Department of Health, Education, and Welfare, Washington, DC.

Hanisch F, Friedemann J, Piro J, Gutmann P (2009) Maintenance electroconvulsive therapy for comorbid pharmacotherapy-refractory obsessive-compulsive and schizoaffective disorder. *European Journal of Medical Research* 14, 367–368.

Hiemke C (1994) Paroxetin: Pharmakokinetik und Pharmakodynamik. [Paroxetine: pharmacokinetics and pharmacodynamics]. *Fortschritte der Neurologie-Psychiatrie* 62 (Suppl. 1), 2–8. [German]

Huber E, Gross G (1982) Zwingssyndrome bei Schizophrenie [Obsessive-compulsive symptoms in schizophrenia]. *Schwerpunktmedizin* 5, 12–19. [German]

Kane JM, Barnes TRE, Corell CU, et al. (2010) Evaluation of akathisia in patients with schizophrenia, schizoaffective disorder, or bipolar I disorder: a post hoc analysis of pooled data from short- and long-term aripiprazole trials. *Journal of Psychopharmacology* 24, 1019–1029.

Ketter TA, Brooks JO, Hoblyn JC, et al. (2008) Effectiveness of lamotrigine in bipolar disorder in a clinical setting. *Journal of Psychiatric Research* 43, 13–23.

Kim SW, Shin IS, Kim JM, *et al.* (2008) Amisulpiride improves obsessive-compulsive symptoms in schizophrenia patients taking atypical antipsychotics: an open-label switch study. *Journal of Clinical Psychopharmacology* **28**, 349–352.

Krüger S, Bräunig P, Höffler J, *et al.* (2000) Prevalence of obsessive-compulsive disorder in schizophrenia and significance of motor symptoms. *Journal of Neuropsychiatry and Clinical Neurosciences* **12**, 16–24.

Krystal JH, Perry EB Jr, Gueorguieva R, *et al.* (2005) Comparative and interactive human psychopharmacologic effects of ketamine and amphetamine: implications for glutamatergic and dopaminergic model psychoses and cognitive function. *Archives of General Psychiatry* **62**, 985–994.

Lavin MR, Halligan P (1996) ECT for comorbid obsessive-compulsive disorder and schizophrenia. *American Journal of Psychiatry* **153**, 1652–1653.

Lecrubier Y, Azorin M, Bottai T, *et al.* (2001) Consensus on the practical use of amisulpiride, an atypical antipsychotic, in the treatment of schizophrenia. *Neuropsychobiology* **44**, 41–46.

Leo R (1998) Movement disturbances associated with the use of selective serotonin-reuptake inhibitors. *Annals of Pharmacotherapy* **32**, 712–714.

Lykouras L, Zervas IM, Gournellis R, Rabavilas A (2000) Olanzapine and obsessive-compulsive symptoms. *European Neuropsychopharmacology* **10**, 385–387.

Mamo D, Graff A, Mizrahi R, *et al.* (2007) Differential effects of aripiprazole on D(2), 5-HT(2), and 5-HT(1A) receptor occupancy in patients with schizophrenia: a triple tracer PET study. *American Journal of Psychiatry* **164**, 1411–1417.

Margetis B (2008) Aggravation of schizophrenia by clomipramine in a patient with comorbid obsessive-compulsive disorder. *Psychopharmacology Bulletin* **41**, 9–11.

McDougle CJ, Barr LC, Goodman WK, *et al.* (1995) Lack of efficacy of clozapine monotherapy in refractory obsessive-compulsive disorder. *American Journal of Psychiatry*, **152**, 1812–1814.

Mouaffak F, Gallarda T, Baylé FJ, Olié JP, Baup N (2007) Worsening of obsessive-compulsive symptoms after treatment with aripiprazole. *Journal of Clinical Psychopharmacology* **27**, 237–238.

Pigott TA, Pato MT, Bernstein SE, *et al.* (1990) Controlled comparisons of clomipramine and fluoxetine in the treatment of obsessive-compulsive disorder: behavioral and biological results. *Archives of General Psychiatry* **47**, 926–932.

Pittenger C, Krystal JH, Coric V (2006) Glutamate-modulating drugs as novel pharmacotherapeutic agents in the treatment of obsessive-compulsive disorder. *Neurotherapeutics* **3**, 69–81.

Plewnia C, Schober F, Rilk A, *et al.* (2008) Sustained improvement of obsessive-compulsive disorder by deep brain stimulation in a woman with residual schizophrenia. *International Journal of Neuropsychopharmacology* **11**, 1181–1183.

Porcelli S, Balzarro B, Serretti A (2012) Clozapine resistance: augmentation strategies. *European Neuropsychopharmacology* **22**, 165–182.

Poyurovsky M, Weizman A (1998) Intravenous clomipramine for a schizophrenic patient with obsessive-compulsive symptoms. *American Journal of Psychiatry* **155**, 993.

Poyurovsky M, Isakov V, Hromnikov S, *et al.* (1999) Fluvoxamine treatment of obsessive-compulsive symptoms in schizophrenic patients: an add-on open study. *International Clinical Psychopharmacology* **14**, 95–100.

Poyurovsky M, Dorfman-Etrog P, Hermesh H, *et al.* (2000) Beneficial effect of olanzapine in schizophrenic patients with obsessive-compulsive symptoms. *International Clinical Psychopharmacology* **15**, 169–173.

Poyurovsky M, Kurs R, Weizman A (2003) Olanzapine-sertraline combination in schizophrenia with obsessive-compulsive disorder. *Journal of Clinical Psychiatry* **64**, 611.

Poyurovsky M, Glick I, Koran LM (2010) Lamotrigine augmentation in schizophrenia and schizoaffective patients with obsessive-compulsive symptoms. *Journal of Psychopharmacology* **24**, 861–866.

Reznik I, Sirota P (2000) Obsessive and compulsive symptoms in schizophrenia: a randomized controlled trial with fluvoxamine and neuroleptics. *Journal of Clinical Psychopharmacology* **20**, 410–416.

Sasson Y, Zohar J, Chopra M, *et al.* (1997) Epidemiology of obsessive-compulsive disorder: a world view. *Journal of Clinical Psychiatry* **58**, 7–10.

Simpson GM, Angus JWS (1970) A rating scale for extrapyramidal side effects. *Acta Psychiatrica Scandinavica* **212** (Suppl.), 11–19.

Tibbo P, Gendemann K (1999) Improvement of obsessions and compulsions with clozapine in an individual with schizophrenia. *Canadian Journal of Psychiatry* **44**, 1049–1050.

Tiihonen J, Wahlbeck K, Kiviniemi V (2009) The efficacy of lamotrigine in clozapine-resistant schizophrenia: a systematic review and meta-analysis. *Schizophrenia Research* **109**, 10–14.

Tundo A, Salvati L, Di Spigno D, *et al.* (2012) Cognitive–behavioral therapy for obsessive-compulsive disorder as a comorbidity with schizophrenia or schizoaffective disorder. *Psychotherapy and Psychosomatics* **81**, 58–60.

van Nimwegen L, de Haan L, van Beveren N, *et al.* (2008) Obsessive-compulsive symptoms in a randomized, double-blind study with olanzapine or risperidone in young patients with early psychosis. *Journal of Clinical Psychopharmacology* **28**, 214–218.

Whiteside SP, Port JD, Deacon BJ, Abramowitz JS (2006) A magnetic resonance spectroscopy investigation of obsessive-compulsive disorder and anxiety. *Psychiatry Research* **146**, 137–147.

Zohar J, Kaplan Z, Benjamin J (1993) Clomipramine treatment of obsessive compulsive symptomatology in schizophrenic patients. *Journal of Clinical Psychiatry* **54**, 385–388.

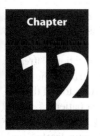

Chapter

Antipsychotic-drug-induced obsessive–compulsive symptoms

Prevalence of antipsychotic-drug-induced obsessive–compulsive symptoms

The complex nature of interactions between the primary schizophrenic disorder, comorbid OCD, and antipsychotic drug treatment is highlighted by the phenomenon of antipsychotic-induced obsessive–compulsive symptoms. There is increasing awareness of researchers and clinicians that atypical antipsychotics might potentially induce *de novo* or exacerbate pre-existing obsessive–compulsive symptoms in schizophrenia patients, though they can be efficacious as adjunctive treatment in OCD patients. The causal relationship between atypical antipsychotics and obsessive–compulsive symptoms is supported by the dose-dependent nature of the interaction, and an abatement of obsessive–compulsive symptoms with withdrawal of atypical agents, followed by their reappearance with reintroduction of the offending agent. Findings that atypical antipsychotics might also induce obsessive–compulsive symptoms in patients with bipolar disorder, mental retardation, delusional disorder, and psychotic depression indicates that this is a drug-specific effect in susceptible patients rather than an illness-related effect. An additional argument concerning the potential of atypical antipsychotics to induce obsessive–compulsive symptoms is that a majority of reported patients experiences *de novo* emergence of obsessive–compulsive symptoms (de Haan *et al.*, 2002; Lykouras *et al.*, 2003; Mahendran *et al.*, 2007; Mukhopadhaya *et al.*, 2009).

The magnitude of the problem is supported by the high incidence of drug-induced obsessive–compulsive symptoms reported in association with virtually all atypical antipsychotic agents. When a strict definition of DSM-IV OCD was employed, an incidence of 3% (nine of 303 patients) was detected (Mahendran *et al.*, 2007). However, relaxing criteria from OCD to obsessive–compulsive symptoms accounted for a substantially higher rate of occurrence. Using a structured interview and the Yale–Brown Obsessive–Compulsive Scale (Y-BOCS), Lim *et al.* (2007) screened 209 patients with schizophrenia and schizoaffective disorder treated with atypical antipsychotic agents, and found obsessive–compulsive symptoms in 44 (21.1%) of the participants, and in 26 (12.4%) of them obsessive–compulsive symptoms were considered antipsychotic-related. Estimates of *de novo* obsessive–compulsive symptoms as high as 20% and 24% in clozapine-treated schizophrenia patients were also reported (Ertugrul *et al.*, 2005; Mukhopadhaya *et al.*, 2009).

Clozapine might have greater potential to induce or exacerbate obsessive–compulsive symptoms than other antipsychotic agents. De Haan *et al.* (1999) conducted a retrospective study using chart reviews to identify patients who experienced emergence or exacerbation of pre-existing obsessive–compulsive symptoms while treated with clozapine ($N = 32$) or other antipsychotics (typical [$N = 57$] or risperidone [$N = 19$]). Clozapine treatment was evaluated

213

over a period of 7.3 ± 1.9 months, and other antipsychotics over 10.1 ± 3.1 months. All patients had recent-onset schizophrenia-spectrum disorders and age at admission was 20.9 ± 2.2 years. Seven out of 32 (21.9%) of the clozapine-treated patients reported the emergence or increase in obsessions, compared to only 1.3% (one of 76 patients) treated with other antipsychotics. Obsessions were diagnosed according to DSM-IV criteria; however, compulsions were not assessed. This limitation might account for underestimation of the rate of antipsychotic-induced obsessive–compulsive symptoms in schizophrenia patients.

Using a cross-sectional comparative study design, Sa and colleagues (2009) assessed the prevalence and severity of OCD in 60 patients with DSM-IV schizophrenia treated with clozapine (40 patients) or haloperidol (20 patients). The prevalence of OCD in patients taking clozapine was twofold higher than in those taking haloperidol (20% vs. 10%). The difference, however, was not statistically significant ($p = 0.54$), most probably due to small sample sizes. Clozapine-treated patients showed substantially greater severity of OCD symptoms than those treated with haloperidol (Y-BOCS total score: 21.5 ± 6.9 vs.12.7 ± 7.9, $p < 0.05$).

In a comparative prospective 6-week study de Haan *et al.* (2002) found no differences between olanzapine and risperidone in the potential to induce/exacerbate obsessive–compulsive symptoms in 113 patients with recent-onset schizophrenia. However, duration of olanzapine, but not risperidone, treatment correlated with the severity of obsessive–compulsive symptoms. A similar positive correlation between the duration of treatment and the severity of obsessions and compulsions also characterizes clozapine (Schirmbeck *et al.*, 2011). With the exception of the de Haan *et al.* (2002) study, cross-sectional and retrospective designs are limiting factors in all reports.

Mechanism of atypical antipsychotic-drug-induced obsessive–compulsive symptoms in schizophrenia

The mechanism underlying the OCD-provoking effect of antipsychotic agents in schizophrenia remains elusive. The serotonergic (5-HT) system is implicated because of its essential role in the pathophysiology of OCD and in the mechanism of action of SSRIs, the treatment of choice for OCD. The 5-HT_2 receptor antagonism has been postulated to play a role in the induction of obsessive–compulsive symptoms by atypical antipsychotics (Dursun and Reveley, 1994; Poyurovsky *et al.*, 1996; Lykouras *et al.*, 2003; Zink *et al.*, 2007). Indeed, agents with the highest affinity to 5-HT_2 receptors seem to possess a stronger potential to induce/aggravate obsessive–compulsive symptoms in schizophrenia. By contrast, quetiapine possesses a much lower 5-HT_2 receptor binding affinity, which may account for its tentatively lower potential to induce OCD (Khullar *et al.*, 2001) (Table 12.1).

The role of 5-HT_2 receptor antagonism in mediating the OCD-provoking effect of atypical antipsychotics was substantiated in a clinical investigation aimed to explicitly compare the rate of occurrence and the severity of obsessive–compulsive symptoms in patients treated with atypical antipsychotics stratified by their affinity to the 5-HT_2 receptor into the "high-affinity" group (clozapine and olanzapine) and the "low-affinity" group (apipiprazole and amisulpiride) (Schirmbeck *et al.*, 2011). Indeed, 28 (71.8%) patients in the "high-affinity" group scored higher than 8 (mild OCD) on the Y-BOCS, in contrast to only three patients (9.7%) in the "low-affinity" group (mean total Y-BOCS score 13.5 ± 8.5 vs. 2.6 ± 4.7). Moreover, 16 (57.1%) patients in the "high-affinity" group in contrast to only one in the comparison group had a total Y-BOCS score ≥ 16, indicating clinically meaningful OCD severity. Remarkably, aripiprazole and amisulpiride with their negligible affinity to

Table 12.1 In vitro receptor binding profiles from animal and human brain tissue of antipsychotic agents

Drug	Receptor binding affinity (K) nmol/L		
	5-HT$_{2A}$ (human cloned receptors)	5-HT$_{2C}$ (pig choroid plexus)	D$_2$ (human cloned receptors)
Haloperidol	200	> 5000	2.2
Quetiapine	96	3820	700
Olanzapine	2.5	7	31
Risperidone	0.52	63	5.6
Clozapine	9.6	13	190

Source: Adapted from Schotte A, Janssen PF, Gommeren W, Luyten WH, Van Gompel P, Lesage AS, De Loore K, Leysen JE (1996) Risperidone compared with new and reference antipsychotic drugs: in vitro and in vivo receptor binding. *Psychopharmacology (Berlin)* **124**, 57–73. Reprinted with permission.

5-HT$_2$ receptors not only exert the lowest risk, but in fact may be effective in the alleviation of clozapine- and olanzapine-induced OCD (Zink *et al.*, 2007; Schönfelder *et al.*, 2011).

An intriguing question is a possible differential effect of atypical antipsychotics on obsessive–compulsive symptoms in schizophrenia. For example, from the pharmacological perspective, olanzapine possesses a lower affinity to the serotonin 5-HT$_{2A}$ receptor than risperidone (Bymaster *et al.*, 1996). A signal attenuation animal model of OCD supports relevance to an anti-obsessive effect of the 5-HT$_{2C}$ rather than the 5-HT$_{2A}$ receptor blockade in the orbitofrontal cortex (Flaisher-Grinberg *et al.*, 2009). Conceivably, olanzapine's lower 5-HT$_{2A}$ antagonism compared to risperidone is associated with a lower propensity to induce or exacerbate obsessive–compulsive symptoms, as shown by van Nimwegen *et al.* (2008), while its greater 5-HT$_{2C}$ blockade accounts for the OCD-ameliorating effect in some schizo-obsessive patients (Sasson *et al.*, 1997; Poyurovsky *et al.*, 2000). A differential drug effect on the glutamatergic neurotransmission, implicated in the pathogenesis of both schizophrenia and OCD, may also be relevant. Olanzapine but not risperidone restores the deficit in pre-pulse inhibition, a model of sensorimotor gating deficits observed in both schizophrenia and OCD, induced by N-methyl-D-aspartate inhibitors (Geyer *et al.*, 2001; Ahmari *et al.*, 2012).

Dopaminergic neurotransmission has a putative role in antipsychotic-induced obsessive–compulsive symptoms as well. The inhibition of the nigrostriatal dopamine system via serotonin 5-HT$_{2A}$ receptors by SSRIs is considered to be related to the improvement of obsessive–compulsive symptoms, and a beneficial effect of adjunctive antipsychotic agents is thought to be related to the dopamine D$_2$ receptor blockade (Denys *et al.*, 2004; Bloch *et al.*, 2006). Clozapine's weak D$_2$ receptor antagonism may be among the properties that account for its propensity to induce obsessive–compulsive symptoms.

On the whole, fine-tuning of the serotonergic, dopaminergic, and glutamatergic neurotransmitter systems seems to be essential in determining whether an antipsychotic will provoke or ameliorate obsessive–compulsive symptoms in susceptible individuals. The primary disorder, schizophrenia or OCD, is an additional key determinant in the interrelationship between antipsychotics and obsessive–compulsive symptoms.

Pharmacokinetic mechanisms and plasma levels of antipsychotic agents may potentially contribute to the induction of obsessive–compulsive symptoms. Among patients treated with clozapine, those with obsessive–compulsive symptoms had a higher plasma drug concentration of clozapine and its metabolite norclozapine than those without (Lin *et al.*, 2006). These findings, however, were not replicated (Schirmbeck *et al.*, 2011).

Pharmacogenetic mechanisms may account for the response complexity to clozapine and other atypical antipsychotics. Thus, clozapine-induced obsessive–compulsive symptoms that emerged concordantly in a pair of monozygotic twins have been described, suggesting the influence of genetic factors on this adverse effect (Hong *et al.*, 2008). The association of the glutamate transporter gene *SLC1A1*, a promising candidate gene for susceptibility to OCD, has also been shown to be associated with atypical antipsychotic-induced obsessive–compulsive symptoms in schizophrenia patients (Kwon *et al.*, 2009).

Diagnosis of antipsychotic-induced obsessive–compulsive symptoms

The diagnosis of antipsychotic-drug-induced obsessive–compulsive symptoms in patients with schizophrenia poses a challenge. Based on the available literature, the following characteristics of antipsychotic-induced obsessive–compulsive symptoms may be informative in their detection (Box 12.1).

1. Most reported cases of drug-induced obsessive–compulsive symptoms occur in men, indicating possible male predominance in susceptibility.
2. Schizophrenia patients with pre-existing obsessive–compulsive symptoms may be at particular risk of drug-induced exacerbation of obsessions and compulsions; however, a majority of reports deals with *de novo* emergence of obsessive–compulsive symptoms.
3. Drug-induced obsessive–compulsive symptoms are characterized by a predominance of compulsions over obsessions, supporting the view that the diagnosis of obsessive–compulsive symptoms in schizophrenia should be validated primarily by the presence of compulsions (Eisen *et al.*, 1997). However, diagnostic difficulties in identification of antipsychotic-induced obsessions may account for their underestimation. In a majority of patients, however, the content of obsessive–compulsive symptoms is clearly different from the content of the psychotic symptoms and quite typical to ordinary OCD. Sexual and aggressive obsessions were the most prevalent obsessions; checking and washing

---

Box 12.1 Clinical characteristics of antipsychotic-drug-induced obsessive–compulsive symptoms

1. Men may be more susceptible than women.
2. Schizophrenia patients with pre-existing obsessive–compulsive symptoms are at particular risk.
3. Obsessive–compulsive symptoms are typical to ordinary OCD and are different from the content of delusions and hallucinations. Drug-induced compulsions are more common than obsessions.
4. Obsessive–compulsive symptoms induced by olanzapine, risperidone, and quetiapine tend to appear during the first weeks of treatment. In contrast, clozapine-induced OCD has early (up to 12 weeks) and delayed (after 12 weeks) onset.
5. Olanzapine provokes obsessive–compulsive symptoms in a wide dose range (5–25 mg/day), in contrast to relatively high doses of risperidone (>3 mg/day) and quetiapine (450–1100 mg/day). Two dose levels of clozapine were identified: low (150–250 mg/day) in early-onset and high (350–900 mg/day) in delayed-onset OCD.

rituals were the most prevalent compulsions in the reported cases of antipsychotic-induced obsessive–compulsive symptoms. In addition, most affected patients show fair-to-good insight into the senseless nature of their obsessive–compulsive symptoms. The use of structured interviews, standardized DSM OCD criteria, and psychometric instruments (e.g., Y-BOCS) may assist in the identification of obsessive–compulsive symptoms in schizophrenia patients.

4. In a majority of the patients with olanzapine-, risperidone-, and quetiapine-induced obsessive–compulsive symptoms, the symptoms appeared during the first weeks of treatment. By contrast, clozapine-treated patients could be divided into two groups according to time of onset of obsessive–compulsive symptoms: early (up to 12 weeks) and delayed (after 12 weeks). The late appearance of obsessive–compulsive symptoms associated with clozapine, however, may be attributed to the gradual up-titration of clozapine in clinical practice.

5. A wide range of doses was associated with the OCD-provoking effect of olanzapine (5–25 mg/day), compared to the relatively high doses associated with risperidone-induced (>3 mg/day) and quetiapine-induced (450–800 mg/day) obsessive–compulsive symptoms. Two dose levels of clozapine were identified: low (150–250 mg/day) in early-onset and high (350–900 mg/day) in delayed-onset obsessive–compulsive symptoms.

Management of antipsychotic-drug-induced obsessive–compulsive symptoms

Three major therapeutic approaches have been used in the treatment of antipsychotic-induced obsessive–compulsive symptoms:

- dose reduction or discontinuation of an offending antipsychotic;
- addition of an SRI;
- combination of antipsychotic dose reduction and addition of an SRI.

Although in some patients clozapine-induced obsessive–compulsive symptoms may resolve spontaneously (Patil, 1992; Poyurovsky et al., 1996), the majority of patients will require clozapine dose reduction and/or addition of an anti-obsessive agent.

The following is a case vignette illustrating transient occurrence of obsessive–compulsive symptoms in a clozapine-treated schizophrenia patient.

Case 12.1. A 29-year-old single man had a 12-year history of DSM-III-R schizophrenic disorder, undifferentiated type. He had been treated unsuccessfully with various neuroleptics for 8 years and continued to display psychotic features with predominant negative symptoms. Owing to treatment resistance clozapine treatment was eventually initiated, and the dosage was gradually increased to 125 mg/day. During the first 4 weeks of clozapine treatment, no changes were observed in his schizophrenic symptomatology, and he experienced side effects including sedation, tachycardia, and hypersalivation. In the fifth week of treatment (clozapine, 125 mg), prominent ego-dystonic obsessive–compulsive symptoms suddenly appeared. The patient began to wash his hands compulsively for long periods at least 15 times per day. He also had repeated obsessive thoughts and persistently touched tables. His schizophrenic signs became grossly aggravated. Negativism, irritability, uncooperativeness, inappropriate affect, and aggressive behavior increased. Despite the apparent deterioration in his condition, the clozapine dose was gradually increased. Six weeks later when his clozapine dosage reached 400 mg/day, his obsessive–compulsive symptoms disappeared, and there was significant improvement in his core schizophrenic symptomatology. His score on the Brief Psychiatric Rating Scale decreased from 52 to 17, the Y-BOCS score from 34 to 4, and the Scale for Assessment of Negative Symptoms decreased from 49 to 19. He was discharged to the outpatient unit, and a rehabilitation program was initiated.

In clinical practice transient occurrence of obsessive–compulsive symptoms during clozapine administration is rare. Therefore, clozapine dose reduction may be required in some cases, while the addition of an anti-obsessive medication is needed in others. The following SRIs have been administered to control clozapine-induced OCD: fluoxetine (20–60 mg/day), fluvoxamine (150–250 mg/day), sertraline (50–200 mg/day), and clomipramine (100 mg/day) (Lykouras *et al.*, 2003). Though there are no reports focused on the therapeutic effect of citalopram or escitalopram in patients with clozapine-induced obsessive–compulsive symptoms, the drugs' well-tolerated side effect profiles and paucity of drug–drug interactions support their therapeutic value for this indication. Notably, a clozapine/SRIs combination was efficacious in a majority of the reported cases. However, in some individuals a second-line SRI may be needed to ameliorate clozapine-induced obsessive–compulsive symptoms. No cases of clozapine discontinuation or switch to another antipsychotic were reported. This is reasonable, since clozapine is reserved for treatment-resistant patients. Side effects of each SRI, along with their pharmacokinetic and pharmacodynamic interactions with clozapine need to be carefully considered (see Chapter 11).

The following is a case vignette illustrating the efficacy of an SRI in treating clozapine-induced obsessive–compulsive symptoms in a schizophrenia patient.

Case 12.2. A 42-year-old single man suffered from DSM-III-R schizophrenic disorder, paranoid type, since age 17 and had been repeatedly admitted to psychiatric hospitals. Various antipsychotic medications and ultimately electroconvulsive therapy had no significant effect. The course of illness was characterized by episodic psychotic exacerbations (hearing voices, thought broadcasting, paranoid delusions) and periods of remission with social withdrawal and apathy. He had exhibited obsessive–compulsive symptoms for many years. Compulsive hand-washing lasted for 1–2 hours per day, and his obsessive fear of contamination led him to avoid contact with people. Clozapine was administered and by the sixth week of treatment the dosage had reached 150 mg/day. The obsessive–compulsive symptoms were grossly aggravated; hand-washing now lasted twice as long as previously and caused signs of dermatitis. Complex rituals accompanied taking medication including tapping the medication glass, changing the glasses, checking the cleanliness of the tablets, and putting the tablets in one side of the mouth and transferring them to the other before swallowing. In addition he would pass through doorways and cross streets a set number of times. The anticholinergic effect of clozapine caused constipation which led to the use of laxatives that in turn caused him to purge and was associated with ritualistic checking and cleaning behaviors in the bathroom. It was decided to add fluvoxamine to his ongoing clozapine treatment. Four weeks after the addition of fluvoxarnine (250 mg/day) a marked reduction in his ritualistic behavior was noted. The Y-BOCS score decreased from 32 to 9, and there was also improvement in his schizophrenic symptoms. Despite the beneficial effect of fluvoxamine, it was gradually discontinued because of gastrointestinal side effects. Five weeks later, compulsive behavior and obsessive thoughts returned to the previous level. Unfortunately, the patient refused the reintroduction of fluvoxamine because of the disabling side effects of the drug.

Another putative pharmacological approach aimed to deal with clozapine-induced obsessive–compulsive symptoms is the addition of aripiprazole. Hence, Englisch and colleagues

(2009) identified seven patients with DSM-IV schizophrenia or schizoaffective disorder (mean age 37 ± 10 years) who experienced distressing obsessive–compulsive symptoms associated with clozapine therapy. Clozapine was used for a mean duration of 9.0 ± 4.3 years, and the mean clozapine dose was 364.3 mg/day (serum level, clozapine 439 ng/L; desmethyl-clozapine, 211 ng/L) when obsessive–compulsive symptoms were detected. Clinically significant obsessive–compulsive symptoms had emerged approximately 4.0 ± 3.7 years after the start of clozapine. Because cognitive–behavioral therapy and anti-obsessive agents failed to ameliorate obsessive–compulsive symptoms, aripiprazole was added. Indeed, aripiprazole addition (mean dose 22.9 mg/day for a mean duration of 9.7 weeks) was associated with a marked reduction of the severity of obsessive–compulsive symptoms (mean total Y-BOCS score decreased from 18.7 to 12.4, $p < 0.01$). A small, statistically non-significant improvement of psychotic symptoms was also observed. Notably, adjunctive aripiprazole facilitated dose reduction of the suggested pro-obsessive agent clozapine by 19.6%, and resulted in reduced serum levels of clozapine by 27.3% and its metabolite desmethyl-clozapine by 23.8%. In addition to pharmacokinetic interactions between the two agents, the beneficial effect of adjunctive aripiprazole might be attributed to pharmacodynamic interactions. Acting as a partial agonist at $5\text{-}HT_{2A}$ and $5\text{-}HT_{2C}$ receptors, aripiprazole might counteract antagonistic effects of clozapine on these receptors (Englisch et al., 2009). Additional potential positive effects of adjunctive aripiprazole include the reduction of body weight and the reversal of metabolic side effects induced by clozapine, as well as further improvement of negative symptoms (Porcelli et al., 2012).

Following is a case vignette illustrating clinical utility of adjunctive aripiprazole in a schizophrenia patient with clozapine-induced obsessive–compulsive symptoms (Villari et al., 2011).

Case 12.3. A 32-year-old single unemployed man with disorganized schizophrenia failed to respond to several antipsychotics including chlorpromazine, clotiapine, haloperidol, quetiapine, and zuclopenthixol at therapeutical doses. The patient showed a very good response to clozapine (200 mg/day), except for the onset of obsessive thinking and control rituals. This patient did not report a history of obsessive thoughts or compulsive behaviors before he began clozapine treatment. His persecutory delusions, bizarre behaviors, and hallucinations appeared approximately 4 weeks after starting clozapine. However, with the initiation of clozapine, he began to experience intrusive and unpleasant thoughts that produced uneasiness and apprehension. Specifically, he began to have thoughts about the possibility that his electrical appliances in general, and the espresso machine in particular, would not work. He clearly understood and recognized that his impressions were baseless, but he felt that he had to act as if his thoughts were real. He described those thoughts as unwanted, paralyzing, severe, and constantly present. He clearly differentiated such thoughts from his previously experienced delusional thoughts. Although he was able to recognize that the obsessive thoughts were irrational, he was unable to stop thinking about the coffee machine and the only way for him to decrease the anxiety was to call the repair service several times per day. The patient was diagnosed with schizophrenia comorbid with medication-induced obsessive symptoms. Given the concomitant presence of residual negative symptoms, aripiprazole 15 mg/day was added, and was then increased to 30 mg/day. Upon starting aripiprazole, the obsessive–compulsive symptoms gradually diminished and completely resolved approximately 5 weeks later.

Figure 12.1 shows a proposed treatment algorithm to control this clozapine-related adverse effect.

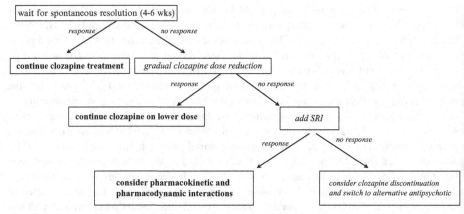

Figure 12.1 Proposed treatment algorithm for clozapine-induced obsessive–compulsive symptoms.

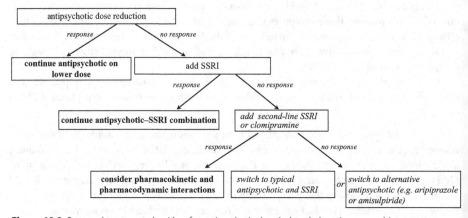

Figure 12.2 Proposed treatment algorithm for antipsychotic-drug-induced obsessive–compulsive symptoms.

The primary approach to control risperidone-, olanzapine-, and quetiapine-induced obsessive–compulsive symptoms is dose reduction. Add-on SSRIs and a combination of a dose reduction and SSRIs co-administration are appropriate next steps. A second-line SSRI or clomipramine may be needed to ameliorate antipsychotic-induced obsessive–compulsive symptoms. Pharmacokinetic and pharmacodynamic drug–drug interactions should be carefully looked after. Discontinuation of the offending compound and switch to a typical antipsychotic agent and a second-line SRI in case of non-response may follow. A switch to an atypical antipsychotic with lower potential to induce obsessive–compulsive symptoms (e.g., aripiprazole, amisulpiride) may be a promising alternative option.

Figure 12.2 shows a proposed treatment algorithm to control antipsychotic-induced obsessive–compulsive symptoms.

Treatment of schizophrenia patients with obsessive–compulsive symptoms is challenging. A great deal of clinical experience is required to identify obsessive–compulsive symptoms in the context of schizophrenia. Considering therapeutic complexity, particularly the potential of atypical antipsychotic agents to both ameliorate and provoke obsessive–compulsive symptoms in schizophrenia patients, the ability to predict response would enable clinicians to tailor treatment more effectively and lead to improved patient outcomes. Individualized pharmacotherapy is the key in the drive towards personalized medicine.

References

Ahmari SE, Risbrough VB, Geyer MA, Simpson HB (2012) Impaired sensorimotor gating in unmedicated adults with obsessive-compulsive disorder. *Neuropsychopharmacology* 37, 1216–1223.

Bloch MH, Landeros-Weisenberger A, Kelmendi B, et al. (2006) A systematic review: antipsychotic augmentation with treatment refractory obsessive-compulsive disorder. *Molecular Psychiatry* 11, 622–632.

Bymaster FP, Calligaro DO, Falcone JF, et al. (1996) Radioreceptor binding profile of the atypical antipsychotic olanzapine. *Neuropsychopharmacology* 14, 87–96.

Chen CH, Chiu CC, Huang MC (2008) Dose-related exacerbation of obsessive-compulsive symptoms with quetiapine treatment. *Progress in Neuropsychopharmacology and Biological Psychiatry* 32, 304–305.

de Haan L, Linszen DH, Gorsira R (1999) Clozapine and obsessions in patients with recent-onset schizophrenia and other psychotic disorders. *Journal of Clinical Psychiatry* 60, 364–365.

de Haan L, Beuk N, Hoogenboom B, Dingemans P, Linszen D (2002) Obsessive-compulsive symptoms during treatment with olanzapine and risperidone: a prospective study of 113 patients with recent-onset schizophrenia or related disorders. *Journal of Clinical Psychiatry* 63, 104–107.

Denys D, Zohar J, Westenberg HG (2004) The role of dopamine in obsessive-compulsive disorder: preclinical and clinical evidence. *Journal of Clinical Psychiatry* 65 (Suppl. 14), 11–17.

Dursun SM, Reveley MA (1994) Obsessive-compulsive symptoms and clozapine. *British Journal of Psychiatry* 165, 267–268.

Eisen JL, Beer DA, Pato MT, Venditto TA, Rasmussen SA (1997) Obsessive-compulsive disorder in patients with schizophrenia or schizoaffective disorder. *American Journal of Psychiatry* 154, 271–273.

Englisch S, Esslinger C, Inta D, et al. (2009) Clozapine-induced obsessive-compulsive syndromes improve in combination with aripiprazole. *Clinical Neuropharmacology* 32, 227–229.

Ertugrul A, Anil Yagcioglu AE, Eni N, Yazici KM (2005) Obsessive-compulsive symptoms in clozapine-treated schizophrenic patients. *Psychiatry and Clinical Neurosciences* 59, 219–222.

Flaisher-Grinberg S, Albelda N, Gitter L, et al. (2009) Ovarian hormones modulate "compulsive" lever-pressing in female rats. *Hormones and Behavior* 55, 356–365.

Geyer MA, Krebs-Thomson K, Braff DL, Swerdlow NR (2001) Pharmacological studies of prepulse inhibition models of sensorimotor gating deficits in schizophrenia: a decade in review. *Psychopharmacology (Berlin)* 156, 117–154.

Hong KS, Nam HJ, Lim M (2008) Emergence of obsessive-compulsive symptoms during clozapine treatment in a pair of monozygotic twins. *British Journal of Psychiatry* 190, 81a.

Khullar A, Chue P, Tibbo P (2001) Quetiapine and obsessive-compulsive symptoms (OCS): case report and review of atypical antipsychotic-induced OCS. *Journal of Psychiatry and Neuroscience* 26, 55–59.

Kwon JS, Joo YH, Nam HJ, et al. (2009) Association of the glutamate transporter gene SLC1A1 with atypical antipsychotics-induced obsessive-compulsive symptoms. *Archives of General Psychiatry* 66, 1233–1241.

Lim M, Park DY, Kwon JS, Joo YH, Hong KS (2007) Prevalence and clinical characteristics of obsessive-compulsive symptoms associated with atypical antipsychotics. *Journal of Clinical Psychopharmacology* 27, 712–713.

Lin SK, Su SF, Pan CH (2006) Higher plasma drug concentration in clozapine-treated schizophrenic patients with side effects of obsessive/compulsive symptoms. *Therapeutic Drug Monitoring* 28, 303–307.

Lykouras L, Alevizos B, Michalopoulou P, Rabavilas A (2003) Obsessive-compulsive symptoms induced by atypical antipsychotics: a review of the reported cases. *Progress in Neuropsychopharmacology and Biological Psychiatry* 27, 333–346.

Mahendran R, Liew E, Subramaniam M (2007) De novo emergence of obsessive-compulsive symptoms with atypical antipsychotics in Asian patients with schizophrenia or schizoaffective disorder: a retrospective, cross-sectional study. *Journal of Clinical Psychiatry* 68, 542–545.

Mukhopadhaya K, Krishnaiah R, Taye T, et al. (2009) Obsessive-compulsive disorder in UK clozapine-treated schizophrenia and schizoaffective disorder: a cause for clinical concern. *Journal of Psychopharmacology* 23, 6–13.

Patil VJ (1992) Development of transient obsessive-compulsive symptoms during treatment with clozapine. *American Journal of Psychiatry* 149, 272.

Porcelli S, Balzarro B, Serretti A (2012) Clozapine resistance: augmentation strategies. *European Neuropsychopharmacology* 22, 165–182.

Poyurovsky M, Hermesh H, Weizman A (1996) Fluvoxamine treatment in clozapine-induced obsessive-compulsive symptoms in schizophrenic patients. *Clinical Neuropharmacology* 19, 305–313.

Poyurovsky M, Dorfman-Etrog P, Hermesh H, et al. (2000) Beneficial effect of olanzapine in schizophrenic patients with obsessive-compulsive symptoms. *International Clinical Psychopharmacology* 15, 169–173.

Sa AR, Hounie AG, Sampaio AS, et al. (2009) Obsessive-compulsive symptoms and disorder in patients with schizophrenia treated with clozapine or haloperidol. *Comprehensive Psychiatry* 50, 437–442.

Sasson Y, Zohar J, Chopra M, et al. (1997) Epidemiology of obsessive-compulsive disorder: a world view. *Journal of Clinical Psychiatry* 58, 7–10.

Schirmbeck F, Esslinger C, Rausch F, et al. (2011) Antiserotonergic antipsychotics are associated with obsessive-compulsive symptoms in schizophrenia. *Psychological Medicine* 41, 2361–2373.

Schönfelder S, Schirmbeck F, Waltereit R, Englisch S, Zink M (2011) Aripiprazole improves olanzapine-associated obsessive compulsive symptoms in schizophrenia. *Clinical Neuropharmacology* 34, 256–257.

Schotte A, Janssen PF, Gommeren W, et al. (1996) Risperidone compared with new and reference antipsychotic drugs: in vitro and in vivo receptor binding. *Psychopharmacology (Berlin)* 124, 57–73.

van Nimwegen L, de Haan L, van Beveren N, et al. (2008) Obsessive-compulsive symptoms in a randomized, double-blind study with olanzapine or risperidone in young patients with early psychosis. *Journal of Clinical Psychopharmacology* 28, 214–218.

Villari V, Frieri T, Fagiolini A (2011) Aripiprazole augmentation in clozapine-associated obsessive-compulsive symptoms. *Journal of Clinical Psychopharmacology* 31, 375–376.

Zink M, Knopf U, Kuwilsky A (2007) Management of clozapine-induced obsessive-compulsive symptoms in a man with schizophrenia. *Australian and New Zealand Journal of Psychiatry* 41, 293–294.

Chapter 13

Conclusions and future directions

This book pinpoints some of the crucial steps in the consolidation of views on the complex interface between schizophrenia and OCD, a schizo-obsessive disorder. The following is a summary of what we now know and what needs to be accomplished in order to extend our understanding of this puzzling psychiatric condition.

Undoubtedly, schizophrenia and obsessive–compulsive disorder (OCD) are distinct nosological entities with discrete underlying brain mechanisms, clinical presentations, and treatments. Nevertheless, they share demographic and clinical characteristics and, apparently, some pathophysiological underpinnings. Both inflictions are characterized by similar distributions between men and women, age of onset during adolescence or early adulthood, and earlier age of onset in men. Increasingly sophisticated translational, neuro-physiological, and neuroimaging research has revealed a substantial overlap between schizophrenia and OCD in structural and functional brain abnormalities and in the involvement of the dopamine, serotonin, and glutamate neurotransmitter systems in the pathophysiology underlying these disorders. Hence, it is not surprising that obsessive–compulsive and schizophrenic symptoms coexist in a substantially greater proportion of patients than would be expected from random co-occurrence of the two disorders.

As discussed in this book, in contrast to positive, negative, and cognitive symptoms, obsessive–compulsive symptoms are not considered primary features of schizophrenia. However, from the early stages of schizophrenia research, founders of modern psychiatry clearly identified obsessive–compulsive symptoms in schizophrenia and deemed them a feature of the disorder's prodromal, active, or residual phases. Initially, obsessive–compulsive symptoms were thought to occur in a minority of schizophrenia patients and were considered to be a "protective" factor. What is more, psychiatric classifications, such as DSM-III, did not allow a diagnosis of OCD in the presence of schizophrenia, since OCD was considered to be "due to" a disorder higher in the hierarchy. Later, however, DSM-IV allowed for the diagnosis of co-occurring schizophrenia and clinically meaningful and potentially treatable secondary syndromes, facilitating studies into the association of schizophrenia and OCD. Contemporary studies challenge the "positive" view of obsessive–compulsive symptoms in schizophrenia by showing a significantly poorer outcome for schizo-obsessive patients than for schizophrenia patients without OCD. It is estimated that roughly 10–15% of schizophrenia patients also exhibit OCD. Relaxing the diagnostic threshold for obsessive–compulsive symptoms leads to an even higher prevalence rate of approximately 25%. Remarkably, as in "pure" OCD, the reported rates of OCD in schizophrenia samples across the globe are consistent. The term "schizo-obsessive" has been suggested in order to draw attention to schizophrenia patients who have clinically signifi-cant obsessive–compulsive symptoms.

We now know that valid and reliable identification of obsessive–compulsive symptoms in schizophrenia patients is feasible, despite a symptomatic overlap between the two disorders. Utilizing instruments developed to evaluate OCD (e.g., the Yale–Brown Obsessive–Compulsive Scale), studies have consistently shown that in a majority of schizo-obsessive patients, obsessive–compulsive symptoms precede initial psychotic symptoms, are associated with fair to good insight, and exhibit symptom dimensions comparable to those seen in "pure" OCD. The documented substantial distress and functional impairment particularly associated with obsessive–compulsive symptoms, lend additional support to their independent nature and clinical significance in schizophrenia.

It has become increasingly clear that obsessive–compulsive symptoms in schizophrenia are not a sequel to chronic illness or to antipsychotic treatment, since a comparable prevalence rate has been revealed in individuals at ultra-high risk for psychosis, in the prodromal phase of schizophrenia, and in drug-naïve first-episode schizophrenia patients. Detection of obsessive–compulsive symptoms across the lifespan in adolescent, adult, and elderly patients further highlights the broad prevalence and persistence of obsessive–compulsive phenomena in schizophrenia.

Compared with schizophrenia patients, schizo-obsessive patients have distinct clinical features. They exhibit an earlier age at onset, more depressive symptoms and suicide attempts, increased rates of hospitalization, decreased likelihood of being employed or married, lower quality of life, and greater disability. The presence of obsessive–compulsive symptoms is associated with higher global, positive, and negative schizophrenia symptom severity. A unique pattern of comorbidity is an additional distinctive feature. Similar to "pure" OCD, schizo-obsessive patients show a preferential aggregation of OCD-spectrum disorders, primarily body dysmorphic disorder and tic disorders. Identification of these "extra" morbidities is indispensable for the provision of adequate care. Conversely, because the presence of OCD-spectrum disorders increases the odds of OCD in schizophrenia, clinicians should be aware that targeting these additional syndromes may improve identification of an obsessive–compulsive component in schizophrenia.

Important differences in psychiatric morbidities are also found in first-degree relatives of schizophrenia patients with and without obsessive–compulsive symptoms. Compared with relatives of schizophrenia patients, relatives of patients with schizo-obsessive disorder have a significantly higher morbid risk for schizo-obsessive disorder, obsessive–compulsive personality disorder, and OCD. Differential familial aggregation of OCD-related disorders further supports the validity of recognizing a distinct schizo-obsessive subgroup in the schizophrenia spectrum. From the clinical perspective, explicit inquiry into the presence of OCD and related disorders in first-degree relatives would apparently aid in the detection of obsessive–compulsive phenomena in schizophrenia patients.

The neurobiological underpinnings of schizo-obsessive disorder are not yet clearly understood but preliminary evidence suggests a distinct neurobiological profile. Initial magnetic resonance imaging studies have identified significantly reduced volumes of some of the brain structures (e.g., hippocampus), while a neurophysiological investigation using event-related potentials (ERPs) during a discriminative response task found a distinct ERP pattern in schizo-obsessive patients. They also exhibit more soft neurological signs and neurocognitive deficits, primarily in abstraction and executive function, than do schizophrenia patients without obsessive–compulsive phenomena.

However, a lack of difference or even better performance of schizo-obsessive patients than of schizophrenia patients, particularly during the initial stages of illness, has also been noted. Obviously further large-scale comparative evaluation of cognitive deficits in schizophrenia patients with and without OCD is imperative, considering the central role of cognitive impairment in schizophrenia and its impact on patients' functional outcome and prognosis.

Treatment of schizo-obsessive patients is a challenging endeavor. Evidence-based data is still lacking. However, there is a general consensus that schizo-obsessive patients are difficult to treat and differentially responsive to specific treatment interventions. Indeed, in contrast to schizophrenia patients without OCD, monotherapy with typical antipsychotics appears to have limited therapeutic value in schizo-obsessive patients and is associated with heightened sensitivity to motor side effects. Second-generation antipsychotics may be effective as monotherapy in the amelioration of both schizophrenic and obsessive–compulsive symptoms in some patients, but a combination with serotonin reuptake inhibitors (SRIs) is usually required. Pharmacotherapeutic complexity is further highlighted by the phenomenon of atypical antipsychotic-drug-induced obsessive–compulsive symptoms. In fact, atypical antipsychotics both improve and induce or exacerbate obsessive–compulsive symptoms in schizophrenia patients. Underlying mechanisms of this bidirectional effect of atypical antipsychotic agents remain unknown.

Overall, substantial bodies of evidence indicate that obsessive–compulsive symptoms represent a clinically meaningful dimension of psychopathology in schizophrenia, and that schizophrenia patients with obsessive–compulsive symptoms have distinct clinical and neurobiological characteristics, family inheritance, treatment response, and prognosis. The following are provisional diagnostic criteria for the identification of an obsessive–compulsive symptom subgroup ("schizo-obsessive") of schizophrenia (Poyurovsky et al., 2012).

Proposed diagnostic criteria for an obsessive–compulsive symptom subgroup ("schizo-obsessive") of schizophrenia

A. Symptoms are present that meet the DSM-IV Criterion A for obsessive–compulsive disorder at some time point during the course of the schizophrenia.

B. If the content of the obsessions and/or compulsions is interrelated with the content of delusions and/or hallucinations (e.g., compulsive hand-washing due to command auditory hallucinations), additional typical OCD obsessions and compulsions recognized by the person as unreasonable and excessive are required.

C. Symptoms of obsessive–compulsive disorder are present for a substantial portion of the total duration of the prodromal, active, and/or the residual period of schizophrenia.

D. The obsessions and compulsions are time-consuming (more than 1 hour a day), cause distress, or significantly interfere with the person's normal routine, in addition to the functional impairment associated with schizophrenia.

E. The obsessions and compulsions in the patient with schizophrenia are not due to the direct effect of antipsychotic agents, a substance of abuse (e.g., cocaine), or an organic factor (e.g., head trauma).

Considering the diagnostic pitfalls in the discrimination between obsessive–compulsive and schizophrenic phenomena, until more studies on the nature and course of OCD

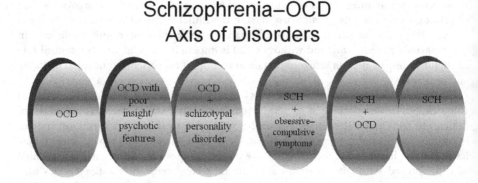

Figure 13.1 Schizophrenia–OCD axis of disorders.

symptoms in schizophrenia become available, the diagnosis of schizo-obsessive disorder, as suggested above, should be confined to those patients who meet full DSM-IV criteria of both disorders. Patients who fail to recognize their obsessive–compulsive symptoms as senseless and unreasonable or have transient psychotic transformation of obsessions, but do not meet the criteria of schizophrenia, can be diagnosed as having OCD with poor insight (DSM-IV) (American Psychiatric Association, 1994) or OCD with psychotic features (Insel and Akiskal, 1986), respectively. Those who exert "full-blown" OCD and "subthreshold" schizophrenia, that is DSM-IV schizotypal personality disorder, may have schizotypal OCD (Figure 13.1). Schematic representations of the major dimensions of the psychopathology may be of practical value in the differentiation of distinct clinical entities within the putative schizophrenia–OCD spectrum (Table 13.1).

What needs to be achieved to further understand the psychopathology, neurobiology, and treatment of patients with schizo-obsessive disorder? First, the definition of obsessions and compulsions in the nosological context of schizophrenia and the differential diagnoses that distinguish these symptoms from delusions and delusionally motivated repetitive behaviors are essential in the study of schizo-obsessive schizophrenia. Prospective studies are required to address course-dependent interrelationships between obsessive–compulsive and schizophrenic symptoms, and diagnostic stability during long-term follow-up. Valid and reliable diagnostic instruments for assessing psychotic-related obsessive–compulsive phenomena (e.g., "obsessive delusions," "obsessive hallucinations") in schizophrenia patients, in addition to typical ego-dystonic obsessive–compulsive symptoms, should be developed to assist clinicians and researchers in their identification. This may facilitate delineation of distinct subgroups of patients on a putative schizophrenia–OCD axis of disorders, namely schizophrenia with obsessive–compulsive symptoms versus primary OCD with poor insight or psychotic features versus schizotypal OCD. Accurate diagnosis has prognostic and treatment implications, given that current treatments for schizophrenia and OCD differ, and first-line medications for one disorder can exacerbate the symptoms of the other; that is, antipsychotics can exacerbate obsessive–compulsive symptoms, and SRIs may exacerbate psychosis.

Table 13.1 Symptomatic dimensions in patients with OCD, schizophrenia, and their associations

	Positive		Negative	Disorganized	Obsessive–compulsive symptoms	
	Delusions	Hallucinations			Obsessions	Compulsions
OCD	−	−	−	−	+	+
OCD with poor insight/ psychotic features	+	−	−	−	+	+
Schizotypal OCD	+/−	+/−	+/−	+/−	+	+
Schizophrenia with obsessive– compulsive symptoms	+	+	+	+	+/−	+/−
Schizo- obsessive disorder	+	+	+	+	+	+
Schizophrenia	+	+	+	+	−	−

+ present; − absent; +/− subsyndromal.

Further studies of brain function are needed to ascertain whether obsessive–compulsive symptoms modify the pattern of brain activation in schizophrenia patients. A further search for intermediate neurophysiological and neurocognitive endophenotypes might also facilitate the delineation of a schizo-obsessive subgroup. Since such endophenotypes seem to represent heritable trait markers, their assessment in relatives of patients with isolated schizophrenia and OCD and with their comorbid forms may contribute to the pathophysiological differentiation of a schizophrenia subgroup exhibiting obsessive–compulsive symptoms.

A search for effective, tolerable, and safe treatment that addresses both schizophrenic and obsessive–compulsive symptoms in schizo-obsessive patients is another important goal. A pharmacogenetic approach is promising for the development of personalized treatment. As mentioned in this book, there is preliminary evidence pointing towards an association of the glutamate transporter gene *SLC1A1* with atypical antipsychotic-induced obsessive–compulsive symptoms in schizophrenia patients. Conceivably, patients who manifest obsessive–compulsive symptoms associated with atypical antipsychotics have a genetic predisposition, which is "unmasked" by treatment. It is also possible that genetic predisposition, albeit with a differential "load," exists in schizophrenia patients who exhibit obsessive–compulsive symptoms that are unrelated to treatment with atypical antipsychotic agents. Finally, large-scale controlled trials to evaluate the therapeutic efficacy of antipsychotic agents alone and in combination with SRIs or other potentially effective compounds (e.g., glutamatergic drugs) are essential to establish evidence-based treatment guidelines for patients with schizo-obsessive disorder, a group that remains diagnostically challenging and difficult to treat.

Overall, growing evidence strongly supports the clinical and neurobiological significance of obsessive–compulsive symptoms in schizophrenia. Substantial advances in our conceptualization of the interface between the two disorders justify its introduction in future psychiatric classifications. In the meantime, awareness of clinicians of the co-occurrence of obsessive–compulsive and schizophrenic phenomena is important for early identification and treatment. This book is the first step towards that goal.

References

American Psychiatric Association (1994) *Diagnostic and Statistical Manual of Mental Disorders*, 4th edn. American Psychiatric Association, Washington, DC

Insel TR, Akiskal HS (1986) Obsessive-compulsive disorder with psychotic features: a phenomenologic analysis. *American Journal of Psychiatry* **143**, 1527–1533.

Poyurovsky M, Zohar J, Glick I, *et al.* (2012) Obsessive-compulsive symptoms in schizophrenia: implications for future psychiatric classifications. *Comprehensive Psychiatry* **53**, 480–483.

Index

Printed in the United States
By Bookmasters